50% OFF Online TEAS 7 Prep Course!

Dear Customer,

We consider it an honor and a privilege that you chose our ATI TEAS Study Guide. As a way of showing our appreciation and to help us better serve you, we have partnered with Mometrix Test Preparation to offer you **50% off their online ATI TEAS 7 Prep Course.** Many TEAS courses are needlessly expensive and don't deliver enough value. With their course, you get access to the best TEAS prep material, and **you only pay half price**.

Mometrix has structured their online course to perfectly complement your printed study guide. This TEAS 7 Prep Course contains **in-depth lessons** that cover all the most important topics, **190+ video reviews** that explain difficult concepts, **over 1,450 practice questions** to ensure you feel prepared, and **digital flashcards** for studying on the go.

Online TEAS 7 Prep Course

Topics Covered:

- Reading
  - Key Ideas and Details
  - Craft and Structure
  - Integration of Knowledge and Ideas
- Mathematics
  - Numbers and Algebra
  - Measurement and Data
- Science
  - Human Anatomy and Physiology
  - Biology
  - Chemistry (**New on TEAS 7**)
  - Scientific Reasoning
- English and Language Usage
  - Conventions of Standard English
  - Knowledge of Language
  - Using Language and Vocabulary to Express Ideas in Writing

Course Features:

- ATI TEAS 7 Study Guide
  - Get content that complements our best-selling study guide.
- 8 Full-Length Practice Tests
  - With over 1,450 practice questions, you can test yourself again and again.
- Mobile Friendly
  - If you need to study on the go, the course is easily accessible from your mobile device.
- TEAS Flashcards
  - Their course includes a flashcard mode with content cards to help you study.

To receive this discount, visit them at mometrix.com/university/teas-test/ or simply scan this QR code with your smartphone. At the checkout page, enter the discount code: **APEX50**

SCAN HERE

If you have any questions or concerns, please don't hesitate to contact Mometrix at universityhelp@mometrix.com.

Sincerely,

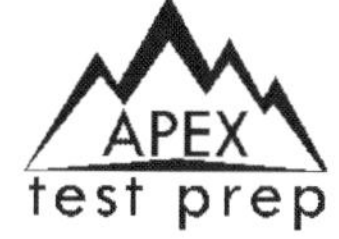

in partnership with

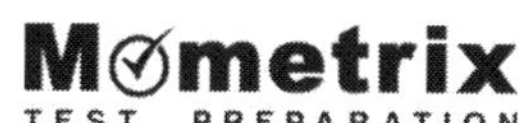

FREE

Free Study Tips Videos/DVD

In addition to this guide, we have created a FREE set of videos with helpful study tips. **These FREE videos provide you with top-notch tips to conquer your exam and reach your goals.**

Our simple request is that you give us feedback about the book in exchange for these strategy-packed videos. We would love to hear what you thought about the book, whether positive, negative, or neutral. It is our #1 goal to provide you with quality products and customer service.

To receive your **FREE Study Tips Videos**, scan the QR code or email freevideos@apexprep.com. Please put "FREE Videos" in the subject line and include the following in the email:

a. The title of the book

b. Your rating of the book on a scale of 1-5, with 5 being the highest score

c. Any thoughts or feedback about the book

Thank you!

ATI TEAS 7th Edition Study Guide

TEAS Exam Prep for Nursing with Practice Test Questions
[Includes Detailed Answer Explanations]

J. M. Lefort

Written and edited by APEX Publishing.

ISBN 13: 9781637757185
ISBN 10: 1637757182

For additional information or for bulk orders, contact info@apexprep.com.

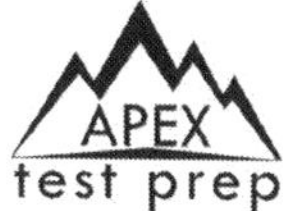

Table of Contents

Test Taking Strategies

1. Reading the Whole Question

A popular assumption in Western culture is the idea that we don't have enough time for anything. We speed while driving to work, we want to read an assignment for class as quickly as possible, or we want the line in the supermarket to dwindle faster. However, speeding through such events robs us from being able to thoroughly appreciate and understand what's happening around us. While taking a timed test, the feeling one might have while reading a question is to find the correct answer as quickly as possible. Although pace is important, don't let it deter you from reading the whole question. Test writers know how to subtly change a test question toward the end in various ways, such as adding a negative or changing focus. If the question has a passage, carefully read the whole passage as well before moving on to the questions. This will help you process the information in the passage rather than worrying about the questions you've just read and where to find them. A thorough understanding of the passage or question is an important way for test takers to be able to succeed on an exam.

2. Examining Every Answer Choice

Let's say we're at the market buying apples. The first apple we see on top of the heap may *look* like the best apple, but if we turn it over we can see bruising on the skin. We must examine several apples before deciding which apple is the best. Finding the correct answer choice is like finding the best apple. Although it's tempting to choose an answer that seems correct at first without reading the others, it's important to read each answer choice thoroughly before making a final decision on the answer. The aim of a test writer might be to get as close as possible to the correct answer, so watch out for subtle words that may indicate an answer is incorrect. Once the correct answer choice is selected, read the question again and the answer in response to make sure all your bases are covered.

3. Eliminating Wrong Answer Choices

Sometimes we become paralyzed when we are confronted with too many choices. Which frozen yogurt flavor is the tastiest? Which pair of shoes look the best with this outfit? What type of car will fill my needs as a consumer? If you are unsure of which answer would be the best to choose, it may help to use process of elimination. We use "filtering" all the time on sites such as eBay® or Craigslist® to eliminate the ads that are not right for us. We can do the same thing on an exam. Process of elimination is crossing out the answer choices we know for sure are wrong and leaving the ones that might be correct. It may help to cover up the incorrect answer choice. Covering incorrect choices is a psychological act that alleviates stress due to the brain being exposed to a smaller amount of information. Choosing between two answer choices is much easier than choosing between all of them, and you have a better chance of selecting the correct answer if you have less to focus on.

4. Sticking to the World of the Question

When we are attempting to answer questions, our minds will often wander away from the question and what it is asking. We begin to see answer choices that are true in the real world instead of true in the world of the question. It may be helpful to think of each test question as its own little world. This world may be different from ours. This world may know as a truth that the chicken came before the egg or may assert that two plus two equals five. Remember that, no matter what hypothetical nonsense may be in the question, assume it to be true. If the question states that the chicken came before the egg, then choose

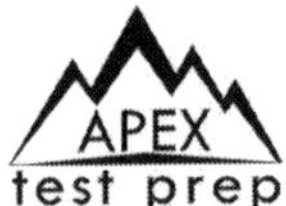

your answer based on that truth. Sticking to the world of the question means placing all of our biases and assumptions aside and relying on the question to guide us to the correct answer. If we are simply looking for answers that are correct based on our own judgment, then we may choose incorrectly. Remember an answer that is true does not necessarily answer the question.

5. Key Words

If you come across a complex test question that you have to read over and over again, try pulling out some key words from the question in order to understand what exactly it is asking. Key words may be words that surround the question, such as *main idea, analogous, parallel, resembles, structured,* or *defines*. The question may be asking for the main idea, or it may be asking you to define something. Deconstructing the sentence may also be helpful in making the question simpler before trying to answer it. This means taking the sentence apart and obtaining meaning in pieces, or separating the question from the foundation of the question. For example, let's look at this question:

> Given the author's description of the content of paleontology in the first paragraph, which of the following is most parallel to what it taught?

The question asks which one of the answers most *parallels* the following information: The *description* of paleontology in the first paragraph. The first step would be to see *how* paleontology is described in the first paragraph. Then, we would find an answer choice that parallels that description. The question seems complex at first, but after we deconstruct it, the answer becomes much more attainable.

6. Subtle Negatives

Negative words in question stems will be words such as *not, but, neither,* or *except*. Test writers often use these words in order to trick unsuspecting test takers into selecting the wrong answer—or, at least, to test their reading comprehension of the question. Many exams will feature the negative words in all caps (*which of the following is NOT an example*), but some questions will add the negative word seamlessly into the sentence. The following is an example of a subtle negative used in a question stem:

> According to the passage, which of the following is *not* considered to be an example of paleontology?

If we rush through the exam, we might skip that tiny word, *not*, inside the question, and choose an answer that is opposite of the correct choice. Again, it's important to read the question fully, and double check for any words that may negate the statement in any way.

7. Spotting the Hedges

The word "hedging" refers to language that remains vague or avoids absolute terminology. Absolute terminology consists of words like *always, never, all, every, just, only, none,* and *must*. Hedging refers to words like *seem, tend, might, most, some, sometimes, perhaps, possibly, probability,* and *often*. In some cases, we want to choose answer choices that use hedging and avoid answer choices that use absolute terminology. It's important to pay attention to what subject you are on and adjust your response accordingly.

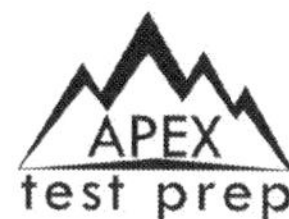

8. Restating to Understand

Every now and then we come across questions that we don't understand. The language may be too complex, or the question is structured in a way that is meant to confuse the test taker. When you come across a question like this, it may be worth your time to rewrite or restate the question in your own words in order to understand it better. For example, let's look at the following complicated question:

> Which of the following words, if substituted for the word *parochial* in the first paragraph, would LEAST change the meaning of the sentence?

Let's restate the question in order to understand it better. We know that they want the word *parochial* replaced. We also know that this new word would "least" or "not" change the meaning of the sentence. Now let's try the sentence again:

> Which word could we replace with *parochial,* and it would not change the meaning?

Restating it this way, we see that the question is asking for a synonym. Now, let's restate the question so we can answer it better:

> Which word is a synonym for the word *parochial*?

Before we even look at the answer choices, we have a simpler, restated version of a complicated question.

9. Predicting the Answer

After you read the question, try predicting the answer *before* reading the answer choices. By formulating an answer in your mind, you will be less likely to be distracted by any wrong answer choices. Using predictions will also help you feel more confident in the answer choice you select. Once you've chosen your answer, go back and reread the question and answer choices to make sure you have the best fit. If you have no idea what the answer may be for a particular question, forego using this strategy.

10. Avoiding Patterns

One popular myth in grade school relating to standardized testing is that test writers will often put multiple-choice answers in patterns. A runoff example of this kind of thinking is that the most common answer choice is "C," with "B" following close behind. Or, some will advocate certain made-up word patterns that simply do not exist. Test writers do not arrange their correct answer choices in any kind of pattern; their choices are randomized. There may even be times where the correct answer choice will be the same letter for two or three questions in a row, but we have no way of knowing when or if this might happen. Instead of trying to figure out what choice the test writer probably set as being correct, focus on what the *best answer choice* would be out of the answers you are presented with. Use the tips above, general knowledge, and reading comprehension skills in order to best answer the question, rather than looking for patterns that do not exist.

FREE Videos/DVD OFFER

Achieving a high score on your exam depends on both understanding the content and applying your knowledge. **Because your success is our primary goal, we offer FREE Study Tips Videos, which provide top-notch test taking strategies to help optimize your testing experience.**

Our simple request is that you email us feedback about our book in exchange for the strategy-packed videos.

To receive your **FREE Study Tips Videos**, scan the QR code or email freevideos@apexprep.com. Please put "FREE Videos" in the subject line and include the following in the email:

a. The title of the book

b. Your rating of the book on a scale of 1-5, with 5 being the highest score

c. Any thoughts or feedback about the book

Thank you!

Introduction to the TEAS 7

Function of the Test

The TEAS test is a standardized Test of Essential Academic Skills given by the Assessment Technologies Institute (ATI) Nursing Education. Those who want to be considered for admissions into nursing school or an allied health school must take the TEAS as part of an overall assessment of qualification for the program. The TEAS test is nationwide and offered in both the United States and Canada. The newest version of the TEAS is called the ATI TEAS 7.

The TEAS test is very important in determining admissions to nursing programs, although the preferred score by nursing schools varies. The TEAS can be taken by students wishing to be considered for a nursing or allied health program, or for professionals already in the industry who want to advance their certification.

Test Administration

The TEAS test is offered by ATI Testing in PSI testing centers or at nursing schools or allied health schools. You can determine where these centers are by visiting the PSI exam's website directly or through beginning registration at atitesting.com. Once you start your registration for the TEAS, you will be shown various testing locations to choose from by city and state, ranging from metropolitan cities to less-populated towns. Administration frequency will vary based on the location, but test dates are offered at regular intervals year-round. Retaking the test is permitted, but the rules vary by school. Disability accommodations can be made available by contacting the testing administration site.

Test Format

Once you present your ID to the staff, you will have a seat in the testing area. The format of the exam can either be computerized or on paper. Keep in mind that proctors will be standing around the room to monitor for disruption. The proctor will provide you with a calculator and scratch paper.

Breaks will begin at the end of each section. Other than these breaks, the testing clock will not stop. The staff at the administration center ask that you raise your hand for any kind of issues with the test. The following table depicts the sections on the TEAS, the number of questions, and the time limit given for each section:

Subject	**Questions**	**Time**
Reading	45 (6 unscored)	55 minutes
Math	38 (4 unscored)	57 minutes
Science	50 (6 unscored)	60 minutes
English and Language Usage	37 (4 unscored)	37 minutes
Total	**170 (20 unscored)**	**209 minutes**

Scoring

Scores are available immediately after taking the online version of the test. For those who take the paper version of the test, ATI Nursing Education will process the scores between 48 and 72 hours of receiving the test. The scores will provide your total scores, the individual content scores, and which specific topic areas were missed. Nursing programs all have a different minimum of TEAS scores required for admission into the program, so you will have to check with the appropriate schools. Nursing programs typically look at the composite score listed at the top of the score report. The report will also show the national mean and the program mean—the national mean composite score is usually between a 65% and a 75%.

Recent/Future Developments

The ATI TEAS is the seventh version of the test and was released in June 2022. Calculators may now be used on the newest version of the test. The ATI TEAS 7 is the same difficulty level as the previous version.

The TEAS 7 includes five types of questions: multiple choice, multiple-select, supply answer, ordering, and hot spot. *Multiple choice* questions provide four answer choices, and the test taker must select the one correct answer. *Multiple-select* are similar to multiple choice, but they may have more than one correct answer. *Supply answer* questions require the test taker to produce the answer without any choices and write it in a blank. *Ordering* questions involve putting a list of items into a given order. Finally, *hot spot* questions present an image and ask the test taker to identify a particular section of the image.

Study Prep Plan for the TEAS 7

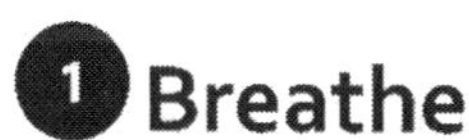

Reducing stress is key when preparing for your test.

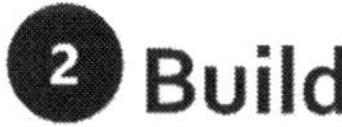

Create a study plan to help you stay on track.

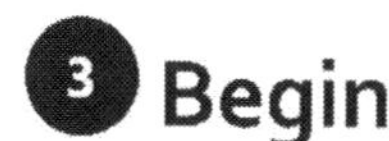

Stick with your study plan. You've got this!

1 Week Study Plan

Day 1	Day 2	Day 3	Day 4	Day 5	Day 6	Day 7
Reading	Mathematics	Science	Biology	English and Language Usage	Practice Test	Take Your Exam!

2 Week Study Plan

Day 1	Day 2	Day 3	Day 4	Day 5	Day 6	Day 7
Reading	Integration of Knowledge and Ideas	Mathematics	Measurement and Data	Science	Reproductive System	Biology
Day 8	**Day 9**	**Day 10**	**Day 11**	**Day 12**	**Day 13**	**Day 14**
Chemistry	Scientific Reasoning	English and Language Usage	Knowledge of Language	Practice Test	Answer Explanations	Take Your Exam!

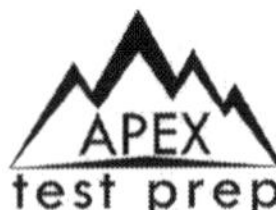

30 Day Study Plan

Day 1	Day 2	Day 3	Day 4	Day 5	Day 6	Day 7
Reading	Craft and Structure	Integration of Knowledge and Ideas	Reading Practice Quiz	Mathematics	Simplifying Rational Algebraic Expressions	Comparing and Ordering Rational Numbers

Day 8	Day 9	Day 10	Day 11	Day 12	Day 13	Day 14
Applying Estimation Strategies and Rounding Rules	Measurement and Data	Data Sets, Tables, Charts, And Graphs Using Statistics	Calculating Geometric Quantities	Mathematics Practice Quiz	Science	Cardiovascular System

Day 15	Day 16	Day 17	Day 18	Day 19	Day 20	Day 21
Nervous System	Endocrine System	Urinary System	Biology	Genetic Material and The Structure of Proteins	Chemistry	Chemical Reactions

Day 22	Day 23	Day 24	Day 25	Day 26	Day 27	Day 28
Scientific Reasoning	Science Practice Quiz	English and Language Usage	Knowledge of Language	Using Language & Vocabulary to Express Ideas in Writing	English & Language Usage Practice Quiz	Practice Test

Day 29	Day 30
Answer Explanations	Take Your Exam!

Reading

Key Ideas and Details

Summarizing a Multi-Paragraph Text

An important skill is the ability to read a complex text and then reduce its length and complexity by focusing on the key events and details. A **summary** is a shortened version of the original text, written by the reader in their own words. The summary should be shorter than the original text, and it must include the most critical points.

In order to effectively summarize a complex text, it's necessary to understand the original source and identify the key points covered. It may be helpful to outline the original text to get the big picture and avoid getting bogged down in the minor details. For example, a summary wouldn't include a statistic from the original source unless it was the major focus of the text. It is also important for readers to use their own words but still retain the original meaning of the passage. The key to a good summary is emphasizing the main idea without changing the focus of the original information.

Complex texts will likely be more difficult to summarize. Readers must evaluate all points from the original source, filter out the unnecessary details, and maintain only the essential ideas. The summary often mirrors the original text's organizational structure. For example, in a problem-solution text structure, the author typically presents readers with a problem and then develops solutions through the course of the text. An effective summary would likely retain this general structure, rephrasing the problem and then reporting the most useful or plausible solutions.

Paraphrasing is somewhat similar to summarizing. It calls for the reader to take a small part of the passage and list or describe its main points. Paraphrasing is more than rewording the original passage, though. As with summary, a paraphrase should be written in the reader's own words, while still retaining the meaning of the original source. The main difference between summarizing and paraphrasing is that a summary would be appropriate for a much larger text, while paraphrase might focus on just a few lines of text. Effective paraphrasing will indicate an understanding of the original source, yet still help the reader expand on their interpretation. A paraphrase should neither add new information nor remove essential facts that change the meaning of the source.

Identifying the Topic, Main Idea, and Supporting Details

The **topic** of a text is the general subject matter. Text topics can usually be expressed in one word, or a few words at most. Additionally, readers should ask themselves what point the author is trying to make. This point is the **main idea** of the text, the one thing the author wants readers to know concerning the topic. Once the author has established the main idea, they will support the main idea by supporting details. **Supporting details** are evidence that support the main idea and include personal testimonies, examples, or statistics.

One analogy for these components and their relationships is that a text is like a well-designed house. The topic is the roof, covering all rooms. The main idea is the frame. The supporting details are the various rooms. To identify the topic of a text, readers can ask themselves what or who the author is writing about in the paragraph. To locate the main idea, readers can ask themselves what one idea the author wants readers to know about the topic. To identify supporting details, readers can put the main idea into question form and ask "what does the author use to prove or explain their main idea?"

Let's look at an example. An author is writing an essay about the Amazon rainforest and trying to convince the audience that more funding should go into protecting the area from deforestation. The author makes the argument stronger by including evidence of the benefits of the rainforest: it provides habitats to a variety of species, it provides much of the earth's oxygen which in turn cleans the atmosphere, and it is the home to medicinal plants that may be the answer to some of the world's deadliest diseases.

Here is an outline of the essay looking at topic, main idea, and supporting details:

Topic: Amazon rainforest
Main Idea: The Amazon rainforest should receive more funding in order to protect it from deforestation.
Supporting Details:

1. It provides habitats to a variety of species
2. It provides much of the earth's oxygen which in turn cleans the atmosphere
3. It is home to medicinal plants that may be the answer to some of the world's deadliest diseases.

Notice that the topic of the essay is listed in a few key words: "Amazon rainforest". The main idea tells us what about the topic is important: that the topic should be funded in order to prevent deforestation. Finally, the supporting details are what author relies on to convince the audience to act or to believe in the truth of the main idea.

Inferences and Conclusions About a Text's Purpose and Meaning

An inference is an educated guess or conclusion based on sound evidence and reasoning within the text. Evidence may either be explicit (directly stated) or implicit (implied). When present, both types of evidence should be used to form conclusions. The test may include multiple-choice questions asking about the logical conclusion that can be drawn from reading a text, and you will have to identify the choice that unavoidably leads to that conclusion. In order to eliminate the incorrect choices, the test-taker should come up with a hypothetical situation wherein an answer choice is true, but the conclusion is not true.

Here is an example:

> Fred purchased the newest PC available on the market. Therefore, he purchased the most expensive PC in the computer store.
>
> What can one assume for this conclusion to follow logically?
>
> a. Fred enjoys purchasing expensive items.
> b. PCs are some of the most expensive personal technology products available.
> c. The newest PC is the most expensive one.

The premise of the text is the first sentence: Fred purchased the newest PC. The conclusion is the second sentence: Fred purchased the most expensive PC. Recent release and price are two different factors; the difference between them is the logical gap. To eliminate the gap, one must connect the new information from the conclusion with the pertinent information from the premise. In this example, there must be a connection between product recency and product price. Therefore, a possible bridge to the logical gap could be a sentence stating that the newest PCs always cost the most.

Written Directions

To follow directions, an individual must hold them in short-term memory while using working memory and language to comprehend the information. Being able to follow a direction requires understanding of the direction's specific words. In addition to language comprehension, the ability to follow directions requires interest in the activity, motivation to follow the directions, and paying attention to them.

Directions are typically given in the order in which they are to be completed. However, it is still a good idea to read the entire set of directions before beginning the first step; this can help provide a higher-level view of the process and the final product. Take note of words like *first, second, third, then, next, after, before,* etc. as these words indicate order. Directions indicate priority through order. For example, if they explicitly say to complete one step before beginning the next, it's very likely that the next step will not even be possible until the previous step is completed. Sometimes it's possible to jump around, but reading the directions fully first will enable the reader to determine whether that is the case.

It is also important to read all the directions before beginning the first step because the directions may contain mistakes, be (or appear to be) contradictory, or be too simplistic and missing important information. When encountering any of these issues, use logical reasoning or additional resources to form a conclusion about what needs to be done.

The following example shows why it's extremely important to read all the directions in a test setting first before acting on any of them. Follow the directions below:

1. Carefully read everything in the directions before you do anything.
2. Write your name on the top of this page.
3. Put your birthday and date underneath your name.
4. Write an "Z" on an empty space anywhere on the page.
5. Circle the "Z" and draw a line below it referring to "Y."
6. Draw a line from "Y" referring to "X."
7. Draw a box at the bottom of this page.
8. Describe the shape you drew around the letters inside the box.
9. Write your name inside the box.
10. Now that you've carefully read everything, follow only directions (1) and (2).

Those who get to direction 10 without having acted on any instructions yet will save a lot of wasted time opposed to those who immediately begin to act on the instructions. Remember, read all the directions before you begin, and you will have a better idea of what the bigger picture entails!

Specific Information in a Text

When utilizing a text to solve a problem, answer a question, or make a decision, it is likely that only certain parts of the text will be relevant. There are many textual features that can direct you to relevant information. If you cannot find the information you seek, asking questions is a helpful tactic that can assist you in refining your research scope as you continue to search elsewhere.

Using Text Features

Table of Contents and Index

When examining a book, a journal article, a monograph, or other publication, the table of contents is in the front. In books, it is typically found following the title page, publication information (often on the facing side of the title page), and dedication page, when one is included. In shorter publications, the table of contents may follow the title page, or the title on the same page. The table of contents in a book lists the number and title of each chapter and its beginning page number. An index, which is most common in books but may also be included in shorter works, is at the back of the publication. Books, especially academic texts, frequently have two: a subject index and an author index. Readers can look alphabetically for specific subjects in the subject index. Likewise, they can look up specific authors cited, quoted, discussed, or mentioned in the author index.

The index in a book offers particular advantages to students. For example, college course instructors typically assign certain textbooks, but do not expect students to read the entire book from cover to cover immediately. They usually assign specific chapters to read in preparation for specific lectures and/or discussions in certain upcoming classes. Reading portions at a time, some students may find references they either do not fully understand or want to know more about. They can look these topics up in the book's subject index to find them in later chapters. When a text author refers to another author, students can also look up the name in the book's author index to find all page numbers of all other references to that author. College students also typically are assigned research papers to write. A book's subject and author indexes can guide students to pages that may help inform them of other books to use for researching paper topics.

Headings

Headings and subheadings concisely inform readers what each section of a paper contains, as well as showing how its information is organized both visually and verbally. Headings are typically up to about five words long. They are not meant to give in-depth analytical information about the topic of their section, but rather an idea of its subject matter. Text authors should maintain consistent style across all headings. Readers should not expect headings if there is not material for more than one heading at each level, just as a list is unnecessary for a single item. Subheadings may be a bit longer than headings because they expand upon them. Readers should skim the subheadings in a paper to use them as a map of how content is arranged. Subheadings are in smaller fonts than headings to mirror relative importance. Subheadings are not necessary for every paragraph. They should enhance content, not substitute for topic sentences.

When a heading is brief, simple, and written in the form of a question, it can have the effect of further drawing readers into the text. An effective author will also answer the question in the heading soon in the following text. Question headings and their text answers are particularly helpful for engaging readers with average reading skills. Both headings and subheadings are most effective with more readers when they are obvious, simple, and get to their points immediately. Simple headings attract readers; simple subheadings allow readers a break, during which they also inform reader decisions whether to continue reading or not. Headings stand out from other text through boldface, but also italicizing and underlining them would be excessive. Uppercase-lowercase headings are easier for readers to comprehend than all capitals. More legible fonts are better. Some experts prefer serif fonts in text, but sans-serif fonts in headings. Brief subheadings that preview upcoming chunks of information reach more readers.

Other Text Features

Textbooks that are designed well employ varied text features for organizing their main ideas, illustrating central concepts, spotlighting significant details, and signaling evidence that supports the ideas and points conveyed. When a textbook uses these features in recurrent patterns that are predictable, it makes it easier for readers to locate information and come up with connections. When readers comprehend how to make use of text features, they will take less time and effort deciphering how the text is organized, leaving them more time and energy for focusing on the actual content in the text. Instructional activities can include not only previewing text through observing main text features, but moreover through examining and deconstructing the text and ascertaining how the text features can aid them in locating and applying text information for learning.

Included among various text features are a table of contents, headings, subheadings, an index, a glossary, a foreword, a preface, paragraphing spaces, bullet lists, footnotes, sidebars, diagrams, graphs, charts, pictures, illustrations, captions, italics, boldface, colors, and symbols. A **glossary** is a list of key vocabulary words and/or technical terminology and definitions. This helps readers recognize or learn specialized terms used in the text before reading it. A **foreword** is typically written by someone other than the text author and appears at the beginning to introduce, inform, recommend, and/or praise the work. A **preface** is often written by the author and also appears at the beginning, to introduce or explain something about the text, like new additions. A **sidebar** is a box with text and sometimes graphics at the left or right side of a page, typically focusing on a more specific issue, example, or aspect of the subject. **Footnotes** are additional comments/notes at the bottom of the page, signaled by superscript numbers in the text.

Navigational Tools on Websites

On the Internet or in computer software programs, text features include URLs, home pages, pop-up menus, drop-down menus, bookmarks, buttons, links, navigation bars, text boxes, arrows, symbols, colors, graphics, logos, and abbreviations. URLs (Universal Resource Locators) indicate the internet "address" or location of a website or web page. They often start with www. (world wide web) or http:// (hypertext transfer protocol) or https:// (the "s" indicates a secure site) and appear in the Internet browser's top address bar. Clickable buttons are often links to specific pages on a website or other external sites. Users can click on some buttons to open pop-up or drop-down menus, which offer a list of actions or departments from which to select. Bookmarks are the electronic versions of physical bookmarks. When users bookmark a website/page, a link is established to the site URL and saved, enabling returning to the site in the future without having to remember its name or URL by clicking the bookmark.

Readers can more easily navigate websites and read their information by observing and utilizing their various text features. For example, most fully developed websites include search bars, where users can type in topics, questions, titles, or names to locate specific information within the large amounts stored on many sites. Navigation bars (software developers frequently use the abbreviation term "navbar") are graphical user interfaces (GUIs) that facilitate visiting different sections, departments, or pages within a website, which can be difficult or impossible to find without these. Typically, they appear as a series of links running horizontally across the top of each page. Navigation bars displayed vertically along the left side of the page are also called sidebars. Links (i.e., hyperlinks) enable hyper-speed browsing by allowing readers to jump to new pages/sites. They may be URLs, words, phrases, images, buttons, etc. They are often but not always underlined and/or blue, or other colors.

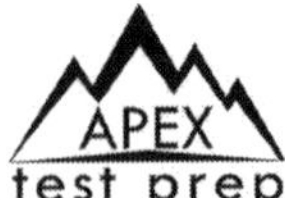

Charts, Graphs, and Other Visuals

Visuals are often used to aid a reader's understanding of a text. Words alone are not always sufficient to explain a concept or prove the truth of a conclusion. Therefore, to strengthen their argument, authors may choose to present supporting data in graphic form. As a reader, be sure to consider the argument and all supporting evidence carefully because it is common for authors to present only information that is favorable to their position. Selective inclusion and exclusion of evidence can be misleading and/or affirm an author's biased position.

Line Graphs

Line graphs are useful for visually representing data that vary continuously over time, like an individual student's test scores. The horizontal or *x*-axis shows dates/times; the vertical or *y*-axis shows point values. A dot is plotted on the point where each horizontal date line intersects each vertical number line, and then these dots are connected, forming a line. Line graphs show whether changes in values over time exhibit trends like ascending, descending, flat, or more variable, like going up and down at different times. For example, suppose a student's scores on the same type of reading test were 75% in October, 80% in November, 78% in December, 82% in January, 85% in February, 88% in March, and 90% in April. A line graph of these scores would look like this.

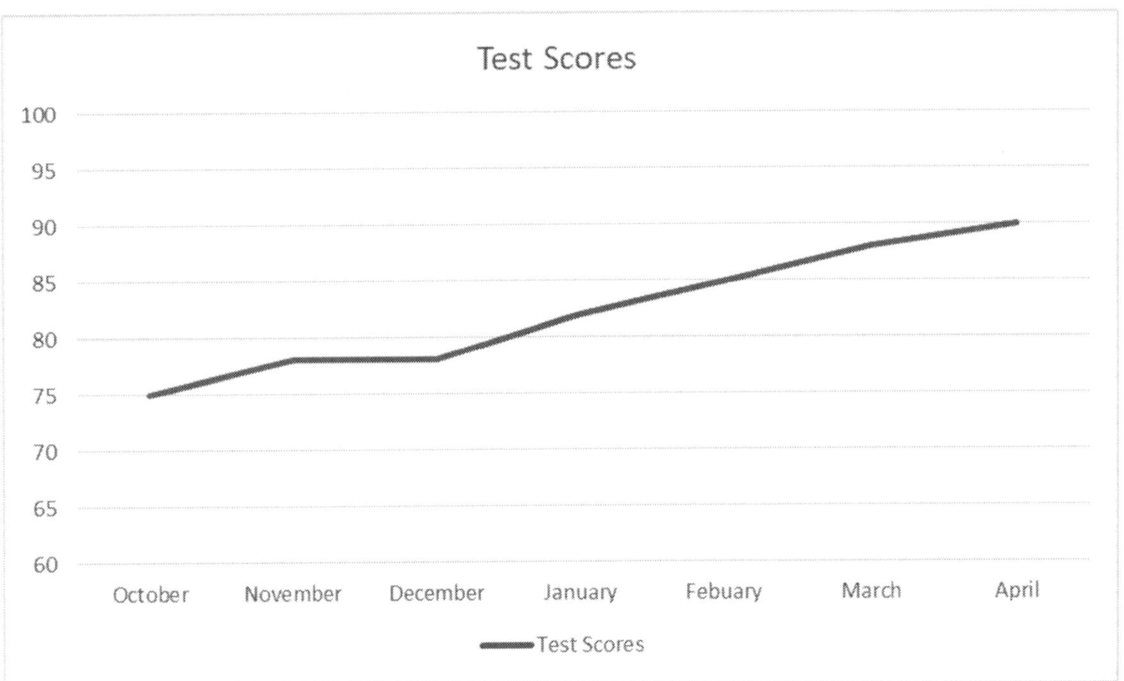

Bar Graphs

Bar graphs feature equally spaced, horizontal or vertical rectangular bars representing numerical values. They can show change over time as line graphs do, but unlike line graphs, bar graphs can also show differences and similarities among values at a single point in time. Bar graphs are also helpful for visually representing data from different categories, especially when the horizontal axis displays some value that is not numerical, like basketball players with their heights:

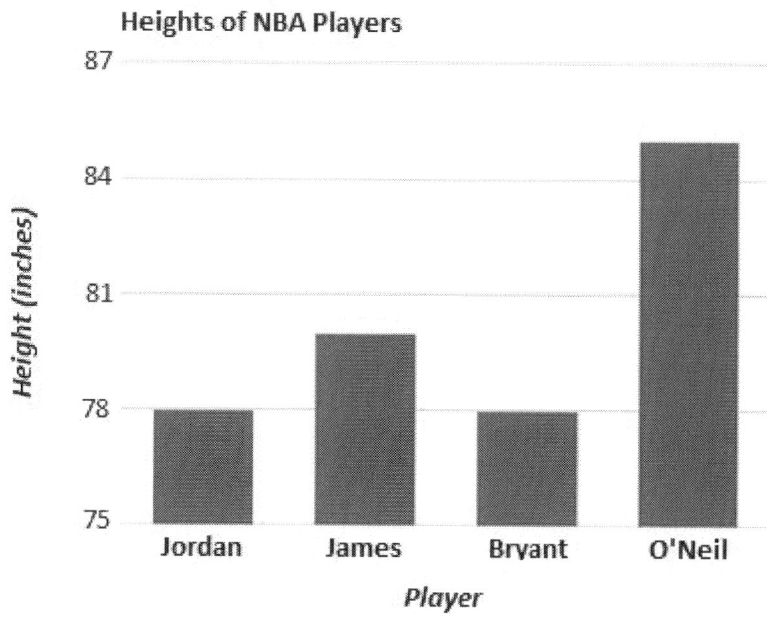

Pie Charts

Pie charts, also called **circle graphs**, are good for representing percentages or proportions of a whole quantity because they represent the whole as a circle or "pie", with the various proportion values shown as "slices" or wedges of the pie. This gives viewers a clear idea of how much of a total each item occupies. For example, biologists may have information that 62% of dogs have brown eyes, 20% have green eyes, and 18% have blue eyes. A pie chart of these distributions would look like this:

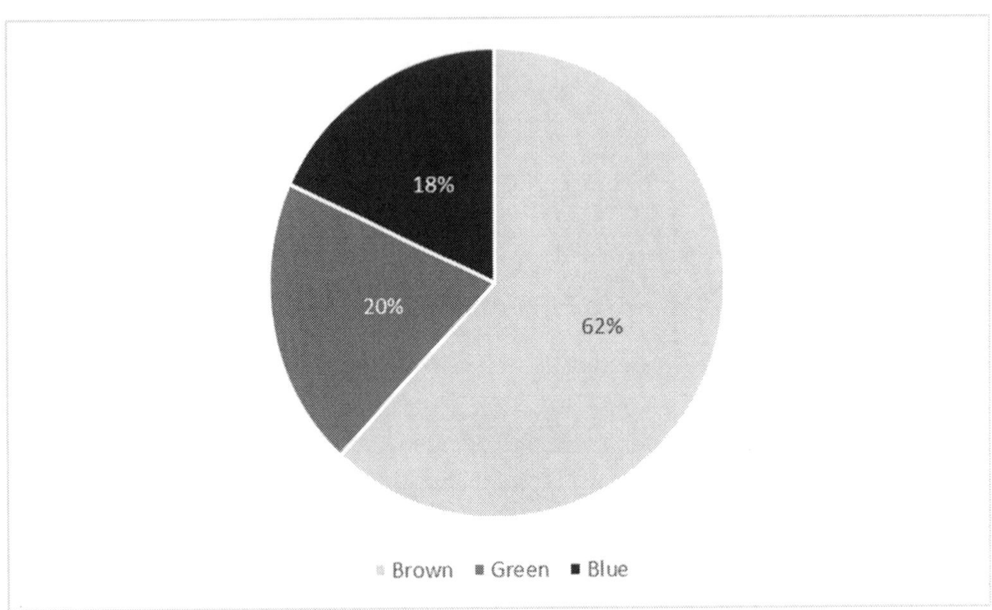

Pictograms

Magazines, newspapers, and other similar publications designed for consumption by the general public often use pictograms to represent data. **Pictograms** feature icons or symbols that look like whatever category of data is being counted, like little silhouettes shaped like human beings commonly used to represent people. If the data involve large numbers, like populations, one person symbol might represent one million people, or one thousand, etc. For smaller values, such as how many individuals out of ten fit a given description, one symbol might equal one person. Male and female silhouettes are used to differentiate gender, and child shapes for children. Little clock symbols are used to represent amounts of time, such as a given number of hours; calendar pages might depict months; suns and moons could show days and nights; hourglasses might represent minutes. While pictogram symbols are easily recognizable and appealing to general viewers, one disadvantage is that it is difficult to display partial symbols for in-between quantities.

Events in a Sequence

Recognizing the Structure of Texts in Various Formats

Text structure is the way in which the author organizes and presents textual information so readers can follow and comprehend it. One kind of text structure is sequence. This means the author arranges the text in a logical order from beginning to middle to end. There are three types of sequences:

- Chronological: ordering events in time from earliest to latest
- Spatial: describing objects, people, or spaces according to their relationships to one another in space

- Order of Importance: addressing topics, characters, or ideas according to how important they are, from either least important to most important

Chronological sequence is the most common sequential text structure. Readers can identify sequential structure by looking for words that signal it, like *first, today, earlier, meanwhile, next, then, later, finally;* verb tense; and specific times and dates the author includes as chronological references.

Sequence Structure in Narratives

Linear Narrative

A narrative is linear when it is told in chronological order. Traditional linear narratives will follow the plot diagram below depicting the narrative arc. The narrative arc consists of the exposition, conflict, rising action, climax, falling action, and resolution.

- Exposition: The exposition is in the beginning of a narrative and introduces the characters, setting, and background information of the story. The exposition provides the context for the upcoming narrative. Exposition literally means "a showing forth" in Latin.

- Conflict: In a traditional narrative, the conflict appears toward the beginning of the story after the audience becomes familiar with the characters and setting. The conflict is a single instance between characters, nature, or the self, in which the central character is forced to make a decision or move forward with some kind of action. The conflict presents something for the main character, or **protagonist**, to overcome.

- Rising Action: The rising action is the part of the story that leads into the climax. The rising action will develop the characters and plot while creating tension and suspense that eventually lead to the climax.

- Climax: The climax is the part of the story where the tension produced in the rising action comes to a culmination. The climax is the peak of the story. In a traditional structure, everything before the climax builds up to it, and everything after the climax falls from it. It is the height of the narrative, and it is usually either the most exciting part of the story or a turning point in the character's journey.

- Falling Action: The falling action happens as a result of the climax. Characters continue to develop, although there is a wrapping up of loose ends here. The falling action leads to the resolution.

- Resolution: The resolution is where the story comes to an end and usually leaves the reader with the satisfaction of knowing what happened within the story and why. However, stories do not always end in this fashion. Sometimes readers can be confused or frustrated at the end from lack of information or the absence of a happy ending.

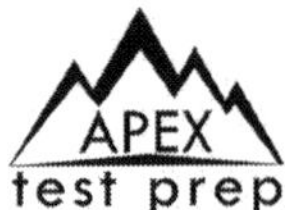

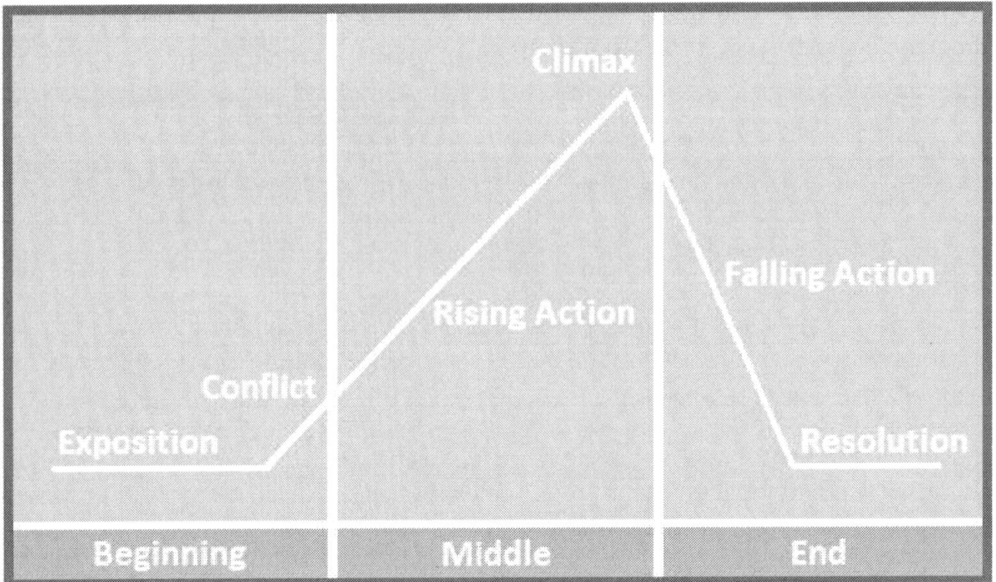

Nonlinear Narrative

A **nonlinear narrative** deviates from the traditional narrative because it does not always follow the traditional plot structure of the narrative arc. Nonlinear narratives may include structures that are disjointed, circular, or disruptive, in the sense that they do not follow chronological order. **In medias res** is an example of a nonlinear structure. ***In medias res*** is Latin for "in the middle of things," which is how many ancient texts, especially epic poems, began their story, such as Homer's *Iliad*. Instead of having a clear exposition with a full development of characters, they would begin right in the middle of the action. To form a chronological timeline when reading nonlinear narratives, readers must pay close attention when the storyline jumps back and forth between the present and the past. They may have to use their imaginations to fill in the gaps or use reasoning to make predictions, inferences, or conclusions.

Many modernist texts in the late nineteenth and early twentieth centuries experimented with disjointed narratives, moving away from traditional linear narrative. Disjointed narratives are depicted in novels like *Catch 22*, where the author, Joseph Heller, structures the narrative based on free association of ideas rather than chronology. Another nonlinear narrative can be seen in the novel *Wuthering Heights*, written by Emily Brontë; after the first chapter, the narrative progresses retrospectively instead of chronologically. There seem to be two narratives in *Wuthering Heights* working at the same time: a present narrative as well as a past narrative. Authors employ disrupting narratives for various reasons; some use it for the purpose of creating situational irony for the readers, while some use it to create a certain effect, such as excitement, discomfort, or fear.

Sequence Structure in Technical Documents

The purpose of technical documents, such as instructions manuals, cookbooks, or "user-friendly" documents, is to provide information to users as clearly and efficiently as possible. In order to do this, the sequence structure in technical documents should be as straightforward as possible. This usually involves some kind of chronological order or a direct sequence of events. For example, someone who is reading an instruction manual on how to set up their Smart TV wants directions in a clear, simple, straightforward manner that does not confuse them or leave them guessing about the proper sequence.

Sequence Structure in Informational Texts

The structure of informational texts depends on the specific genre. For example, a newspaper article may start by stating an exciting event that happened, then talk about that event in chronological order. Many informational texts also use **cause and effect structure**, which describes an event and then identifies reasons for why that event occurred. Some essays may write about their subjects by way of **comparison and contrast**, which is a structure that compares two things or contrasts them to highlight their differences. Other documents, such as proposals, will have a **problem to solution structure**, where the document highlights some kind of problem and then offers a solution. Finally, some informational texts are written with lush details and description in order to captivate the audience, allowing them to visualize the information presented to them. This type of structure is known as **descriptive.**

Craft and Structure

Fact and Opinion

Facts and Opinions

A fact is a statement that is true empirically or an event that has actually occurred in reality and can be proven or supported by evidence; it is generally objective. In contrast, an **opinion** is subjective, representing something that someone believes rather than something that exists in the absolute. People's individual understandings, feelings, and perspectives contribute to variations in opinion. Though facts are typically objective in nature, in some instances, a statement of fact may be both factual and yet also subjective. For example, emotions are individual subjective experiences. If an individual says that they feel happy or sad, the feeling is subjective, but the statement is factual; hence, it is a subjective fact. In contrast, if one person tells another that the other is feeling happy or sad—whether this is true or not—that is an assumption or an opinion.

Biases

Biases usually occur when someone allows their personal preferences or ideologies to interfere with what should be an objective decision. In personal situations, someone is biased towards someone if they favor them in an unfair way. In academic writing, being biased in your sources means leaving out objective information that would turn the argument one way or the other. The evidence of bias in academic writing makes the text less credible, so be sure to present all viewpoints when writing, not just your own, so to avoid coming off as biased. Bias can also show up in the tone of writing. For example, when an author speaks only positively or negatively about a certain subject (even if all statements are factual), the tone indicates a bias. It is important to be objective by presenting multiple sides of an argument and presenting facts with an unbiased tone; doing so usually allows the person to gain more credibility.

Stereotypes

Stereotypes are preconceived notions that place a particular rule or characteristics on an entire group of people. Stereotypes are usually offensive to the group they refer to or allies of that group and often have negative connotations. The reinforcement of stereotypes isn't always obvious. Sometimes stereotypes can be very subtle and are still widely used in order for people to understand categories within the world. For example, saying that women are more emotional and intuitive than men is a stereotype, although this is still an assumption used by many in order to understand the differences between one another.

Using Context to Determine Meaning

When readers encounter an unfamiliar word in text, they can use the surrounding context to help determine the word's meaning. The text's overall subject matter, the specific chapter or section, and the immediate sentence context can all provide clues to help the reader understand the word. Among others, one category of context clues is grammar. For example, the position of a word in a sentence and its relationship to the other words can help the reader establish whether the unfamiliar word is a verb, a noun, an adjective, an adverb, etc. This narrows down the possible meanings of the word to one part of speech. However, this may be insufficient. In the sentence, "Many birds migrate twice yearly," the reader can determine that the italicized word is a verb. While it probably does not mean eat or drink (because birds would need to do those actions more than twice each year), it could mean travel, mate, lay eggs, hatch, molt, etc.

Some words can have a number of different meanings depending on how they are used. For example, the word *fly* has a different meaning in each of the following sentences:

- "His trousers have a fly on them."
- "He swatted the fly on his trousers."
- "Those are some fly trousers."
- "They went fly fishing."
- "She hates to fly."
- "If humans were meant to fly, they would have wings."

As strategies, readers can try substituting a familiar word for an unfamiliar one and see whether it makes sense in the sentence. They can also identify other words in a sentence, offering clues to an unfamiliar word's meaning.

Word Choice

An author's word choice can also affect the style, tone, and mood of the text. Word choices, grammatical choices, and syntactical choices can help the audience figure out the scope, purpose, and emphasis. These choices—embedded in the words and sentences of the passage (i.e., the "parts")—help paint the intentions and goals of the author (i.e., the "whole"). For instance, if an author is using strong language like *enrage*, *ignite*, *infuriate*, and *antagonize*, then they may be cueing the reader into their own rage or they may be trying to incite anger in other. Likewise, if an author is continually using rapid, simple sentences, he or she might be trying to incite excitement and nervousness. These different choices and styles affect the overall message, or purpose. Sometimes the subject matter or audience will be discussed explicitly, but often readers have to decode the passage, or "break it down," to find the target audience and intentions. Meanwhile, the impact of the article can be personal or historical, for example, depending upon the passage—it can either "speak" to you personally or "capture" an historical era.

Denotation and Connotation

Denotation, a word's explicit definition, is often set in comparison to connotation, the emotional, cultural, social, or personal implications associated with a word. Denotation is more of an objective definition, whereas connotation can be more subjective, although many connotative meanings of words are similar for certain cultures. The denotative meanings of words are usually based on facts, and the connotative meanings of words are usually based on emotion. Here are some examples of words and their denotative and connotative meanings in Western culture:

Word	Denotative Meaning	Connotative Meaning
Home	A permanent place where one lives, usually as a member of a family.	A place of warmth; a place of familiarity; comforting; a place of safety and security. "Home" usually has a positive connotation.
Snake	A long reptile with no limbs and strong jaws that moves along the ground; some snakes have a poisonous bite.	An evil omen; a slithery creature (human or nonhuman) that is deceitful or unwelcome. "Snake" usually has a negative connotation.
Winter	A season of the year that is the coldest, usually from December to February in the northern hemisphere and from June to August in the southern hemisphere.	Circle of life, especially that of death and dying; cold or icy; dark and gloomy; hibernation, sleep, or rest. Winter can have a negative connotation, although many who have access to heat may enjoy the snowy season from their homes.

Literal Language

Literal language uses words in accordance with their actual definition. Many informational texts employ literal language because it is straightforward and precise. Documents such as instructions, proposals, technical documents, and workplace documents use literal language for the majority of their writing, so there is no confusion or complexity of meaning for readers to decipher. The information is best communicated through clear and precise language. The following are brief examples of literal language:

- I cook with olive oil.
- There are 365 days in a year.
- My grandma's name is Barbara.
- Yesterday we had some scattered thunderstorms.
- World War II began in 1939.
- Blue whales are the largest species of whale.

Figurative Language

Not meant to be taken literally, **figurative language** is useful when the author of a text wants to produce an emotional effect in the reader or add a heightened complexity to the meaning of the text. Figurative language is used more heavily in texts such as literary fiction, poetry, critical theory, and speeches. It goes beyond literal language, allowing readers to form associations they wouldn't normally form. Using language in a figurative sense appeals to the imagination of the reader. It is important to remember that words signify objects and ideas and are not the objects and ideas themselves. Figurative language can highlight this detachment by creating multiple associations, but it also points to the fact that language is fluid and capable of creating a world full of linguistic possibilities. It can be argued that figurative language is the heart of communication even outside of fiction and poetry. People connect through humor, metaphors, cultural allusions, puns, and symbolism in their everyday rhetoric. The following are terms associated with figurative language:

Simile

A **simile** is a comparison of two things using *like*, *than*, or *as*. A simile usually takes objects that have no apparent connection, such as a mind and an orchid, and compares them:

> His mind was as complex and rare as a field of ghost orchids.

Similes encourage new, fresh perspectives on objects or ideas that would not otherwise occur. Unlike similes, **metaphors** are comparisons that do not use *like*, *than*, or *as*. So, a metaphor from the above example would be:

> His mind was a field of ghost orchids.

Thus, similes highlight the comparison by focusing on the figurative side of the language, elucidating the author's intent. Metaphors, however, provide a beautiful yet somewhat equivocal comparison.

Metaphor

A popular use of figurative language, **metaphors** compare objects or ideas directly, asserting that something *is* a certain thing, even if it isn't. The following is an example of a metaphor used by writer Virginia Woolf:

> Books are the mirrors of the soul.

Metaphors have a vehicle and a tenor. The tenor is "books" and the vehicle is "mirrors of the soul." That is, the tenor is what is meant to be described, and the vehicle is that which carries the weight of the comparison. In this metaphor, perhaps the author means to say that written language (books) reflect a person's most inner thoughts and desires.

Dead metaphors are phrases that have been overused to the point where the figurative language has taken on a literal meaning, like "crystal clear." This phrase is in such popular use that the meaning seems literal ("perfectly clear") even when it is not.

Finally, an **extended metaphor** is one that goes on for several paragraphs, or even an entire text. "On First Looking into Chapman's Homer," a poem by John Keats, begins, "Much have I travell'd in the realms of gold," and goes on to explain the first time he hears Chapman's translation of Homer's writing. We see the extended metaphor begin in the first line. Keats is comparing travelling into "realms of gold" and exploration of new lands to the act of hearing a certain kind of literature for the first time. The extended metaphor goes on until the end of the poem where Keats stands "Silent, upon a peak in Darien," having heard the end of Chapman's translation. Keats has gained insight into new lands (new text) and is the richer for it.

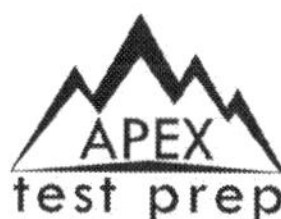

The following are brief definitions and examples of popular figurative language:

Onomatopoeia: A word that, when spoken, imitates the sound to which it refers. Ex: "We heard a loud *boom* while driving to the beach yesterday."

Personification: When human characteristics are given to animals, inanimate objects, or abstractions. An example would be in William Wordsworth's poem "Daffodils" where he sees a "crowd . . . / of golden daffodils . . . / Fluttering and dancing in the breeze." Dancing is usually a characteristic attributed solely to humans, but Wordsworth personifies the daffodils here as a crowd of people dancing.

Juxtaposition: Juxtaposition places two objects side by side for comparison or contrast. For example, Milton juxtaposes God and Satan in "Paradise Lost."

Paradox: A paradox is a statement that appears self-contradictory but is actually true. One example of a paradox is when Socrates said, "I know one thing; that I know nothing." Seemingly, if Socrates knew nothing, he wouldn't know that he knew nothing. However, he is using figurative language not to say that he literally knows nothing, but that true wisdom begins with casting all presuppositions about the world aside.

Hyperbole: A hyperbole is an exaggeration. Ex: "I'm so tired I could sleep for centuries."

Allusion: An allusion is a reference to a character or event that happened in the past. T.S. Eliot's "The Waste Land" is a poem littered with allusions, including, "I will show you fear in a handful of dust," alluding to Genesis 3:19: "For you are dust, and to dust you shall return."

Pun: Puns are used in popular culture to invoke humor by exploiting the meanings of words. They can also be used in literature to give hints of meaning in unexpected places. In "Romeo and Juliet," Mercutio makes a pun after he is stabbed by Tybalt: "look for me tomorrow and you will find me a grave man."

Imagery: This is a collection of images given to the reader by the author. If a text is rich in imagery, it is easier for the reader to imagine themselves in the author's world. One example of a poem that relies on imagery is William Carlos Williams' "The Red Wheelbarrow":

> so much depends
> upon
>
> a red wheel
> barrow
>
> glazed with rain
> water
>
> beside the white
> chickens

The starkness of the imagery and the placement of the words in this poem bring to life the images of a purely simple world. Through its imagery, this poem tells a story in just sixteen words.

Symbolism: A symbol is used to represent an idea or belief system. For example, poets in Western civilization have been using the symbol of a rose for hundreds of years to represent love. In Japan, poets have used the firefly to symbolize passionate love, and sometimes even spirits of those who have died. Symbols can also express powerful political commentary and can be used in propaganda.

Irony: There are three types of irony: verbal, dramatic, and situational. **Verbal irony** is when a person states one thing and means the opposite. For example, a person is probably using irony when they say, "I can't wait to study for this exam next week." **Dramatic irony** occurs in a narrative and happens when the audience knows something that the characters do not. In the modern TV series Hannibal, the audience knows that Hannibal Lecter is a serial killer, but most of the main characters do not. This is dramatic irony. Finally, **situational irony** is when one expects something to happen, and the opposite occurs. For example, we can say that a fire station burning down would be an instance of situational irony.

Author's Purpose

Authors may have many purposes for writing a specific text. They could be imparting information, entertaining their audience, expressing their own feelings, or trying to persuade their readers of a particular position. Authors' purposes are their reasons for writing something. A single author may have one overriding purpose for writing or multiple reasons. An author may explicitly state their intention in the text, or the reader may need to infer that intention. When readers can identify the author's purpose, they are better able to analyze information in the text. By knowing why the author wrote the text, readers can glean ideas for how to approach it.

The following is a list of questions readers can ask in order to discern an author's purpose for writing a text:

- Does the title of the text give you any clues about its purpose?
- Was the purpose of the text to give information to readers?
- Did the author want to describe an event, issue, or individual?
- Was it written to express emotions and thoughts?
- Did the author want to convince readers to consider a particular issue?
- Do you think the author's primary purpose was to entertain?
- Why do you think the author wrote this text from a certain point of view?
- What is your response to the text as a reader?
- Did the author state their purpose for writing it?

Rather than simply consuming the text, readers should attempt to interpret the information being presented and identify the information/evidence that is most relevant to the author's purpose. Being able to identify an author's purpose efficiently improves reading comprehension, develops critical thinking, and makes students more likely to consider issues in depth before accepting writer viewpoints. Authors of fiction frequently write to entertain readers. Another purpose for writing fiction is making a political statement; for example, Jonathan Swift wrote "A Modest Proposal" (1729) as a political satire. Another purpose for writing fiction as well as nonfiction is to persuade readers to take some action or further a particular cause. Fiction authors and poets both frequently use the tone of their writing to evoke certain moods; for example, Edgar Allan Poe wrote novels, short stories, and poems that evoke moods of gloom, guilt, terror, and dread. Another purpose of poets is evoking certain emotions: love is popular, as in Shakespeare's sonnets and numerous others. In "The Waste Land" (1922), T.S. Eliot evokes society's alienation, disaffection, sterility, and fragmentation.

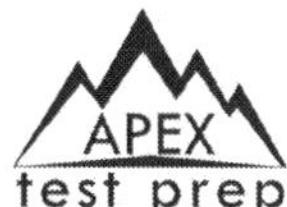

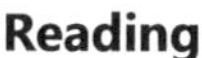

Authors seldom directly state their purposes in texts. Some students may be confronted with nonfiction texts such as biographies, histories, magazine and newspaper articles, and instruction manuals, among others. To identify the purpose in nonfiction texts, students can ask the following questions:

- Is the author trying to teach something?
- Is the author trying to persuade the reader?
- Is the author imparting factual information only?
- Is this a reliable source?
- Does the author have some kind of hidden agenda?

To apply author purpose in nonfictional passages, students can also analyze sentence structure, word choice, and transitions to answer the aforementioned questions and to make inferences. For example, authors wanting to convince readers to view a topic negatively often choose words with negative connotations.

Narrative Writing

Narrative writing tells a story. The most prominent type of narrative writing is the fictional novel. Here are some examples:

- Mark Twain's The Adventures of Tom Sawyer and The Adventures of Huckleberry Finn
- Victor Hugo's *Les Misérables*
- Charles Dickens' Great Expectations, David Copperfield, and A Tale of Two Cities
- Jane Austen's Northanger Abbey, Mansfield Park, Pride and Prejudice, Sense and Sensibility, and Emma
- Toni Morrison's Beloved, The Bluest Eye, and Song of Solomon
- Gabriel García Márquez's One Hundred Years of Solitude and Love in the Time of Cholera

Nonfiction works can also appear in narrative form. For example, some authors choose a narrative style to convey factual information about a topic, such as a specific animal, country, geographic region, and scientific or natural phenomenon.

Narrative writing tells a story, and the one telling the story is called the narrator. The narrator may be a fictional character telling the story from their own viewpoint. This narrator uses the first person (*I, me, my, mine* and *we, us, our,* and *ours*). The narrator may also be the author; for example, when Louisa May Alcott writes "Dear reader" in *Little Women*, she (the author) addresses us as readers. In this case, the novel is typically told in third person, referring to the characters as he, she, they, or them. Another more common technique is the omniscient narrator; in other words, the story is told by an unidentified individual who sees and knows everything about the events and characters—not only their externalized actions, but also their internalized feelings and thoughts. Second person narration, which addresses readers as you throughout the text, is more uncommon than the first and third person options.

Expository Writing

Expository writing is also known as informational writing. Its purpose is not to tell a story as in narrative writing, to paint a picture as in descriptive writing, or to persuade readers to agree with something as in argumentative writing. Rather, its point is to communicate information to the reader. As such, the point of view of the author will necessarily be more objective. ***Expository writing*** does not appeal to emotions or reason, nor does it use subjective descriptions to sway the reader's opinion or thinking; rather, expository writing simply provides facts, evidence, observations, and objective descriptions of the subject matter. Some examples of expository writing include research reports, journal articles, books about history, academic textbooks, essays, how-to articles, user instruction manuals, news articles, and other factual journalistic reports.

Technical Writing

Technical writing is similar to expository writing because it provides factual and objective information. Indeed, it may even be considered a subcategory of expository writing. However, technical writing differs from expository writing in two ways: (1) it is specific to a particular field, discipline, or subject, and (2) it uses technical terminology that belongs only to that area. Writing that uses technical terms is intended only for an audience familiar with those terms. An example of technical writing would be a manual on computer programming and use.

Persuasive Writing

Persuasive writing, or ***argumentative writing***, attempts to convince the reader to agree with the author's position. Some writers may respond to other writers' arguments by making reference to those authors or texts and then disagreeing with them. However, another common technique is for the author to anticipate opposing viewpoints, both from other authors and from readers. The author brings up these opposing viewpoints, and then refutes them before they can even be raised, strengthening the author's argument. Writers persuade readers by appealing to the readers' reason and emotion, as well as to their own character and credibility. Aristotle called these appeals ***logos***, ***pathos***, and ***ethos***, respectively.

Author's Point of View or Perspective

When a writer tells a story using the first person, readers can identify this by the use of first-person pronouns, like *I, me, we, us,* etc. However, first-person narratives can be told by different people or from different points of view. For example, some authors write in the first person to tell the story from the main character's viewpoint, as Charles Dickens did in his novels *David Copperfield* and *Great Expectations.* Some authors write in the first person from the viewpoint of a fictional character in the story, but not necessarily the main character. For example, F. Scott Fitzgerald wrote *The Great Gatsby* as narrated by Nick Carraway, a character in the story, about the main characters, Jay Gatsby and Daisy Buchanan. Other authors write in the first person, but as the omniscient narrator—an often unnamed person who knows all of the characters' inner thoughts and feelings. Writing in first person as oneself is more common in nonfiction.

First Person

First-person singular point of view becomes apparent when the author uses the pronouns "I," "me," "my," and "mine." The use of pronouns "we," "us," "our," and "ours" indicates the use of the first-person plural. Authors often choose first-person point of view to develop a close connection with the audience. First-person point of view brings a familiar and human feel to the writing, to which many readers relate. Often filled with subjective messaging, first-person point of view strives to connect with the readers on a personal level. Consider the following first-person point of view:

> "It was Sunday, the best day of the week. After church, Mama would take me straight to Grandma's house for cookies and tea. We would rock on the rocking chair on the front porch as if we didn't have a care in the world—truth be told, we really didn't have a care in the world."

This example demonstrates a clear example of how an author strives to pull in the reader with the use of first-person point of view. Readers connect to the sentimentality and develop a sense of nostalgia.

Second Person

Second-person point of view employs the pronouns "you," "your," and "yours." Only occasionally used in fiction, second-person point of view requires a lot more effort to develop. When authors want to fully immerse their audience in the experiences unfolding in the story, or when they wish for the audience to imagine themselves in that exact place and time, feeling that exact way, they may choose a second-person point of view. Consider the following passage:

> "Imagine you were at the site when the first thunderbolt fell from the sky. You look up and cannot believe your eyes. At first, you are mesmerized, but that feeling quickly morphs into shock. You look to your left, then to your right, because in that moment, you do not want to be alone. You want nothing more than to share these sensations with someone you love."

Second-person point of view, however, is difficult to sustain for a long period of time, especially in fiction, and it is better used for only brief moments when authors wish to plunge their audience directly into the storyline.

Third Person

When written from the third-person point of view, the writing can sometimes feel distant. The reader is somewhat removed from the experiences taking place. In literature, third-person points of view are developed with the use of a narrator who acts as a person on the outside looking in and giving play-by-play accounts of what is taking place. Pronouns "he," "she," "they," and even "it" can be used to describe the scenes in the story. Consider the following passage:

> "Emily knew it was just a matter of time before she would have to leave. She heard the clock ticking in the big, empty hallway, and it seemed as loud as a thousand church bells. She sat—completely still—until the clock struck twelve. Then she drew a deep breath, stood, picked up her bags, and left. 'Soon, it will all be over', she whispered to herself."

Although the narrator is describing Emily from a distance, and readers also feel somewhat removed, they can still feel that sense of fear, or perhaps anxiety, as Emily awaits the moment when she must leave.

Analyzing point of view is an essential skill for readers to develop in order to gain a deeper understanding of the storyline, as well as the different characters who all play a role in the story's development.

Interpreting Authorial Decisions Rhetorically

One of the freedoms in reading is to derive a unique perspective on the author's intent. Writing is an art form and can have many different interpretations. Often, readers who read the same literary work may have varying opinions regarding the author's intent. In fact, their varying interpretations might also differ from the author's intended message. Reading literature is less about being right than about striving to derive meaning from the message. The beauty of literature, as in any art form, is that it is open to interpretation.

There have been many theories about the intended meaning of Lewis Carroll's *Alice's Adventures in Wonderland*, from a bizarre take on the world brought on by drug use, to an obsession with food and drink—and many other interpretations as well. However, the author himself said that the intent was nothing more than to entertain a child friend by creating a dreamlike, fantastical tale. Does that mean, then, that readers should stop imagining, should stop analyzing, and should simply accept the author's intended meaning? Although it should be respected, the author's intended meaning may not be the only interpretation.

Literature can often take on a life of its own, and each reader is free to interpret literature in their own unique way, while keeping an open mind on other perspectives, particularly that of the author. Authors may learn a great deal about their work of art through the eyes of their readers, and authors may develop different perspectives based on their readers' keen observations and discoveries. True artists appreciate different interpretations of their work of art, and they regard the varied interpretations as something to be celebrated. Readers and authors affect one another, learn from one another, and become more skilled in their art when they allow their own interpretations to be analyzed.

Differentiating Between Various Perspectives

"Point of view" refers to the type of narration the author employs in a given story. "Perspective" refers to how characters perceive what is happening within the story. The characters' perspectives reveal their attitudes and help to shape their unique personalities. Consider the following scenario:

> "The family grabbed their snacks and blankets, loaded up the van, and headed out to the neighborhood park, even though Suki would have preferred to stay home. Once they settled in at their spot on the grass, the celebration was about to start. Within minutes, the fireworks began—crack, bang, pop! Hendrix jumped up and down with glee, Suki angrily put down her phone, and the dog yelped and buried its head under the blankets."

Each character was experiencing the same event—fireworks—and yet each character had a different reaction. Hendrix seems excited, Suki, angry, and the dog, frightened. No *one* perspective is the "right" perspective, just as no particular perspective is wrong; they are simply perspectives. What makes characters unique within a story are their unique perspectives. When authors develop characters with unique personalities and differing perspectives, stories are not only more believable, but they are more alive, more colorful, and more interesting. If all characters had the same one-dimensional perspective, the story would likely be quite dull.

There would never be a protagonist or antagonist, and there would be no reason to examine why each character acts and reacts to situations in such unique ways. Differentiating between various perspectives in a story can also lead to a much deeper understanding. For instance, it seems relatively easy to consider the perspective of the protagonist in any story since most readers connect with good and reject evil. But readers might wish to explore the story through the eyes of the antagonist. They might want to discover how the antagonist ended up so villainous, what events led to their corruption, and what, if anything, might lead them back to truth and justice.

Perspectives are how individuals see the world in which they live, and they are often formed from the individual's unique life experiences, their morals, and their values. Differentiating between various perspectives in literature helps readers to develop a greater appreciation for the story and for each character that helps to shape that story.

Evaluating Texts

When evaluating a text, readers should first identify the credentials of the author and publisher. For example, an author is more credible if he or she has education and/or experience in the field of their subject matter. The publisher should have measures in place to ensure validity of their content too. Depending on the text's format and subject matter, the publication may have had to go through a peer review process to double check veracity.

Readers should also evaluate content with a critical eye. Authors may include distracting information that sounds good but is not truly relevant. Additionally, it is possible for authors to misrepresent data or research in order to prove their point. Readers should take everything they read with a grain of salt and get in the habit of conduct their own research if something doesn't seem right.

Integration of Knowledge and Ideas

Using Evidence from the Text

One technique authors often use to make their fictional stories more interesting is not giving away too much information by providing hints and description. It is then up to the reader to draw a conclusion about the author's meaning by connecting textual clues with the reader's own pre-existing experiences and knowledge. Making interpretations and drawing conclusions are important reading strategies for understanding what is occurring in a text. Rather than directly stating who, what, where, when, or why, authors often describe story elements. Then, readers must draw conclusions to understand significant story components. As they go through a text, readers can think about the setting, characters, plot, problem, and solution; whether the author provided any clues for consideration; and combine any story clues with their existing knowledge and experiences to draw conclusions about what occurs in the text. Interpretations, predictions, and conclusions should always be supported by supporting evidence within the text.

Making Predictions

Before and during reading, readers can apply the reading strategy of making predictions about what they think may happen next. For example, what plot and character developments will occur in fiction? What points will the author discuss in nonfiction? Making predictions about portions of text they have not yet read prepares readers mentally for reading, and also gives them a purpose for reading. To inform and make predictions about text, the reader can do the following:

- Consider the title of the text and what it implies
- Look at the cover of the book
- Look at any illustrations or diagrams for additional visual information
- Analyze the structure of the text
- Apply outside experience and knowledge to the text

Readers may adjust their predictions as they read. Reader predictions may or may not come true in text.

Making Inferences

Authors describe settings, characters, character emotions, and events. Readers must infer to understand text fully. Inferring enables readers to figure out meanings of unfamiliar words, make predictions about upcoming text, draw conclusions, and reflect on reading. Readers can infer about text before, during, and after reading. In everyday life, we use sensory information to infer. Readers can do the same with text. When authors do not answer all readers' questions, readers must infer by saying "I think....This could be....This is because....Maybe....This means....I guess..." etc. Looking at illustrations, considering characters' behaviors, and asking questions during reading facilitate inference. Taking clues from text and connecting text to prior knowledge help to draw conclusions. Readers can infer word meanings, settings, reasons for occurrences, character emotions, pronoun referents, author messages, and answers to questions unstated in text. To practice inference, students can read sentences written/selected by the instructor, discuss the setting and character, draw conclusions, and make predictions.

Making inferences and drawing conclusions involve skills that are quite similar: both require readers to fill in information the author has omitted. Authors may omit information as a technique for inducing readers to discover the outcomes themselves; or they may consider certain information unimportant; or they may assume their reading audience already knows certain information. To make an inference or draw a conclusion about text, readers should observe all facts and arguments the author has presented and consider what they already know from their own personal experiences. Reading students taking multiple-choice tests that refer to text passages can determine correct and incorrect choices based on the information in the passage. For example, from a text passage describing an individual's signs of anxiety while unloading groceries and nervously clutching their wallet at a grocery store checkout, readers can infer or conclude that the individual may not have enough money to pay for everything.

Comparing and Contrasting Themes

The **theme** of a piece of text is the central idea the author communicates. Whereas the topic of a passage of text may be concrete in nature, the theme is always conceptual. For example, while the topic of Mark Twain's novel *The Adventures of Huckleberry Finn* might be described as something like the coming-of-age experiences of a poor, illiterate, functionally orphaned boy around and on the Mississippi River in 19th-century Missouri, one theme of the book might be that human beings are corrupted by society. Another might be that slavery and "civilized" society itself are hypocritical. Whereas the main idea in a text is the most important single point that the author wants to make, the theme is the concept or view around which the author centers the text.

Throughout time, humans have told stories with similar themes. Some themes are universal across time, space, and culture. These include themes of the individual as a hero, conflicts of the individual against nature, the individual against society, change vs. tradition, the circle of life, coming-of-age, and the complexities of love. Themes involving war and peace have featured prominently in diverse works, like Homer's *Iliad*, Tolstoy's *War and Peace* (1869), Stephen Crane's *The Red Badge of Courage* (1895), Hemingway's *A Farewell to Arms* (1929), and Margaret Mitchell's *Gone with the Wind* (1936). Another universal literary theme is that of the quest. These appear in folklore from countries and cultures worldwide, including the Gilgamesh Epic, Arthurian legend's Holy Grail quest, Virgil's *Aeneid*, Homer's *Odyssey*, and the *Argonautica*. Cervantes' *Don Quixote* is a parody of chivalric quests. J.R.R. Tolkien's *The Lord of the Rings* trilogy (1954) also features a quest.

Similar themes across cultures often occur in countries that share a border or are otherwise geographically close together. For example, a folklore story of a rabbit in the moon using a mortar and pestle is shared among China, Japan, Korea, and Thailand—making medicine in China, making rice cakes in Japan and Korea, and hulling rice in Thailand. Another instance is when cultures are more distant geographically, but their languages are related. For example, East Turkestan's Uighurs and people in Turkey share tales of folk hero Effendi Nasreddin Hodja. Another instance, which may either be called cultural diffusion or simply reflect commonalities in the human imagination, involves shared themes among geographically and linguistically different cultures: both Cameroon's and Greece's folklore tell of centaurs; Cameroon, India, Malaysia, Thailand, and Japan, of mermaids; Brazil, Peru, China, Japan, Malaysia, Indonesia, and Cameroon, of underwater civilizations; and China, Japan, Thailand, Vietnam, Malaysia, Brazil, and Peru, of shape-shifters.

Two prevalent literary themes are love and friendship, which can end happily, sadly, or both. William Shakespeare's *Romeo and Juliet*, Emily Brontë's *Wuthering Heights*, Leo Tolstoy's *Anna Karenina*, and both *Pride and Prejudice* and *Sense and Sensibility* by Jane Austen are famous examples. Another theme recurring in popular literature is of revenge, an old theme in dramatic literature, e.g. Elizabethans Thomas

Kyd's *The Spanish Tragedy* and Thomas Middleton's *The Revenger's Tragedy.* Some more well-known instances include Shakespeare's tragedies *Hamlet* and *Macbeth,* Alexandre Dumas' *The Count of Monte Cristo,* John Grisham's *A Time to Kill,* and Stieg Larsson's *The Girl Who Kicked the Hornet's Nest.*

Themes are underlying meanings in literature. For example, if a story's main idea is a character succeeding against all odds, the theme is overcoming obstacles. If a story's main idea is one character wanting what another character has, the theme is jealousy. If a story's main idea is a character doing something they were afraid to do, the theme is courage. Themes differ from topics in that a topic is a subject matter; a theme is the author's opinion about it. For example, a work could have a topic of war and a theme that war is a curse. Authors present themes through characters' feelings, thoughts, experiences, dialogue, plot actions, and events. Themes function as "glue" holding other essential story elements together. They offer readers insights into characters' experiences, the author's philosophy, and how the world works.

Evaluating an Argument

When authors write text for the purpose of persuading others to agree with them, they assume a position with the subject matter about which they are writing. Rather than presenting information objectively, the author treats the subject matter subjectively so that the information presented supports their position. In their argumentation, the author presents information that refutes or weakens opposing positions. Another technique authors use in persuasive writing is to anticipate arguments against the position. When students learn to read subjectively, they gain experience with the concept of persuasion in writing, and learn to identify positions taken by authors. This enhances their reading comprehension and develops their skills for identifying pro and con arguments and biases.

Argument Structure

There are five main parts of the classical argument that writers employ in a well-designed stance:

- Introduction: In the introduction to a classical argument, the author establishes goodwill and rapport with the reading audience, warms up the readers, and states the thesis or general theme of the argument.

- Narration: In the narration portion, the author gives a summary of pertinent background information, informs the readers of anything they need to know regarding the circumstances and environment surrounding and/or stimulating the argument, and establishes what is at risk or the stakes in the issue or topic. Literature reviews are common examples of narrations in academic writing.

- Confirmation: The confirmation states all claims supporting the thesis and furnishes evidence for each claim, arranging this material in logical order—e.g. from most obvious to most subtle or strongest to weakest.

- Refutation and Concession: The refutation and concession discuss opposing views and anticipate reader objections without weakening the thesis, yet permitting as many oppositions as possible.

- Summation: The summation strengthens the argument while summarizing it, supplying a strong conclusion and showing readers the superiority of the author's solution.

Introduction

A classical argument's introduction must pique reader interest, get readers to perceive the author as a writer, and establish the author's position. Shocking statistics, new ways of restating issues, or quotations or anecdotes focusing the text can pique reader interest. Personal statements, parallel instances, or analogies can also begin introductions—so can bold thesis statements if the author believes readers will agree. Word choice is also important for establishing author image with readers.

The introduction should typically narrow down to a clear, sound thesis statement. If readers cannot locate one sentence in the introduction explicitly stating the writer's position or the point they support, the writer probably has not refined the introduction sufficiently.

Narration and Confirmation

The narration part of a classical argument should create a context for the argument by explaining the issue to which the argument is responding, and by supplying any background information that influences the issue. Readers should understand the issues, alternatives, and stakes in the argument by the end of the narration to enable them to evaluate the author's claims equitably. The confirmation part of the classical argument enables the author to explain why they believe in the argument's thesis. The author builds a chain of reasoning by developing several individual supporting claims and explaining why that evidence supports each claim and also supports the overall thesis of the argument.

Refutation and Concession and Summation

The classical argument is the model for argumentative/persuasive writing, so authors often use it to establish, promote, and defend their positions. In the refutation aspect of the refutation and concession part of the argument, authors disarm reader opposition by anticipating and answering their possible objections, persuading them to accept the author's viewpoint. In the concession aspect, authors can concede those opposing viewpoints with which they agree. This can avoid weakening the author's thesis while establishing reader respect and goodwill for the author: all refutation and no concession can antagonize readers who disagree with the author's position. In the conclusion part of the classical argument, a less skilled writer might simply summarize or restate the thesis and related claims; however, this does not provide the argument with either momentum or closure. More skilled authors revisit the issues and the narration part of the argument, reminding readers of what is at stake.

Determining Whether Evidence is Relevant and Sufficient

Selecting the most relevant material to support a written text is a necessity in producing quality writing and for the credibility of an author. Arguments lacking in reasons or examples won't work in persuading the audience later on, because their hearts have not been pulled. Using examples to support ideas also gives the writing rhetorical devices such as pathos (appeal to emotion), logos (appeal to logic), or ethos (appeal to credibility), all three of which are necessary for a successful text.

An author needs to think about the audience. Are they indifferent? An author might use a personal story or example in order stir empathy. Are they resistant? If so, an author might use logical reasoning based in factual evidence so they will be convinced. Personal stories or testimonials, statistics, or documentary evidence are various types of examples that one can use for their writing.

Assessing Whether an Argument is Valid

Not all arguments are valid. Authors sometimes have one or more flaws in their argument's reasoning. In order to identify flaws in an argument, it will help to know of various argumentative flaws, such as red herring, false choice, and correlation vs. causation.

Here are some examples of what this type of question looks like:

- The reasoning in the argument is flawed because the argument . . .

- The argument is most vulnerable to criticism on the grounds that it . . .
- Which one of the following is an error in the argument's reasoning?
- A flaw in the reasoning of the argument is that . . .
- Which one of the following most accurately describes X's criticism of the argument made by Y?

Bait/Switch

One common flaw that is good to know is called the "bait and switch." It occurs when the test makers will provide an argument that offers evidence about X, and ends the argument with a conclusion about Y. A "bait and switch" answer choice will look like this:

> The argument assumes that X does in fact address Y without providing justification.

Let's look at an example:

> Hannah will most likely always work out and maintain a healthy physique. After all, Hannah's IQ is extremely high.

The correct answer will look like this:

> The argument assumes that Hannah's high IQ addresses her likelihood of always working out without providing justification.

Ascriptive Error

The ascriptive argument will begin the argument with something a third party has claimed. Usually, it will be something very general, like "Some people say that . . ." or "Generally, it has been said . . ." Then, the arguer will follow up that claim with a refutation or opposing view. The problem here is that when the arguer phrases something in this general sense without a credible source, their refutation of that evidence doesn't really matter. Here's an example:

It has been said that peppermint oil has been proven to relieve stomach issues and, in some cases, prevent cancer. I can attest to the relief in stomach issues; however, there is just not enough evidence to prove whether or not peppermint oil has the ability to prevent any kind of cancerous cells from forming in the body.

The correct answer will look like this:

> The argument assumes that the refuting evidence matters to the position that is being challenged.
>
> We have no credible source in this argument, so the refutation is senseless.

Prescriptive Error

First, let's take a look at what "prescriptive" means. Prescriptive means to give directions, or to say something *ought to* or *should* do something else. Sometimes an argument will be a descriptive premise (simply describing) that leads to a prescriptive conclusion, which makes for a very weak argument. This is like saying "There is a hurricane coming; therefore, we should leave the state." Even though this seems like common sense, the logical soundness of this argument is missing. A valid argument is when the truth of the premise leads absolutely to the truth of the conclusion. It's when the conclusion *is* something, not when the conclusion *should* be or do something. The flaw here is the assumption that the conclusion is going to work out; something prescriptive is not ever guaranteed to work out in a logical argument.

False Choice

A false choice, or false dilemma, flaw is a statement that assumes only the object it lists in the statement is the solution, or the only options that exist, for that problem. Here is an example:

> I didn't get the grade I want in Chemistry class. I must either be really stupid, I didn't get enough sleep, or I didn't eat enough that day.

This is a false choice error. We are offered only three options for why the speaker did not get the grade he or she wanted in Chemistry class. However, there is potentially more options why the grade was not achieved other than the three listed. The speaker could have been fighting a cold, or the professor may not have taught the material in a comprehensive way. It is our job as test takers to recognize that there are more options other than the choices we are given, although it appears that the only three choices are listed in the example.

Red Herring

A red herring is a point offered in an argument that is only meant to distract or mislead. A red herring will throw something out after the argument that is unrelated to the argument, although it still commands attention, thus taking attention away from the relevant issue. The following is an example of a red herring fallacy:

> Kirby: It seems like therapy is moving toward a more holistic model rather than something prescriptive, where the space between a therapist and client is seen more organic rather than a controlled space. This helps empower the client to reach their own conclusions about what should be done rather than having someone tell them what to do.
>
> Barlock: What's the point of therapy anyway? It seems like "talking out" problems with a stranger is a waste of time and always has been. Is it even successful as a profession?

We see Kirby present an argument about the route therapy is taking toward the future. Instead of responding to the argument by presenting their own side regarding where therapy is headed, Barlock questions the overall point of therapy. Barlock throws out a red herring here: Kirby cannot proceed with the argument because now Kirby must defend the existence of therapy instead of its future.

Correlation Versus Causality

Test takers should be careful when reviewing causal conclusions because the reasoning is often flawed, incorrectly classifying correlation as causality. Two events that may or may not be associated with one another are said to be linked such that one was the cause or reason for the other, which is considered the effect. To be a true "cause-and-effect" relationship, one factor or event must occur first (the cause) and be the sole reason (unless others are also listed) that the other occurred (the effect). The cause serves as the initiator of the relationship between the two events.

For example, consider the following argument:

> Last weekend, the local bakery ran out of blueberry muffins and some customers had to select something else instead. This week, the bakery's sales have fallen. Therefore, the blueberry muffin shortage last weekend resulted in fewer sales this week.

In this argument, the author states that the decline in sales this week (the effect) was caused by the shortage of blueberry muffins last weekend. However, there are other viable alternate causes for the decline in sales this week besides the blueberry muffin shortage. Perhaps it is summer and many normal patrons are away this week on vacation, or maybe another local bakery just opened or is running a special sale this week. There might be a large construction project or road work in town near the bakery, deterring customers from navigating the detours or busy roads. It is entirely possible that the decline this week is just a random coincidence and not attributable to any factor other than chance, and that next week, sales will return to normal or even exceed typical sales. Insufficient evidence exists to confidently assert that the blueberry muffin shortage was the sole reason for the decline in sales, thus mistaking correlation for causation.

Comparing Information that Differs Between Sources

A **primary source** is a piece of original work. This can include books, musical compositions, recordings, movies, works of visual art (paintings, drawings, photographs), jewelry, pottery, clothing, furniture, and other artifacts. Within books, primary sources may be of any genre. Whether nonfiction based on actual events or a fictional creation, the primary source relates the author's firsthand view of some specific event, phenomenon, character, place, process, ideas, field of study or discipline, or other subject matter. Whereas primary sources are original treatments of their subjects, **secondary sources** are a step removed from the original subjects; they analyze and interpret primary sources. These include journal articles, newspaper or magazine articles, works of literary criticism, political commentaries, and academic textbooks.

In the field of history, primary sources frequently include documents that were created around the same time period that they were describing, and most often produced by someone who had direct experience or knowledge of the subject matter. In contrast, secondary sources present the ideas and viewpoints of other authors about the primary sources; in history, for example, these can include books and other written works about the particular historical periods or eras in which the primary sources were produced. Primary sources pertinent in history include diaries, letters, statistics, government information, and original journal articles and books. In literature, a primary source might be a literary novel, a poem or book of poems, or a play. Secondary sources addressing primary sources may be criticism, dissertations, theses, and journal articles. **Tertiary sources,** typically reference works referring to primary and secondary sources, include encyclopedias, bibliographies, handbooks, abstracts, and periodical indexes.

In scientific fields, when scientists conduct laboratory experiments to answer specific research questions and test hypotheses, lab reports and reports of research results constitute examples of primary sources. When researchers produce statistics to support or refute hypotheses, those statistics are primary sources. When a scientist is studying some subject longitudinally or conducting a case study, they may keep a journal or diary. For example, Charles Darwin kept diaries of extensive notes on his studies during sea voyages on the *Beagle*, visits to the Galápagos Islands, etc.; Jean Piaget kept journals of observational notes for case studies of children's learning behaviors. Many scientists, particularly in past centuries, shared and discussed discoveries, questions, and ideas with colleagues through letters, which also constitute primary sources. When a scientist seeks to replicate another's experiment, the reported results, analysis, and commentary on the original work is a secondary source, as is a student's dissertation if it analyzes or discusses others' work rather than reporting original research or ideas.

Evaluating and Integrating Data

Organizing, Analyzing, and Synthesizing Various Data Sources

There is a myriad of possible research sources, and it is the job of a critical reader to select relevant information from various sources, synthesize them, and evaluate them together to form conclusions. When conducting research, it is important to pick and choose only information that is relevant to the

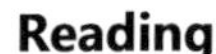

claim in question. When additional information is needed, further research should be conducted so that the argument can be as clear as possible.

Books

When a student has an assignment to research and write a paper, one of the first steps after determining the topic is to select research sources. The student may begin by conducting an Internet or library search of the topic, may refer to a reading list provided by the instructor, or may use an annotated bibliography of works related to the topic. To evaluate the worth of the book for the research paper, the student first considers the book title to get an idea of its content. Then the student can scan the book's table of contents for chapter titles and topics to get further ideas of their applicability to the topic. The student may also turn to the end of the book to look for an alphabetized index. Most academic textbooks and scholarly works have these; students can look up key topic terms to see how many are included and how many pages are devoted to them.

Journal Articles

Like books, journal articles are primary or secondary sources the student may need to use for researching any topic. To assess whether a journal article will be a useful source for a particular paper topic, a student can first get some idea about the content of the article by reading its title and subtitle, if any exists. Many journal articles, particularly scientific ones, include abstracts. These are brief summaries of the content. The student should read the abstract to get a more specific idea of whether the experiment, literature review, or other work documented is applicable to the paper topic. Students should also check the references at the end of the article, which today often contain links to related works for exploring the topic further.

Encyclopedias and Dictionaries

Dictionaries and encyclopedias are both reference books for looking up information alphabetically. Dictionaries are more exclusively focused on vocabulary words. They include each word's correct spelling, pronunciation, variants, part(s) of speech, definitions of one or more meanings, and examples used in a sentence. Some dictionaries provide illustrations of certain words when these inform the meaning. Some dictionaries also offer synonyms, antonyms, and related words under a word's entry. Encyclopedias, like dictionaries, often provide word pronunciations and definitions. However, they have broader scopes: one can look up entire subjects in encyclopedias, not just words, and find comprehensive, detailed information about historical events, famous people, countries, disciplines of study, and many other things. Dictionaries are for finding word meanings, pronunciations, and spellings; encyclopedias are for finding breadth and depth of information on a variety of topics.

Card Catalogs

A card catalog is a means of organizing, classifying, and locating the large numbers of books found in libraries. Without being able to look up books in library card catalogs, it would be virtually impossible to find them on library shelves. Card catalogs may be on traditional paper cards filed in drawers, or electronic catalogs accessible online; some libraries combine both. Books are shelved by subject area; subjects are coded using formal classification systems—standardized sets of rules for identifying and labeling books by subject and author. These assign each book a call number: a code indicating the classification system, subject, author, and title. Call numbers also function as bookshelf "addresses" where books can be located. Most public libraries use the Dewey Decimal Classification System. Most university, college, and research libraries use the Library of Congress Classification. Nursing students will also encounter the National Institute of Health's National Library of Medicine Classification System, which major collections of health sciences publications utilize.

Databases

A database is a collection of digital information organized for easy access, updating, and management. Users can sort and search databases for information. One way of classifying databases is by content, i.e. full-text, numerical, bibliographical, or images. Another classification method used in computing is by organizational approach. The most common approach is a relational database, which is tabular and defines data so they can be accessed and reorganized in various ways. A distributed database can be reproduced or interspersed among different locations within a network. An object-oriented database is organized to be aligned with object classes and subclasses defining the data. Databases usually collect files like product inventories, catalogs, customer profiles, sales transactions, student bodies, and resources. An associated set of application programs is a database management system or database manager. It enables users to specify which reports to generate, control access to reading and writing data, and analyze database usage. Structured Query Language (SQL) is a standard computer language for updating, querying, and otherwise interfacing with databases.

Reading Practice Quiz

The next three questions are based off the following passage.

> What a lark! What a plunge! For so it had always seemed to her, when, with a little squeak of the hinges, which she could hear now, she had burst open the French windows and plunged at Bourton into the open air. How fresh, how calm, stiller than this of course, the air was in the early morning; like the flap of a wave; the kiss of a wave; chill and sharp and yet (for a girl of eighteen as she then was) solemn, feeling as she did, standing there at the open window, that something awful was about to happen; looking at the flowers, at the trees with the smoke winding off them and the rooks rising, falling; standing and looking until Peter Walsh said, "Musing among the vegetables?"—was that it?—"I prefer men to cauliflowers"—was that it? He must have said it at breakfast one morning when she had gone out on to the terrace—Peter Walsh. He would be back from India one of these days, June or July, she forgot which, for his letters were awfully dull; it was his sayings one remembered; his eyes, his pocket-knife, his smile, his grumpiness and, when millions of things had utterly vanished—how strange it was!—a few sayings like this about cabbages.

Excerpt from Virginia Woolf's *Mrs. Dalloway*

1. The passage is reflective of which of the following types of writing?
   a. Persuasive
   b. Expository
   c. Technical
   d. Narrative

2. What was the narrator feeling right before Peter Walsh's voice distracted her?
   a. A spark of excitement for the morning
   b. Anger at the larks
   c. A sense of foreboding
   d. Confusion at the weather

3. What is the main point of the passage?
   a. To present the events leading up to a party.
   b. To show the audience that the narrator is resentful towards Peter.
   c. To introduce Peter Walsh back into the narrator's memory.
   d. To reveal what mornings are like in the narrator's life.

The next question is based on the following directions.

Follow these instructions to transform the word into something new.

1. Start with the word AUDITORIUM.
2. Eliminate all vowels except for the letter O.
3. Eliminate the "T."

4. Which of the following is the new word?
   a. Door
   b. Torn
   c. Dorm
   d. Tram

5. Felicia knew she had to be prudent if she was going to cross the bridge over the choppy water; one wrong move and she would be falling toward the rocky rapids.

Which of the following is the definition of the underlined word based on the context of the sentence above?

   a. Patient
   b. Afraid
   c. Dangerous
   d. Careful

See answers on next page.

Answer Explanations

1. D: The passage is reflective of a narrative. A narrative is used to tell a story, as we see the narrator trying to do in this passage by using memory and dialogue. Choice *A*, persuasive writing, uses rhetorical devices to try to convince the audience of something, and there is no persuasion or argument within this passage. Choice *B*, expository, is a type of writing used to inform the reader. Choice *C*, technical writing, is usually used within business communications and uses technical language to explain procedures or concepts to someone within the same technical field.

2. C: A sense of foreboding. The narrator, after feeling excitement for the morning, feels "that something awful was about to happen," which is considered foreboding. The narrator mentions larks and weather in the passage, but there is no proof of anger or confusion at either of them.

3. C: To introduce Peter Walsh back into the narrator's memory. Choice *A* is incorrect because, although the novel *Mrs. Dalloway* is about events leading up to a party, the passage does not mention anything about a party. Choice *B* is incorrect; the narrator calls Peter *dull* at one point, but the rest of her memories of him are more positive. Choice *D* is incorrect; although morning is described within the first few sentences of the passage, the passage quickly switches to a description of Peter Walsh and the narrator's memories of him.

4. C: Dorm. Eliminating all vowels but the "O" makes Choice *D* incorrect. The "T" is also eliminated, which makes Choice *B* incorrect. *A* is incorrect because there is only one "O" in "auditorium."

5. D: Felicia had to be prudent, or careful, if she was going to cross the bridge over the choppy water. Choice *A*, patient, is close to the word careful. However, careful makes more sense here. Choices *B* and *C* don't make sense within the context—Felicia wasn't hoping to be *afraid* or *dangerous* while crossing over the bridge, but was hoping to be careful to avoid falling.

Mathematics

Numbers and Algebra

Definitions

Whole numbers are the numbers 0, 1, 2, 3, ... Examples of other whole numbers would be 413 and 8,431. Notice that numbers such as 4.13 and $\frac{1}{4}$ are not included in whole numbers. **Counting numbers**, also known as **natural numbers**, consist of all whole numbers except for the zero. In set notation, the natural numbers are the set $\{1, 2, 3, \ldots\}$. The entire set of whole numbers and negative versions of those same numbers comprise the set of numbers known as **integers.** Therefore, in set notation, the integers are $\{\ldots, -3, -2, -1, 0, 1, 2, 3, \ldots\}$. Examples of other integers are −4,981 and 90,131. A number line is a great way to visualize the integers. Integers are labeled on the following number line:

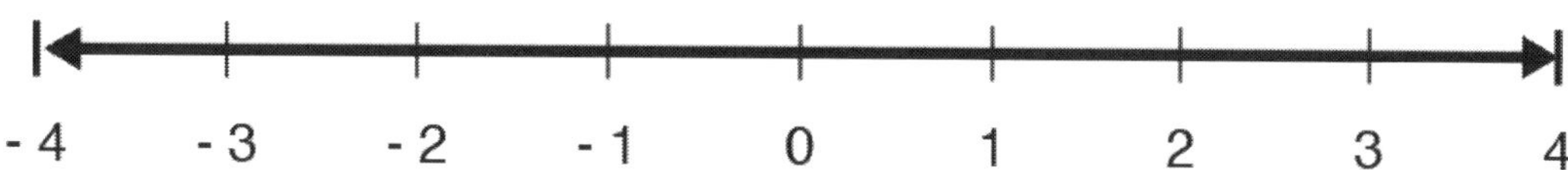

The arrows on the right- and left-hand sides of the number line show that the line continues indefinitely in both directions.

Fractions also exist on the number line as parts of a whole. For example, if an entire pie is cut into two pieces, each piece is half of the pie, or $\frac{1}{2}$. The top number in any fraction, known as the **numerator,** defines how many parts there are. The bottom number, known as the **denominator,** states how many pieces the whole is divided into. Fractions can also be negative or written in their corresponding decimal form.

A **decimal** is a number that uses a decimal point and numbers to the right of the decimal point representing the part of the number that is less than 1. For example, 3.5 is a decimal and is equivalent to the fraction $\frac{7}{2}$ or the mixed number $3\frac{1}{2}$. The decimal is found by dividing 2 into 7. Other examples of fractions are $\frac{2}{7}, \frac{-3}{14}$, and $\frac{14}{27}$.

Any number that can be expressed as a fraction is known as a **rational number.** Basically, if a and b are any integers and $b \neq 0$, then $\frac{a}{b}$ is a rational number. Any integer can be written as a fraction where the denominator is 1, so therefore the rational numbers consist of all fractions and all integers.

Any number that is not rational is known as an **irrational number.** Consider the number $\pi = 3.141592654 \ldots$. The decimal portion of that number extends indefinitely. In that situation, a number can never be written as a fraction. Another example of an irrational number is $\sqrt{2} = 1.414213662 \ldots$. Again, this number cannot be written as a ratio of two integers.

Together, the set of all rational and irrational numbers makes up the real numbers**.** The number line contains all real numbers. To graph a number other than an integer on a number line, it needs to be plotted between two integers. For example, 3.5 would be plotted halfway between 3 and 4.

Even numbers are integers that are divisible by 2. For example, 6, 100, 0, and −200 are all even numbers. Odd numbers are integers that are not divisible by 2. If an odd number is divided by 2, the result is a fraction. For example, −5, 11, and −121 are odd numbers.

Prime numbers consist of natural numbers greater than 1 that are not divisible by any other natural numbers other than themselves and 1. For example, 3, 5, and 7 are prime numbers. If a natural number is not prime, it is known as a **composite number**. 8 is a composite number because it is divisible by both 2 and 4, which are natural numbers other than itself and 1.

The **absolute value** of any real number is the distance from that number to 0 on the number line. The absolute value of a number can never be negative. For example, the absolute value of both 8 and −8 is 8 because they are both 8 units away from 0 on the number line. This is written as:

$$|8| = |-8| = 8$$

Factorization

Factorization is the process of breaking up a mathematical quantity, such as a number or polynomial, into a product of two or more factors. For example, a factorization of the number 16 is:

$$16 = 8 \times 2$$

If multiplied out, the factorization results in the original number. A **prime factorization** is a specific factorization when the number is factored completely using prime numbers only. For example, the prime factorization of 16 is:

$$16 = 2 \times 2 \times 2 \times 2$$

A factor tree can be used to find the prime factorization of any number. Within a factor tree, pairs of factors are found until no other factors can be used, as in the following factor tree of the number 84:

A factor tree

```
        84
       /  \
      4    21
     / \   / \
    2   2 3   7
```

84 = 2 x 2 x 3 x 7

It first breaks 84 into 21×4, which is not a prime factorization. Then, both 21 and 4 are factored into their primes. The final numbers on each branch consist of the numbers within the prime factorization. Therefore:

$$84 = 2 \times 2 \times 3 \times 7$$

Factorization can be helpful in finding greatest common divisors and least common denominators.

Also, a factorization of an algebraic expression can be found. Throughout the process, a more complicated expression can be decomposed into products of simpler expressions. To factor a polynomial, first determine if there is a greatest common factor. If there is, factor it out. For example, $2x^2 + 8x$ has a greatest common factor of $2x$ and can be written as $2x(x + 4)$. Once the greatest common monomial factor is factored out, if applicable, count the number of terms in the polynomial. If there are two terms, is it a difference of squares, a sum of cubes, or a difference of cubes?

If so, the following rules can be used:

$$a^2 - b^2 = (a + b)(a - b)$$

$$a^3 + b^3 = (a + b)(a^2 - ab + b^2)$$

$$a^3 - b^3 = (a - b)(a^2 + ab + b^2)$$

If there are three terms, and if the trinomial is a perfect square trinomial, it can be factored into the following:

$$a^2 + 2ab + b^2 = (a + b)^2$$

$$a^2 - 2ab + b^2 = (a - b)^2$$

If not, try factoring into a product of two binomials in the form of $(x + p)(x + q)$. For example, to factor $x^2 + 6x + 8$, determine what two numbers have a product of 8 and a sum of 6. Those numbers are 4 and 2, so the trinomial factors into $(x + 2)(x + 4)$.

Finally, if there are four terms, try factoring by grouping. First, group terms together that have a common monomial factor. Then, factor out the common monomial factor from the first two terms. Next, look to see if a common factor can be factored out of the second set of two terms that results in a common binomial factor. Finally, factor out the common binomial factor of each expression, for example:

$$xy - x + 5y - 5 = x(y - 1) + 5(y - 1)$$

$$(y - 1)(x + 5)$$

After the expression is completely factored, check the factorization by multiplying it out; if this results in the original expression, then the factoring is correct. Factorizations are helpful in solving equations that consist of a polynomial set equal to zero. If the product of two algebraic expressions equals zero, then at least one of the factors is equal to zero. Therefore, factor the polynomial within the equation, set each factor equal to zero, and solve. For example, $x^2 + 7x - 18 = 0$ can be solved by factoring into:

$$(x + 9)(x - 2) = 0$$

Set each factor equal to zero, and solve to obtain $x = -9$ and $x = 2$.

Algebraic Expressions

An *algebraic expression* is a mathematical phrase that may contain numbers, variables, and mathematical operations. An expression represents a single quantity. For example, $3x + 2$ is an algebraic expression.

An *algebraic equation* is a mathematical sentence with two expressions that are equal to each other. That is, an equation must contain an equals sign, as in $3x + 2 = 17$. This statement says that the value of the expression on the left side of the equals sign is equivalent to the value of the expression on the right side. In an expression, there are not two sides because there is no equals sign. The equals sign (=) is the difference between an expression and an equation.

To distinguish an expression from an equation, just look for the equals sign.

Example: Determine whether each of these is an expression or an equation.

- $16 + 4x = 9x - 7$ Solution: Equation
- $-27x - 42 + 19y$ Solution: Expression
- $4 = x + 3$ Solution: Equation

Using Mathematical Terms to Identify Parts of Expressions and Describe Expressions

A *variable* is a symbol used to represent a number. Letters, like x, y, and z, are often used as variables in algebra.

A *constant* is a number that cannot change its value. For example, 18 is a constant.

A *term* is a constant, variable, or the product of constants and variables. In an expression, terms are separated by + and – signs. Examples of terms are $24x$, -32, and $15xyz$.

Like terms are terms that contain the same variables. For example, $6z$ and $-8z$ are like terms, and $9xy$ and $17xy$ are like terms. Constants, like 23 and 51, are like terms as well.

A *factor* is something that is multiplied by something else. A factor may be a constant, a variable, or a sum of constants or variables.

A *coefficient* is the numerical factor in a term that has a variable. In the term $16x$, the coefficient is 16.

Example: Given the expression, $6x - 12y + 18$, answer the following questions.

- How many terms are in the expression?
- Solution: 3
- Name the terms.
- Solution: 6x, –12y, and 18 (Notice that the minus sign preceding the 12 is interpreted to represent negative 12)
- Name the factors.
- Solution: 6, x, –12, y
- What are the coefficients in this expression?
- Solution: 6 and –12
- What is the constant in this expression?
- Solution: 18

Simplifying expressions is a way of condensing numerical and algebraic information into equivalent forms that are shorter or easier to read. To simplify a mathematical expression such as $4 + 7$ is just adding the numbers to get 11. Any expression can be simplified by just performing all PEMDAS (parentheses, exponents, multiplication, division, addition, and subtraction) operations until no operator symbols remain.

Adding and Subtracting Linear Algebraic Expressions

To add and subtract linear algebraic expressions, you must combine like terms. Like terms are terms that have the same variable with the same exponent. In the following example, the x-terms can be added because the variable and exponent are the same. These terms add to be $9x$. Terms without a variable component are called constants. These terms will add to be nine.

Example: Add $(3x - 5) + (6x + 14)$

$3x - 5 + 6x + 14$	Rewrite without parentheses
$3x + 6x - 5 + 14$	Commutative property of addition
$9x + 9$	Combine like terms

When subtracting linear expressions, be careful to add the opposite when combining like terms. Do this by distributing -1, which is multiplying each term inside the second parentheses by negative one. Remember that distributing -1 changes the sign of each term.

Example: Subtract $(17x + 3) - (27x - 8)$

$17x + 3 - 27x + 8$	Distributive Property
$17x - 27x + 3 + 8$	Commutative property of addition
$-10x + 11$	Combine like terms

Example: Simplify by adding or subtracting:

$(6m + 28z - 9) + (14m + 13) - (-4z + 8m + 12)$

$6m + 28z - 9 + 14m + 13 + 4z - 8m - 12$	Distributive Property
$6m + 14m - 8m + 28z + 4z - 9 + 13 - 12$	Commutative Property of Addition
$12m + 32z - 8$	Combine like terms

Using the Distributive Property to Generate Equivalent Linear Algebraic Expressions

The Distributive Property: $a(b + c) = ab + ac$

The *distributive property* is a way of taking a factor and multiplying it through a given expression in parentheses. Each term inside the parentheses is multiplied by the outside factor, eliminating the parentheses. The following example shows how to distribute the number 3 to all the terms inside the parentheses.

Example: Use the distributive property to write an equivalent algebraic expression:

$3(2x + 7y + 6)$	
$3(2x) + 3(7y) + 3(6)$	Distributive property
$6x + 21y + 18$	Simplify

Because $a - b$ can be written $a + (-b)$, the distributive property can be applied in the following example.

Example: Use the distributive property to write an equivalent algebraic expression.

$7(5m - 8)$	
$7[5m + (-8)]$	Rewrite subtraction as addition of -8
$7(5m) + 7(-8)$	Distributive property
$35m - 56$	Simplify

In the following example, note that the factor of 2 is written to the right of the parentheses but is still distributed as before.

Example: Use the distributive property to write an equivalent algebraic expression:

$(3m + 4x - 10)2$	
$(3m)2 + (4x)2 + (-10)2$	Distributive property
$6m + 8x - 20$	Simplify

Example: $-(-2m + 6x)$

In this example, the negative sign in front of the parentheses can be interpreted as $-1(-2m + 6x)$

$-1(-2m + 6x)$	
$-1(-2m) + (-1)(6x)$	Distributive property
$2m - 6x$	Simplify

Evaluating Simple Algebraic Expressions for Given Values of Variables

To evaluate an algebra expression for a given value of a variable, replace the variable with the given value. Then perform the given operations to simplify the expression.

Example: Evaluate $12 + x$ for $x = 9$

$12 + (9)$	Replace x with the value of 9 as given in the problem. It is a good idea to always use parentheses when substituting this value. This will be particularly important in the following examples.
21	Add

Now see that when x is 9, the value of the given expression is 21.

Example: Evaluate $4x + 7$ for $x = 3$

$4(3) + 7$	Replace the x in the expression with 3
$12 + 7$	Multiply (remember order of operations)
19	Add

Therefore, when x is 3, the value of the given expression is 19.

Example: Evaluate $-7m - 3r - 18$ for $m = 2$ and $r = -1$

$-7(2) - 3(-1) - 18$	Replace m with 2 and r with -1
$-14 + 3 - 18$	Multiply
-29	Add

So, when m is 2 and r is -1, the value of the given expression is -29.

Simplifying Rational Algebraic Expressions

When given a problem, it is necessary to determine the best form of an expression or equation to use, given the context. Usually this involves some algebraic manipulation. If an equation is given, the simplest form of the equation is best. Simplifying involves using the distributive property, collecting like terms, etc. If an equation is needed to be solved, properties involving performing the same operation on both sides of the equation must be used. For instance, if a number is added to one side of the equals sign, it must be added to the other side as well. This maintains a true equation.

If an expression is given, simplifying can only involve properties allowing to rewrite the expression as an equivalent form. If there is no equals sign, mathematical operations cannot be performed on the expression, unless it is a rational expression. A *rational expression* can be written in the form of a fraction, in which the numerator and denominator are both polynomials and the denominator is not equal to zero. Rational expressions can always be multiplied times a form of 1. For example, consider the following rational expression involving radicals: $\frac{2}{\sqrt{2}}$. It is incorrect to write a fraction with a root in the denominator, and therefore the expression must be rationalized. Multiply the fraction times $\frac{\sqrt{2}}{\sqrt{2}}$, a form of 1. This results in $\frac{2}{\sqrt{2}} \times \frac{\sqrt{2}}{\sqrt{2}} = \frac{2\sqrt{2}}{\sqrt{4}} = \frac{2\sqrt{2}}{2} = \sqrt{2}$, which is the most suitable form of the expression.

Creating an Equivalent Form of an Algebraic Expression

Two algebraic expressions are equivalent if they represent the same value, even if they look different. To obtain an equivalent form of an algebraic expression, follow the laws of algebra. For instance, addition and multiplication are both commutative and associative. Therefore, terms in an algebraic expression can be added in any order and multiplied in any order. For instance, $4x + 2y$ is equivalent to $2y + 4x$ and $y \times 2 + x \times 4$. Also, the distributive law allows a number to be distributed throughout parentheses, as in the following:

$$a(b + c) = ab + ac$$

The expressions on both sides of the equals sign are equivalent. Collecting like terms is also important when working with equivalent forms because the simplest version of an expression is always the easiest one to work with.

Note that an expression is not an equation, and therefore expressions cannot be multiplied times numbers, divided by numbers, or have numbers added to them or subtracted from them and still have equivalent expressions. These processes can only happen in equations when the same step is performed on both sides of the equals sign.

Converting Fractions, Decimals, And Percentages

Within the number system, different forms of numbers can be used. It is important to be able to recognize each type, as well as work with, and convert between, the given forms. The **real number system** comprises natural numbers, whole numbers, integers, rational numbers, and irrational numbers. Natural numbers, whole numbers, integers, and irrational numbers typically are not represented as fractions, decimals, or percentages. Rational numbers, however, can be represented as any of these three forms. A **rational number** is a number that can be written in the form $\frac{a}{b}$, where a and b are integers, and b is not equal to zero. In other words, rational numbers can be written in a fraction form. The value a is the **numerator,** and b is the **denominator.** If the numerator is equal to zero, the entire fraction is equal to zero. Non-negative fractions can be less than 1, equal to 1, or greater than 1. Fractions are less than 1 if the numerator is smaller (less than) than the denominator.

For example, $\frac{3}{4}$ is less than 1. A fraction is equal to 1 if the numerator is equal to the denominator. For instance, $\frac{4}{4}$ is equal to 1. Finally, a fraction is greater than 1 if the numerator is greater than the denominator: the fraction $\frac{11}{4}$ is greater than 1. When the numerator is greater than the denominator, the fraction is called an **improper fraction**. An improper fraction can be converted to a **mixed number**, a combination of both a whole number and a fraction. To convert an improper fraction to a mixed number, divide the numerator by the denominator. Write down the whole number portion, and then write any remainder over the original denominator. For example, $\frac{11}{4}$ is equivalent to $2\frac{3}{4}$. Conversely, a mixed number can be converted to an improper fraction by multiplying the denominator by the whole number and adding that result to the numerator.

Fractions can be converted to decimals. With a calculator, a fraction is converted to a decimal by dividing the numerator by the denominator. For example:

$$\frac{2}{5} = 2 \div 5 = 0.4$$

Sometimes, rounding might be necessary. Consider:

$$\frac{2}{7} = 2 \div 7 = 0.28571429$$

This decimal could be rounded for ease of use, and if it needed to be rounded to the nearest thousandth, the result would be 0.286. If a calculator is not available, a fraction can be converted to a decimal manually. First, find a number that, when multiplied by the denominator, has a value equal to 10, 100, 1,000, etc. Then, multiply both the numerator and denominator times that number. The decimal form of the fraction is equal to the new numerator with a decimal point placed as many place values to the left as there are zeros in the denominator. For example, to convert $\frac{3}{5}$ to a decimal, multiply both the numerator and denominator times 2, which results in $\frac{6}{10}$.

The decimal is equal to 0.6 because there is one zero in the denominator, and so the decimal place in the numerator is moved one unit to the left. In the case where rounding would be necessary while working without a calculator, an approximation must be found. A number close to 10, 100, 1,000, etc. can be used. For example, to convert $\frac{1}{3}$ to a decimal, the numerator and denominator can be multiplied by 33 to turn the denominator into approximately 100, which makes for an easier conversion to the equivalent decimal. This process results in $\frac{33}{99}$ and an approximate decimal of 0.33. Once in decimal form, the number can be converted to a percentage. Multiply the decimal by 100 and then place a percent sign after the number. For example, 0.614 is equal to 61.4%. In other words, move the decimal place two units to the right and add the percentage symbol.

Arithmetic Operations

The four basic operations include addition, subtraction, multiplication, and division. The result of addition is a sum, the result of subtraction is a difference, the result of multiplication is a product, and the result of division is a quotient. Each type of operation can be used when working with rational numbers; however, the basic operations need to be understood first while using simpler numbers before working with fractions and decimals.

These operations should first be learned using whole numbers. Addition needs to be done column by column. To add two whole numbers, add the ones column first, then the tens columns, then the hundreds, etc. If the sum of any column is greater than 9, a one must be carried over to the next column. For example, the following is the result of $482 + 924$:

$$\begin{array}{r} {}^{1} \\ 482 \\ +924 \\ \hline 1406 \end{array}$$

Notice that the sum of the tens column was 10, so a one was carried over to the hundreds column. Subtraction is also performed column by column. Subtraction is performed in the ones column first, then the tens, etc. If the number on top is less than the number below, a one must be borrowed from the column to the left. For example, the following is the result of $5{,}424 - 756$:

$$\begin{array}{cccc} 4 & 13 & 11 & 14 \\ \not{5} & \not{4} & \not{2} & \not{4} \\ - & 7 & 5 & 6 \\ \hline 4 & 6 & 6 & 8 \end{array}$$

Notice that a one is borrowed from the tens, hundreds, and thousands place. After subtraction, the answer can be checked through addition. A check of this problem would be to show that $756 + 4{,}668 = 5{,}424$.

In multiplication, the number on top is known as the multiplicand, and the number below is the multiplier. Complete the problem by multiplying the multiplicand by each digit of the multiplier. Make sure to place the ones value of each result under the multiplying digit in the multiplier. The final product is found by adding each partial product.

The following example shows the process of multiplying 46 times 37:

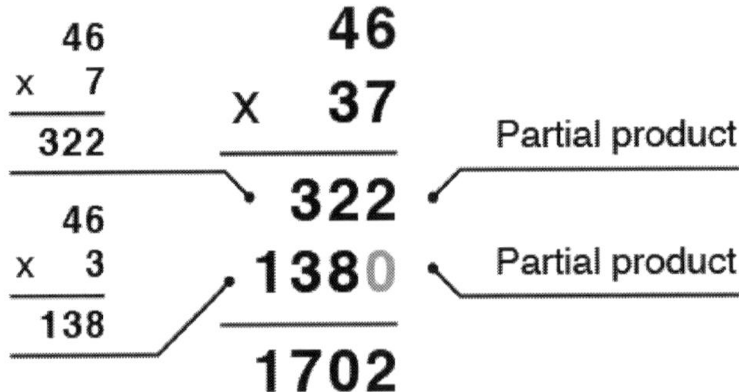

Finally, division can be performed using long division. When dividing, the first number is known as the **dividend,** and the second is the **divisor.** For example, with $a \div b = c$, a is the dividend, b is the divisor, and c is the quotient. For long division, place the dividend within the division bar and the divisor on the outside. For example, with $8{,}764 \div 4$, refer to the first problem in the diagram below. The first digit, 8, is divisible by 4 two times. Therefore, 2 goes above the division bar over the 8. Then, multiply 4 times 2 to get 8, and that product goes below the 8. Subtract to get 0, and then carry down the second digit, 7. Continue the same steps. $7 \div 4 = 1 \text{ R } 3$, so 1 is written above the 7. Multiply 4 times 1 to get 4, and write it below the 7. Subtract to get 3, and carry the 6 down next to the 3. Continuing this process for the next two digits results in a 9 and a 1. The final subtraction results in a 0, which means that 8,764 is evenly divisible by 4 with no remaining numbers.

The second example shows that:

$$4{,}536 \div 216 = 21$$

The steps are a little different because 216 cannot be contained in 4 or 5, so the first step is placing a 2 above the 3 because there are two 216's in 453. Finally, the third example shows that:

$$546 \div 31 = 17 \text{ R } 19$$

The 19 is a remainder. Notice that the final subtraction does not result in a 0, which means that 546 is not divisible by 31. The remainder can also be written as a fraction over the divisor to say that:

$$546 \div 31 = 17\frac{19}{31}$$

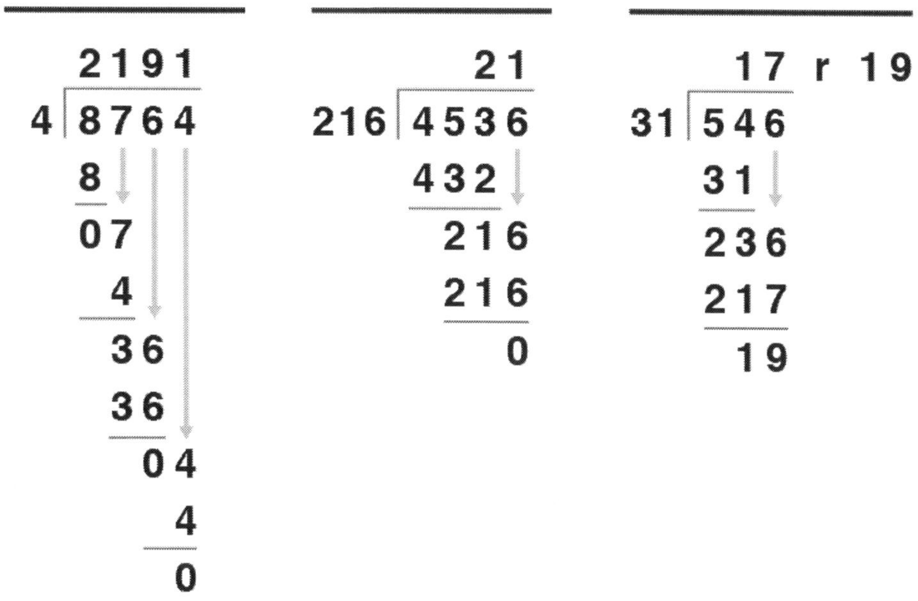

```
    2191              21            17 r 19
4 | 8764      216 | 4536       31 | 546
    8                 432             31
    07                 216            236
     4                 216            217
     36                  0             19
     36
      04
       4
       0
```

A remainder can have meaning in a division problem with real-world application. For example, consider the third example:

$$546 \div 31 = 17 \text{ R } 19$$

Let's say that we had $546 to spend on calculators that cost $31 each, and we wanted to know how many we could buy. The division problem would answer this question. The result states that 17 calculators could be purchased, with $19 left over. Notice that the remainder will never be greater than or equal to the divisor.

Once the operations are understood with whole numbers, they can be used with negative numbers. There are many rules surrounding operations with negative numbers. First, consider addition with integers. The sum of two numbers can first be shown using a number line. For example, to add $-5 + (-6)$, plot the point −5 on the number line. Adding a negative number is the same as subtracting, so move 6 units to the left. This process results in landing on −11 on the number line, which is the sum of −5 and −6. If adding a positive number, move to the right. Visualizing this process using a number line is useful for understanding; however, it is not efficient.

A quicker process is to learn the rules. When adding two numbers with the same sign, add the absolute values of both numbers, and use the common sign of both numbers as the sign of the sum. For example, to add $-5 + (-6)$, add their absolute values:

$$5 + 6 = 11$$

Then, introduce a negative number because both addends are negative. The result is −11. To add two integers with unlike signs, subtract the lesser absolute value from the greater absolute value, and apply the sign of the number with the greater absolute value to the result. For example, the sum $-7 + 4$ can be computed by finding the difference $7 - 4 = 3$ and then applying a negative because the value with the larger absolute value is negative. The result is −3. Similarly, the sum $-4 + 7$ can be found by computing the same difference but leaving it as a positive result because the addend with the larger absolute value is positive. Also, recall that any number plus 0 equals that number. This is known as the **Addition Property of 0.**

Subtracting two integers with opposite signs can be computed by changing to addition to avoid confusion. The rule is to add the first number to the opposite of the second number. The opposite of a number is the number with the same value on the other side of 0 on the number line. For example, −2 and 2 are opposites. Consider $4 - 8$. Change this to adding the opposite as follows: $4 + (-8)$. Then, follow the rules of addition of integers to obtain −4. Secondly, consider $-8 - (-2)$. Change this problem to adding the opposite as $-8 + 2$, which equals −6. Notice that subtracting a negative number functions the same as adding a positive number.

Multiplication and division of integers are actually less confusing than addition and subtraction because the rules are simpler to understand. If two factors in a multiplication problem have the same sign, the result is positive. If one factor is positive and one factor is negative, the result, known as the **product,** is negative. For example, $(-9)(-3) = 27$ and $9(-3) = -27$. Also, any number times 0 always results in 0. If a problem consists of several multipliers, the result is negative if it contains an odd number of negative factors, and the result is positive if it contains an even number of negative factors. For example:

$$(-1)(-1)(-1)(-1) = 1$$

and

$$(-1)(-1)(-1)(-1)(-1) = -1$$

These two problems are also examples of repeated multiplication, which can be written in a more compact notation using exponents. The first example can be written as $(-1)^4 = 1$, and the second example can be written as $(-1)^5 = -1$. Both are exponential expressions; −1 is the base in both instances, and 4 and 5 are the respective exponents. Note that a negative number raised to an odd power is always negative, and a negative number raised to an even power is always positive. Also, $(-1)^4$ is not the same as -1^4. In the first expression, the negative is included in the parentheses, but it is not in the second expression. The second expression is found by evaluating 1^4 first to get 1 and then by applying the negative sign to obtain −1.

Similar rules apply within division. First, consider some vocabulary. When dividing 14 by 2, it can be written in the following ways: $14 \div 2 = 7$ or $\frac{14}{2} = 7$. 14 is the **dividend,** 2 is the **divisor,** and 7 is the **quotient.** If two numbers in a division problem have the same sign, the quotient is positive. If two numbers in a division problem have different signs, the quotient is negative. For example:

$$14 \div (-2) = -7$$

and

$$-14 \div (-2) = 7$$

To check division, multiply the quotient times the divisor to obtain the dividend. Also, remember that 0 divided by any number is equal to 0. However, any number divided by 0 is undefined. It just does not make sense to divide a number by 0 parts.

If more than one operation is to be completed in a problem, follow the **Order of Operations**. The mnemonic device, PEMDAS, for the order of operations states the order in which addition, subtraction, multiplication, and division need to be done. It also includes when to evaluate operations within grouping symbols and when to incorporate exponents. PEMDAS, which some remember by thinking "please excuse my dear Aunt Sally," refers to parentheses, exponents, multiplication, division, addition, and subtraction. First, complete any operation within parentheses or any other grouping symbol like brackets, braces, or absolute value symbols. Note that this does not refer to when parentheses are used to represent multiplication like $(2)(5)$. An operation is not within parentheses like it is in (2×5). Then, any exponents must be computed. Next, multiplication and division are performed from left to right.

Finally, addition and subtraction are performed from left to right. The following is an example in which the operations within the parentheses need to be performed first, so the order of operations must be applied to the exponent, subtraction, addition, and multiplication within the grouping symbol:

$$9-3(3^2-3+4\cdot 3)$$

$$\begin{aligned} & 9-3(3^2-3+4\cdot 3) \\ &= 9-3(9-3+12) \\ &= 9-3(18) \\ &= 9-54 \\ &= -45 \end{aligned}$$

Work within the parentheses first

Once the rules for integers are understood, move on to learning how to perform operations with fractions and decimals. Recall that a rational number can be written as a fraction and can be converted to a decimal through division. If a rational number is negative, the rules for adding, subtracting, multiplying, and dividing integers must be used. If a rational number is in fraction form, performing addition, subtraction, multiplication, and division is more complicated than when working with integers. First, consider addition. To add two fractions having the same denominator, add the numerators and then reduce the fraction. When an answer is a fraction, it should always be in lowest terms. **Lowest terms** means that every common factor, other than 1, between the numerator and denominator is divided out. For example:

$$\frac{2}{8}+\frac{4}{8}=\frac{6}{8}=\frac{6\div 2}{8\div 2}=\frac{3}{4}$$

Both the numerator and denominator of $\frac{6}{8}$ have a common factor of 2, so 2 is divided out of each number to put the fraction in lowest terms. If denominators are different in an addition problem, the fractions must be converted to have common denominators. The **least common denominator (LCD)** of all the given denominators must be found, and this value is equal to the **least common multiple (LCM)** of the denominators. This non-zero value is the smallest number that is a multiple of both denominators. Then, rewrite each original fraction as an equivalent fraction using the new denominator. Once in this form, apply the process of adding with like denominators. For example, consider $\frac{1}{3}+\frac{4}{9}$. The LCD is 9 because it is the smallest multiple of both 3 and 9. The fraction $\frac{1}{3}$ must be rewritten with 9 as its denominator. Therefore, multiply both the numerator and denominator by 3.

Multiplying times $\frac{3}{3}$ is the same as multiplying times 1, which does not change the value of the fraction. Therefore, an equivalent fraction is $\frac{3}{9}$, and $\frac{1}{3}+\frac{4}{9}=\frac{3}{9}+\frac{4}{9}=\frac{7}{9}$, which is in lowest terms. Subtraction is performed in a similar manner; once the denominators are equal, the numerators are then subtracted. The following is an example of addition of a positive and a negative fraction:

$$-\frac{5}{12}+\frac{5}{9}=-\frac{5\times 3}{12\times 3}+\frac{5\times 4}{9\times 4}$$

$$-\frac{15}{36}+\frac{20}{36}=\frac{5}{36}$$

Common denominators are not used in multiplication and division. To multiply two fractions, multiply the numerators together and the denominators together. Then, write the result in lowest terms. For example:

$$\frac{2}{3}\times\frac{9}{4}=\frac{18}{12}=\frac{3}{2}$$

Alternatively, the fractions could be factored first to cancel out any common factors before performing the multiplication. For example:

$$\frac{2}{3}\times\frac{9}{4}=\frac{2}{3}\times\frac{3\times 3}{2\times 2}=\frac{3}{2}$$

This second approach is helpful when working with larger numbers, as common factors might not be obvious. Multiplication and division of fractions are related because the division of two fractions is changed into a multiplication problem. This means that dividing a fraction by another fraction is the same as multiplying the first fraction by the reciprocal of the second fraction, so that second fraction must be inverted, or "flipped," to be in reciprocal form. For example:

$$\frac{11}{15}\div\frac{3}{5}=\frac{11}{15}\times\frac{5}{3}=\frac{55}{45}=\frac{11}{9}$$

The fraction $\frac{5}{3}$ is the reciprocal of $\frac{3}{5}$. It is possible to multiply and divide numbers containing a mix of integers and fractions. In this case, convert the integer to a fraction by placing it over a denominator of 1. For example, a division problem involving an integer and a fraction is:

$$3\div\frac{1}{2}=\frac{3}{1}\times\frac{2}{1}=\frac{6}{1}=6$$

Finally, when performing operations with rational numbers that are negative, the same rules apply as when performing operations with integers. For example, a negative fraction times a negative fraction results in a positive value, and a negative fraction subtracted from a negative fraction results in a negative value.

Operations can be performed on rational numbers in decimal form. Recall that to write a fraction as an equivalent decimal expression, divide the numerator by the denominator. For example:

$$\frac{1}{8} = 1 \div 8 = 0.125$$

With the case of decimals, it is important to keep track of place value. To add decimals, make sure the decimal places are in alignment and add vertically. If the numbers do not line up because there are extra or missing place values in one of the numbers, then zeros may be used as placeholders. For example, $0.123 + 0.23$ becomes:

$$\begin{array}{r} 0.123 \\ +\underline{0.230} \\ 0.353 \end{array}$$

Subtraction is done the same way. Multiplication and division are more complicated. To multiply two decimals, place one on top of the other as in a regular multiplication process and do not worry about lining up the decimal points. Then, multiply as with whole numbers, ignoring the decimals. Finally, in the solution, insert the decimal point as many places to the left as there are total decimal values in the original problem. Here is an example of a decimal multiplication problem:

$$\begin{array}{rl} 0.52 & \textit{2 decimal places} \\ \underline{\text{x} \quad 0.2} & \textit{1 decimal place} \\ 0.104 & \textit{3 decimal places} \end{array}$$

The answer to 52 times 2 is 104, and because there are three decimal values in the problem, the decimal point is positioned three units to the left in the answer.

The decimal point plays an integral role throughout the whole problem when dividing with decimals. First, set up the problem in a long division format. If the divisor is not an integer, move the decimal to the right as many units as needed to make it an integer. The decimal in the dividend must be moved to the right the same number of places to maintain equality. Then, complete division normally. Here is an example of long division with decimals:

Long division with decimals

$$\begin{array}{r|l} & 212 \\ \hline 6 & 1272 \\ & \underline{12} \\ & \ \ 07 \\ & \ \ \ \underline{6} \\ & \ \ \ 12 \end{array}$$

The decimal point in 0.06 needed to move two units to the right to turn it into an integer (6), so it also needed to move two units to the right in 12.72 to make it 1,272. The quotient is 212. To check a division problem, multiply the answer by the divisor to see if the result is equal to the dividend.

Sometimes it is helpful to round answers that are in decimal form. First, find the place to which the rounding needs to be done. Then, look at the digit to the right of it. If that digit is 4 or less, the number in the place value to its left stays the same, and everything to its right becomes a 0. This process is known as **rounding down**. If that digit is 5 or higher, the number in the place value to its left increases by 1, and every number to its right becomes a 0. This is called rounding up. Excess 0s at the end of a decimal can be dropped. For example, 0.145 rounded to the nearest hundredth place would be rounded up to 0.15, and 0.145 rounded to the nearest tenth place would be rounded down to 0.1.

Another operation that can be performed on rational numbers is the square root. Dealing with real numbers only, the positive square root of a number is equal to one of the two repeated positive factors of that number. For example:

$$\sqrt{49} = \sqrt{7 \times 7} = 7$$

A **perfect square** is a number that has a whole number as its square root. Examples of perfect squares are 1, 4, 9, 16, 25, etc. If a number is not a perfect square, an approximation can be used with a calculator. For example, $\sqrt{67} = 8.185$, rounded to the nearest thousandth place. Taking the square root of a fraction that includes perfect squares involves breaking up the problem into the square root of the numerator separate from the square root of the denominator. For example:

$$\sqrt{\frac{16}{25}} = \frac{\sqrt{16}}{\sqrt{25}} = \frac{4}{5}$$

If the fraction does not contain perfect squares, a calculator can be used. Therefore, $\sqrt{\frac{2}{5}} = 0.632$, rounded to the nearest thousandth place. A common application of square roots involves the Pythagorean theorem. Given a right triangle, the sum of the squares of the two legs equals the square of the hypotenuse.

For example, consider the following right triangle:

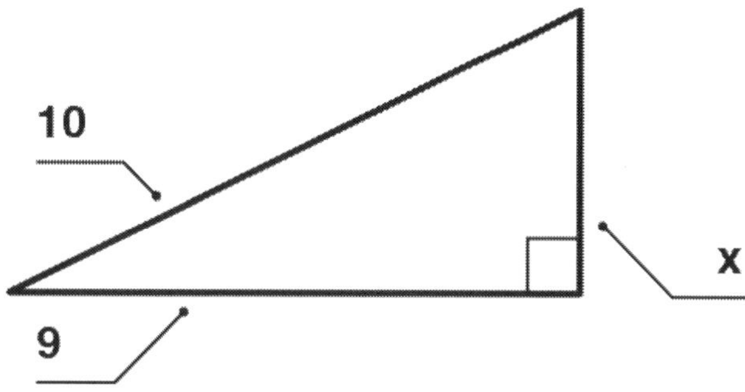

The missing side, *x*, can be found using the Pythagorean theorem.

$$9^2 + x^2 = 10^2$$

$$81 + x^2 = 100$$

$$x^2 = 19$$

To solve for *x*, take the square root of both sides. Therefore, $x = \sqrt{19} = 4.36$, which has been rounded to two decimal places.

In addition to the square root, the cube root is another operation. If a number is a **perfect cube**, the cube root of that number is equal to one of the three repeated factors. For example:

$$\sqrt[3]{27} = \sqrt[3]{3 \times 3 \times 3} = 3$$

A negative number has a cube root, which will also be a negative number. For example:

$$\sqrt[3]{-27} = \sqrt[3]{(-3)(-3)(-3)} = -3$$

Similar to square roots, if the number is not a perfect cube, a calculator can be used to find an approximation. Therefore, $\sqrt[3]{\frac{2}{3}} = 0.873$, rounded to the nearest thousandth place.

Higher-order roots also exist. The number relating to the root is known as the **index.** Given the following root, $\sqrt[3]{64}$, 3 is the index, and 64 is the **radicand.** The entire expression is known as the **radical.** Higher-order roots exist when the index is larger than 3. They can be broken up into two groups: even and odd roots. Even roots, when the index is an even number, follow the properties of square roots. They are found by finding the number that, when multiplied by itself the number of times indicated by the index, results in the radicand.

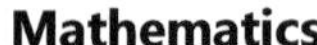

For example, the fifth root of 32 is equal to 2 because:

$$\sqrt[5]{32} = \sqrt[5]{2 \times 2 \times 2 \times 2 \times 2} = 2$$

Odd roots, when the index is an odd number, follow the properties of cube roots. A negative number has an odd root. Similarly, an odd root is found by finding the single factor that is repeated that many times to obtain the radicand. For example, the 4th root of 81 is equal to 3 because $3^4 = 81$. This radical is written as $\sqrt[4]{81} = 3$.

When performing operations with rational numbers, it might be helpful to round the numbers in the original problem to get a rough idea of what the answer should be. For example, if you walked into a grocery store and had a $20 bill, you could round each item to the nearest dollar and add up all the items to make sure that you will have enough money when you check out. This process involves obtaining an estimation of what the exact total would be. In other situations, it might be helpful to round to the nearest $\$10$ amount or $\$100$ amount. **Front-end rounding** might be helpful as well in many situations. In this type of rounding, the first digit of a number is rounded to the highest possible place value. Then, all digits following the first become 0. Consider a situation in which you are at the furniture store and want to estimate your total on three pieces of furniture that cost $434.99, $678.99, and $129.99. Front-end rounding would round these three amounts to $500, $700, and $200.

Therefore, the estimate of your total would be $\$500 + \$700 + \$200 = \$1{,}400$, compared to the exact total of $1,243.97. In this situation, the estimate is not that far off the exact answer. Rounding is useful both for approximation when an exact answer is not needed and for comparison when an exact answer is needed. For instance, if you had a complicated set of operations to complete and your estimate was $1,000, but you obtained an exact answer of $100,000, then you know something is off. You might want to check your work to see if you made a mistake because an estimate should not be that different from an exact answer. Estimates can also be helpful with square roots. If the square root of a number is unknown, then you can use the closest perfect square to help you approximate. For example, $\sqrt{50}$ is not equal to a whole number, but 50 is close to 49, which is a perfect square, and $\sqrt{49} = 7$. Therefore, $\sqrt{50}$ is a little bit larger than 7. The actual approximation, rounded to the nearest thousandth, is 7.071.

Comparing and Ordering Rational Numbers

Ordering rational numbers is a way to compare two or more different numerical values. Determining whether two amounts are equal, less than, or greater than is the basis for comparing both positive and negative numbers. Also, a group of numbers can be compared by ordering them from the smallest amount to the largest amount. A few symbols are necessary to use when ordering rational numbers. The equals sign, $=$, shows that the two quantities on either side of the symbol have the same value. For example, $\frac{12}{3} = 4$ because both values are equivalent. Another symbol that is used to compare numbers is $<$, which represents "less than." With this symbol, the smaller number is placed on the left and the larger number is placed on the right. Always remember that the symbol's "mouth" opens up to the larger number.

When comparing negative and positive numbers, it is important to remember that the number occurring to the left on the number line is always smaller and is placed to the left of the symbol. This idea might seem confusing because some values could appear at first glance to be larger, even though they are not. For example, $-5 < 4$ is read "negative 5 is less than 4." Here is an image of a number line for help:

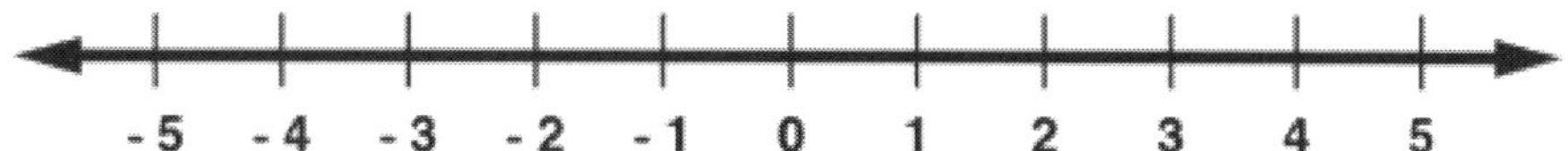

The symbol $\leq$ represents "less than or equal to," and it joins $<$ with equality. Therefore, both $-5 \leq 4$ and $-5 \leq -5$ are true statements and "-5 is less than or equal to both 4 and -5." Other symbols are $>$ and $\geq$, which represent "greater than" and "greater than or equal to." Both $4 \geq -1$ and $-1 \geq -1$ are correct ways to use these symbols.

Here is a chart of these four inequality symbols:

Symbol	Definition
$<$	less than
$\leq$	less than or equal to
$>$	greater than
$\geq$	greater than or equal to

Comparing integers is a straightforward process, especially when using the number line, but the comparison of decimals and fractions is not as obvious. When comparing two non-negative decimals, compare digit by digit, starting from the left. The larger value contains the first larger digit. For example, 0.1456 is larger than 0.1234 because the value 4 in the hundredths place in the first decimal is larger than the value 2 in the hundredths place in the second decimal. When comparing a fraction with a decimal, convert the fraction to a decimal and then compare in the same manner. Finally, there are a few options when comparing fractions. If two non-negative fractions have the same denominator, the fraction with the larger numerator is the larger value.

If they have different denominators, they can be converted to equivalent fractions with a common denominator to be compared, or they can be converted to decimals to be compared. When comparing two negative decimals or fractions, a different approach must be used. It is important to remember that the smaller number exists to the left on the number line. Therefore, when comparing two negative decimals by place value, the number with the larger first place value is smaller due to the negative sign. Whichever value is closer to 0 is larger. For instance, -0.456 is larger than -0.498 because of the values in the hundredth places. If two negative fractions have the same denominator, the fraction with the larger numerator is smaller because of the negative sign.

Solving Equations with One Variable

An **equation in one variable** is a mathematical statement where two algebraic expressions in one variable, usually x, are set equal. To solve the equation, the variable must be isolated on one side of the equals sign. The addition and multiplication principles of equality are used to isolate the variable. The **addition principle of equality** states that the same number can be added to or subtracted from both sides of an equation. Because the same value is being used on both sides of the equals sign, equality is maintained. For example, the equation $2x = 5x$ is equivalent to both $2x + 3 = 5x + 3$, and $2x - 5 = 5x - 5$. This principle can be used to solve the following equation:

$$x + 5 = 4$$

The variable x must be isolated, so to move the 5 from the left side, subtract 5 from both sides of the equals sign. Therefore:

$$x + 5 - 5 = 4 - 5$$

So, the solution is $x = -1$.

This process illustrates the idea of an **additive inverse** because subtracting 5 is the same as adding -5. Basically, add the opposite of the number that must be removed to both sides of the equals sign. The multiplication principle of equality states that equality is maintained when both sides of an equation are multiplied or divided by the same number. For example, $4x = 5$ is equivalent to both $16x = 20$ and $x = \frac{5}{4}$. Multiplying both sides times 4 and dividing both sides by 4 maintains equality. Solving the equation $6x - 18 = 5$ requires the use of both principles. First, apply the addition principle to add 18 to both sides of the equals sign, which results in $6x = 23$. Then use the multiplication principle to divide both sides by 6, giving the solution $x = \frac{23}{6}$. Using the multiplication principle in the solving process is the same as involving a multiplicative inverse. A **multiplicative inverse** is a value that, when multiplied by a given number, results in 1. Dividing by 6 is the same as multiplying by $\frac{1}{6}$, which is both the reciprocal and multiplicative inverse of 6.

When solving linear equations, check the answer by plugging the solution back into the original equation. If the result is a false statement, something was done incorrectly during the solution procedure. Checking the example above gives the following:

$$6 \times \frac{23}{6} - 18 = 23 - 18 = 5$$

Therefore, the solution is correct.

Some equations in one variable involve fractions or the use of the distributive property. In either case, the goal is to obtain only one variable term and then use the addition and multiplication principles to isolate that variable. Consider the equation $\frac{2}{3}x = 6$. To solve for x, multiply each side of the equation by the reciprocal of $\frac{2}{3}$, which is $\frac{3}{2}$. This step results in $\frac{3}{2} \times \frac{2}{3}x = \frac{3}{2} \times 6$, which simplifies into the solution $x = 9$. Now consider the equation:

$$3(x + 2) - 5x = 4x + 1$$

Use the distributive property to clear the parentheses. Therefore, multiply each term inside the parentheses by 3. This step results in:

$$3x + 6 - 5x = 4x + 1$$

Next, collect like terms on the left-hand side. **Like terms** are terms with the same variable or variables raised to the same exponent(s). Only like terms can be combined through addition or subtraction. After collecting like terms, the equation is:

$$-2x + 6 = 4x + 1$$

Finally, apply the addition and multiplication principles. Add $2x$ to both sides to obtain:

$$6 = 6x + 1$$

Then, subtract 1 from both sides to obtain $5 = 6x$. Finally, divide both sides by 6 to obtain the solution:

$$\frac{5}{6} = x$$

Two other types of solutions can be obtained when solving an equation in one variable. There could be no solution, or the solution set could contain all real numbers. Consider the equation:

$$4x = 6x + 5 - 2x$$

First, the like terms can be combined on the right to obtain $4x = 4x + 5$. Next, subtract $4x$ from both sides. This step results in the false statement $0 = 5$. There is no value that can be plugged into x that will ever make this equation true. Therefore, there is no solution. The solution procedure contained correct steps, but the result of a false statement means that no value satisfies the equation. The symbolic way to denote that no solution exists is $\emptyset$. Next, consider the equation:

$$5x + 4 + 2x = 9 + 7x - 5$$

Combining the like terms on both sides results in:

$$7x + 4 = 7x + 4$$

The left-hand side is exactly the same as the right-hand side. Using the addition principle to move terms, the result is $0 = 0$, which is always true. Therefore, the original equation is true for any number, and the solution set is all real numbers. The symbolic way to denote such a solution set is $\mathbb{R}$, or in interval notation, $(-\infty, \infty)$.

Using One- Or Multi-Step Operations

One-step problems take only one mathematical step to solve. For example, solving the equation $5x = 45$ is a one-step problem because the one step of dividing both sides of the equation by 5 is the only step necessary to obtain the solution $x = 9$. The **multiplication principle of equality** is the one step used to isolate the variable. The equation is of the form $ax = b$, where a and b are rational numbers. Similarly, the **addition principle of equality** could be the one step needed to solve a problem. In this case, the equation would be of the form $x + a = b$ or $x - a = b$, for real numbers a and b.

A **multi-step problem** involves more than one step to find the solution, or it could consist of solving more than one equation. An equation that involves both the addition principle and the multiplication principle is a two-step problem, and an example of such an equation is $2x - 4 = 5$. To solve, add 4 to both sides and then divide both sides by 2. An example of a two-step problem involving two separate equations is $y = 3x$, $2x + y = 4$. The two equations form a system that must be solved together in two variables. The system can be solved by the substitution method. Since y is already solved for in terms of x, replace y with $3x$ in the equation $2x + y = 4$, resulting in $2x + 3x = 4$. Therefore, $5x = 4$ and $x = \frac{4}{5}$. Because there are two variables, the solution consists of a value for both x and for y. Substitute $x = \frac{4}{5}$ into either original equation to find y. The easiest choice is $y = 3x$. Therefore:

$$y = 3 \times \frac{4}{5} = \frac{12}{5}$$

The solution can be written as the ordered pair $\left(\frac{4}{5}, \frac{12}{5}\right)$.

Real-world problems can be translated into both one-step and multi-step problems. In either case, the word problem must be translated from the verbal form into mathematical expressions and equations that can be solved using algebra. An example of a one-step real-world problem is the following: A cat weighs half as much as a dog living in the same house. If the dog weighs 14.5 pounds, how much does the cat weigh? To solve this problem, an equation can be used. In any word problem, the first step must be defining variables that represent the unknown quantities. For this problem, let x be equal to the unknown weight of the cat. Because two times the weight of the cat equals 14.5 pounds, the equation to be solved is: $2x = 14.5$. Use the multiplication principle to divide both sides by 2. Therefore, $x = 7.25$, and the cat weighs 7.25 pounds.

Most of the time, real-world problems require multiple steps. The following is an example of a multi-step problem: The sum of two consecutive page numbers is equal to 437. What are those page numbers? First, define the unknown quantities. If x is equal to the first page number, then $x + 1$ is equal to the next page number because they are consecutive integers. Their sum is equal to 437. Putting this information together results in the equation:

$$x + x + 1 = 437$$

To solve, first collect like terms to obtain:

$$2x + 1 = 437$$

Then, subtract 1 from both sides and then divide by 2. The solution to the equation is $x = 218$. Therefore, the two consecutive page numbers that satisfy the problem are 218 and 219. It is always important to make sure that answers to real-world problems make sense. For instance, it should be a red flag if the solution to this same problem resulted in decimals, which would indicate the need to check the work. Page numbers are whole numbers; therefore, if decimals are found to be answers, the solution process should be double-checked for mistakes.

Using Percentages

Percentages are defined as parts per one hundred. To convert a decimal to a percentage, move the decimal point two units to the right and place the percent sign after the number. Percentages appear in many scenarios in the real world. It is important to make sure the statement containing the percentage is translated to a correct mathematical expression. Be aware that it is extremely common to make a mistake when working with percentages within word problems.

An example of a word problem containing a percentage is the following: 35% of people speed when driving to work. In a group of 5,600 commuters, how many would be expected to speed on the way to their place of employment? The answer to this problem is found by finding 35% of 5,600. First, change the percentage to the decimal 0.35. Then compute the product: $0.35 \times 5{,}600 = 1{,}960$. Therefore, it would be expected that 1,960 of those commuters would speed on their way to work based on the data given. In this situation, the word "of" signals to use multiplication to find the answer. Another way percentages are used is in the following problem: Teachers work 8 months out of the year. What percent of the year do they work? To answer this problem, find what percent of 12 the number 8 is, because there are 12 months in a year.

Therefore, divide 8 by 12, and convert that number to a percentage:

$$\frac{8}{12} = \frac{2}{3} = 0.66\overline{6}$$

The percentage rounded to the nearest tenth place tells us that teachers work 66.7% of the year. Percentage problems can also find missing quantities like in the following question: 60% of what number is 75? To find the missing quantity, turn the question into an equation. Let x be equal to the missing quantity. Therefore, $0.60x = 75$. Divide each side by 0.60 to obtain 125. Therefore, 60% of 125 is equal to 75.

Sales tax is an important application relating to percentages because tax rates are usually given as percentages. For example, a city might have an 8% sales tax rate. Therefore, when an item is purchased with that tax rate, the real cost to the customer is 1.08 times the price in the store. For example, a $25 pair of jeans costs the customer:

$$\$25 \times 1.08 = \$27$$

If the sales tax rate is unknown, it can be determined after an item is purchased. If a customer visits a store and purchases an item for $21.44, but the price in the store was $19, they can find the tax rate by first subtracting $\$21.44 - \$19$ to obtain $2.44, the sales tax amount. The sales tax is a percentage of the in-store price. Therefore, the tax rate is $\frac{2.44}{19} = 0.128$, which has been rounded to the nearest thousandths place. In this scenario, the actual sales tax rate given as a percentage is 12.8%.

Applying Estimation Strategies and Rounding Rules

Sometimes it is helpful to find an estimated answer to a problem rather than working out an exact answer. An estimation might be much quicker to find, and it might be all that is required given the scenario. For example, if Aria goes grocery shopping and has only a $100 bill to cover all of her purchases, it might be appropriate for her to estimate the total of the items she is purchasing to determine if she has enough money to cover them. Also, an estimation can help determine if an answer makes sense. For instance, if you estimate that an answer should be in the 100s, but your result is a fraction less than 1, something is probably wrong in the calculation.

The first type of estimation involves rounding. As mentioned, **rounding** consists of expressing a number in terms of the nearest decimal place like the tenth, hundredth, or thousandth place, or in terms of the nearest whole number unit like tens, hundreds, or thousands place. When rounding to a specific place value, look at the digit to the right of the place. If it is 5 or higher, round the number to its left up to the next value, and if it is 4 or lower, keep that number at the same value. For instance, 1,654.2674 rounded to the nearest thousand is 2,000, and the same number rounded to the nearest thousandth is 1,654.267. Rounding can make it easier to estimate totals at the store. Items can be rounded to the nearest dollar. For example, a can of corn that costs $0.79 can be rounded to $1.00, and then all other items can be rounded in a similar manner and added together.

When working with larger numbers, it might make more sense to round to higher place values. For example, when estimating the total value of a dealership's car inventory, it would make sense to round the car values to the nearest thousands place. The price of a car that is on sale for $15,654 can be estimated at $16,000. All other cars on the lot could be rounded in the same manner and then added together. Depending on the situation, it might make sense to calculate an over-estimate. For example, to make sure Aria has enough money at the grocery store, rounding up for each item would ensure that she will have enough money when it comes time to pay. A $0.40 item rounded up to $1.00 would ensure that there is a dollar to cover that item. Traditional rounding rules would round $0.40 to $0, which does not make sense in this particular real-world setting. Aria might not have a dollar available at checkout to pay for that item if she uses traditional rounding. It is up to the customer to decide the best approach when estimating.

Estimating is also very helpful when working with measurements. Bryan is updating his kitchen and wants to retile the floor. Again, an over-measurement might be useful. Also, rounding to nearest half-unit might be helpful. For instance, one side of the kitchen might have an exact measurement of 14.32 feet, and the most useful measurement needed to buy tile could be estimating this quantity to be 14.5 feet. If the kitchen was rectangular and the other side measured 10.9 feet, Bryan might round the other side to 11 feet. Therefore, Bryan would find the total tile necessary according to the following area calculation: $14.5 \times 11 = 159.5$ square feet. To make sure he purchases enough tile, Bryan would probably want to purchase at least 160 square feet of tile. This is a scenario in which an estimation might be more useful than an exact calculation. Having more tile than necessary is better than having an exact amount, in case any tiles are broken or otherwise unusable.

Finally, estimation is helpful when exact answers are necessary. Consider a situation in which Sabina has many operations to perform on numbers with decimals, and she is allowed a calculator to find the result. Even though an exact result can be obtained with a calculator, there is always a possibility that Sabina could make an error while inputting the data. For example, she could miss a decimal place, or misuse the parentheses, causing a problem with the actual order of operations.

A quick estimation at the beginning could help ensure that her final answer is within the correct range. Sabina has to find the exact total of 10 cars listed for sale at the dealership. Each price has two decimal places included to account for both dollars and cents. If one car is listed at $21,234.43 but Sabina incorrectly inputs into the calculator the price of $2,123.443, this error would throw off the final sum by almost $20,000. A quick estimation at the beginning, by rounding each price to the nearest thousands place and finding the sum of the prices, would give Sabina an amount to compare the exact amount to. This comparison would let Sabina see if an error was made in her exact calculation.

Using Proportions

Fractions appear in everyday situations, and in many scenarios, they appear in the real-world as ratios and in proportions. A **ratio** is formed when two different quantities are compared. For example, in a group of 50 people, if there are 33 females and 17 males, the ratio of females to males is 33 to 17. This expression can be written in the fraction form as $\frac{33}{50}$, where the denominator is the sum of females and males, or by using the ratio symbol, 33:17. The order of the number matters when forming ratios. In the same setting, the ratio of males to females is 17 to 33, which is equivalent to $\frac{17}{50}$ or 17:33.

A **proportion** is an equation involving two ratios. The equation $\frac{a}{b}=\frac{c}{d}$, or $a{:}b = c{:}d$ is a proportion, for real numbers a, b, c, and d. Usually, in one ratio, one of the quantities is unknown, and cross-multiplication is used to solve for the unknown. Consider $\frac{1}{4}=\frac{x}{5}$. To solve for x, cross-multiply to obtain $5 = 4x$. Divide each side by 4 to obtain the solution $x=\frac{5}{4}$. It is also true that percentages are ratios in which the second term is 100 minus the first term. For example, 65% is 65:35 or $\frac{65}{100}$. Therefore, when working with percentages, one is also working with ratios.

Real-world problems frequently involve proportions. For example, consider the following problem: If 2 out of 50 pizzas are usually delivered late from a local Italian restaurant, how many would be late out of 235 orders? The following proportion would be solved with x as the unknown quantity of late pizzas: $\frac{2}{50}=\frac{x}{235}$. Cross multiplying results in $470 = 50x$. Divide both sides by 50 to obtain $x=\frac{470}{50}$, which in lowest terms is equal to $\frac{47}{5}$. In decimal form, this improper fraction is equal to 9.4. Because it does not make sense to answer this question with decimals (portions of pizzas do not get delivered) the answer must be rounded. Traditional rounding rules would say that 9 pizzas would be expected to be delivered late. However, to be safe, rounding up to 10 pizzas out of 235 would probably make more sense.

Using Ratios and Rates of Change

Recall that a **ratio** is the comparison of two different quantities. Comparing 2 apples to 3 oranges results in the ratio 2:3, which can be expressed as the fraction $\frac{2}{5}$. Note that order is important when discussing ratios. The number mentioned first is the antecedent, and the number mentioned second is the consequent. Note that the consequent of the ratio and the denominator of the fraction are *not* the same. When there are 2 apples to 3 oranges, there are five fruit total; two fifths of the fruit are apples, while three fifths are oranges. The ratio 2:3 represents a different relationship than the ratio 3:2. Also, it is important to make sure that when discussing ratios that have units attached to them, the two quantities use the same units. For example, to think of 8 feet to 4 yards, it would make sense to convert 4 yards to feet by multiplying by 3. Therefore, the ratio would be 8 feet to 12 feet, which can be expressed as the fraction $\frac{8}{20}$. Also, note that it is proper to refer to ratios in lowest terms. Therefore, the ratio of 8 feet to 4 yards is equivalent to the fraction $\frac{2}{5}$.

Many real-world problems involve ratios. Often, problems with ratios involve proportions, as when two ratios are set equal to find the missing amount. However, some problems involve deciphering single ratios. For example, consider an amusement park that sold 345 tickets last Saturday. If 145 tickets were sold to adults and the rest of the tickets were sold to children, what would the ratio of the number of adult tickets to children's tickets be? A common mistake would be to say the ratio is 145:345. However, 345 is the total number of tickets sold, not the number of children's tickets. There were $345 - 145 = 200$ tickets sold to children. The correct ratio of adult to children's tickets is 145:200. As a fraction, this expression is written as $\frac{145}{345}$, which can be reduced to $\frac{29}{69}$.

While a ratio compares two measurements using the same units, rates compare two measurements with different units. Examples of rates would be $200 for 8 hours of work, or 500 miles traveled per 20 gallons. Because the units are different, it is important to always include the units when discussing rates. Key words in rate problems include for, per, on, from, and in. Just as with ratios, it is important to write rates in lowest terms. A common rate in real-life situations is cost per unit, which describes how much one item/unit costs. When evaluating the cost of an item that comes in several sizes, the cost per unit rate can help buyers determine the best deal. For example, if 2 quarts of soup was sold for $3.50 and 3 quarts was sold for $4.60, to determine the best buy, the cost per quart should be found. $\frac{\$3.50}{2\text{ qt}} = \$1.75$ per quart, and $\frac{\$4.60}{3\text{ qt}} = \$1.53$ per quart. Therefore, the better deal would be the 3-quart option.

Rate of change problems involve calculating a quantity per some unit of measurement. Usually the unit of measurement is time. For example, meters per second is a common rate of change. To calculate this measurement, find the amount traveled in meters and divide by total time traveled. The result is the average speed over the entire time interval. Another common rate of change used in the real world is miles per hour. Consider the following problem that involves calculating an average rate of change in temperature. Last Saturday, the temperature at 1:00 a.m. was 34 degrees Fahrenheit, and at noon, the temperature had increased to 75 degrees Fahrenheit. What was the average rate of change over that time interval? The average rate of change is calculated by finding the change in temperature and dividing by the total hours elapsed. Therefore, the rate of change was equal to $\frac{75-34}{12-1} = \frac{41}{11}$ degrees per hour. This quantity rounded to two decimal places is equal to 3.73 degrees per hour.

A common rate of change that appears in algebra is the slope calculation. Given a linear equation in one variable, $y = mx + b$, the **slope**, m, is equal to $\frac{rise}{run}$ or $\frac{change\ in\ y}{change\ in\ x}$. In other words, slope is equivalent to the ratio of the vertical and horizontal changes between any two points on a line. The vertical change is known as the **rise**, and the horizontal change is known as the **run**. Given any two points on a line (x_1, y_1) and (x_2, y_2), slope can be calculated with the formula:

$$m = \frac{y_2 - y_1}{x_2 - x_1} = \frac{\Delta y}{\Delta x}$$

Common real-world applications of slope include determining how steep a staircase should be, calculating how steep a road is, and determining how to build a wheelchair ramp.

Many times, problems involving rates and ratios involve proportions. A proportion states that two ratios (or rates) are equal. The property of cross products can be used to determine if a proportion is true, meaning both ratios are equivalent. If $\frac{a}{b} = \frac{c}{d}$, then to clear the fractions, multiply both sides by the least common denominator, bd. This results in $ad = bc$, which is equal to the result of multiplying along both diagonals. For example, $\frac{4}{40} = \frac{1}{10}$ grants the cross product $4 \times 10 = 40 \times 1$, which is equivalent to $40 = 40$ and shows that this proportion is true. Cross products are used when proportions are involved in real-world problems. Consider the following: If 3 pounds of fertilizer will cover 75 square feet of grass, how many pounds are needed for 375 square feet? To solve this problem, set up a proportion using two ratios. Let x equal the unknown quantity, pounds needed for 375 feet. Setting the two ratios equal to one another yields the equation:

$$\frac{3}{75} = \frac{x}{375}$$

Cross-multiplication gives $3 \times 375 = 75x$. Therefore, $1{,}125 = 75x$. Divide both sides by 75 to get $x = 15$. Therefore, 15 pounds of fertilizer are needed to cover 375 square feet of grass.

Another application of proportions involves similar triangles. If two triangles have corresponding angles with the same measurements and corresponding sides with proportional measurements, the triangles are said to be similar. If two angles are the same, the third pair of angles are equal as well because the sum of all angles in a triangle is equal to 180 degrees. Each pair of equivalent angles are known as **corresponding angles. Corresponding sides** face the corresponding angles, and it is true that corresponding sides are in proportion. For example, consider the following set of similar triangles:

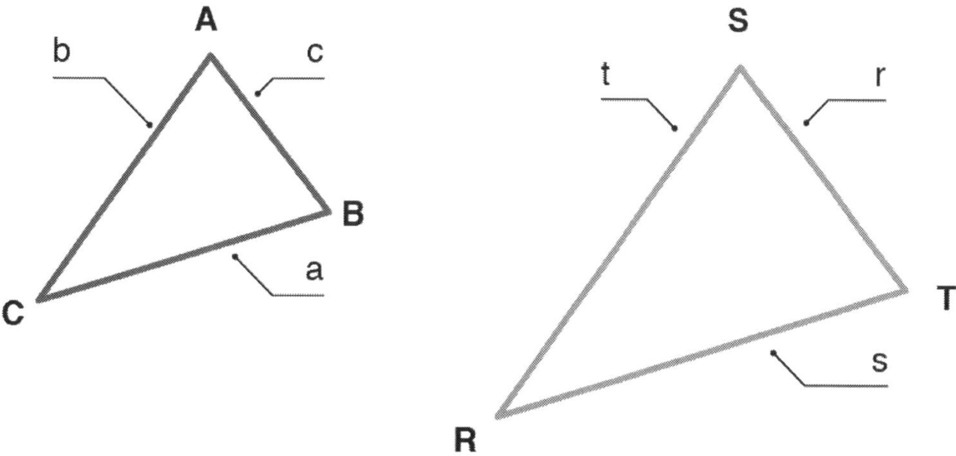

Angles A and S have the same measurement, angles C and R have the same measurement, and angles B and T have the same measurement. Therefore, the following proportion can be set up from the sides:

$$\frac{c}{r} = \frac{a}{s} = \frac{b}{t}$$

This proportion can be helpful in finding missing lengths in pairs of similar triangles. For example, if the following triangles are similar, a proportion can be used to find the missing side lengths, a and b.

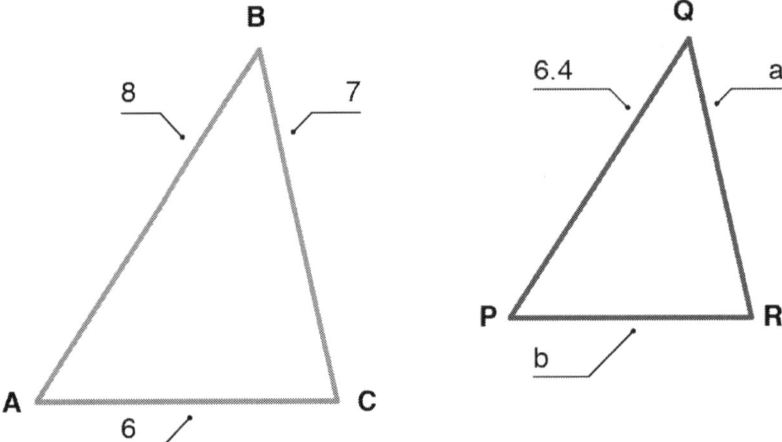

The proportions $\frac{8}{6.4} = \frac{6}{b}$ and $\frac{8}{6.4} = \frac{7}{a}$ can both be cross multiplied and solved to obtain $a = 5.6$ and $b = 4.8$.

A real-life situation that uses similar triangles involves measuring shadows to find heights of unknown objects. Consider the following problem: A building casts a shadow that is 120 feet long, and at the same time, another building that is 80 feet high casts a shadow that is 60 feet long. How tall is the first building? Each building, together with the sun rays and shadows casted on the ground, forms a triangle. They are similar because each building forms a right angle with the ground, and the sun rays form equivalent angles. Therefore, these two pairs of angles are both equal. Because all angles in a triangle add up to 180 degrees, the third angles are equal as well. Both shadows form corresponding sides of the triangle, the buildings form corresponding sides, and the sun rays form corresponding sides. Therefore, the triangles are similar, and the following proportion can be used to find the missing building length:

$$\frac{120}{x} = \frac{60}{80}$$

Cross-multiply to obtain the equation $9{,}600 = 60x$. Then, divide both sides by 60 to obtain $x = 160$. This means that the first building is 160 feet high.

Using Expressions, Equations, and Inequalities

When presented with a real-world problem that must be solved, the first step is always to determine what the unknown quantity is that must be solved for. Use a variable, such as x or t, to represent that unknown quantity. Sometimes there can be two or more unknown quantities. In this case, either choose an additional variable, or if a relationship exists between the unknown quantities, express the other quantities in terms of the original variable. After choosing the variables, form algebraic expressions and/or equations that represent the verbal statement in the problem.

The following table shows examples of vocabulary used to represent the different operations.

Addition	Sum, plus, total, increase, more than, combined, in all
Subtraction	Difference, less than, subtract, reduce, decrease, fewer, remain
Multiplication	Product, multiply, times, part of, twice, triple
Division	Quotient, divide, split, each, equal parts, per, average, shared

The combination of operations and variables form both mathematical expression and equations. The difference between expressions and equations are that there is no equals sign in an expression, and that expressions are evaluated to find an unknown quantity, while equations are solved to find an unknown quantity. Also, inequalities can exist within verbal mathematical statements. Instead of a statement of equality, expressions state quantities are *less than, less than or equal to, greater than*, or *greater than or equal to*. Another type of inequality is when a quantity is said to be *not equal to* another quantity. The symbol used to represent "not equal to" is $\neq$.

The steps for solving inequalities in one variable are the same steps for solving equations in one variable. The addition and multiplication principles are used. However, to maintain a true statement when using the $<$, $\leq$, $>$, and $\geq$ symbols, if a negative number is either multiplied times both sides of an inequality or divided from both sides of an inequality, the sign must be flipped. For instance, consider the following inequality: $3 - 5x \leq 8$. First, 3 is subtracted from each side to obtain $-5x \leq 5$. Then, both sides are divided by -5, while flipping the sign, to obtain $x \geq -1$. Therefore, any real number greater than or equal to -1 satisfies the original inequality.

Measurement and Data

Tables, Charts, And Graphs

They all organize, categorize, and compare data, and they come in different shapes and sizes. Each type has its own way of showing information, whether through a column, shape, or picture. To answer a question relating to a table, chart, or graph, some steps should be followed. First, the problem should be read thoroughly to determine what is being asked to determine what quantity is unknown. Then, the title of the table, chart, or graph should be read. The title should clarify what data is actually being summarized in the table. Next, look at the key and labels for both the horizontal and vertical axes, if they are given. These items will provide information about how the data is organized. Finally, look to see if there is any more labeling inside the table. Taking the time to get a good idea of what the table is summarizing will be helpful as it is used to interpret information.

Tables are a good way of showing a lot of information in a small space. The information in a table is organized in columns and rows. For example, a table may be used to show the number of votes each candidate received in an election. By interpreting the table, one may observe which candidate won the election and which candidates came in second and third. In using a bar chart to display monthly rainfall amounts in different countries, rainfall can be compared between countries at different times of the year. Graphs are also a useful way to show change in variables over time, as in a line graph, or percentages of a whole, as in a pie graph.

The table below relates the number of items to the total cost. The table shows that one item costs \$5. By looking at the table further, five items cost \$25, ten items cost \$50, and fifty items cost \$250. This cost can be extended for any number of items. Since one item costs $5, then two items would cost $10. Though this information is not in the table, the given price can be used to calculate unknown information.

Number of Items	1	5	10	50
Cost ($)	5	25	50	250

A **bar graph** is a graph that summarizes data using bars of different heights. It is useful when comparing two or more items or when seeing how a quantity changes over time. It has both a horizontal and vertical axis. To interpret bar graphs, recognize what each bar represents and connect that to the two variables. The bar graph below shows the scores for six people during three different games. The different colors of the bars distinguish between the three games, and the height of the bar indicates their score for that game. William scored 25 on game 3, and Abigail scored 38 on game 3. By comparing the bars, it is obvious that Williams scored lower than Abigail.

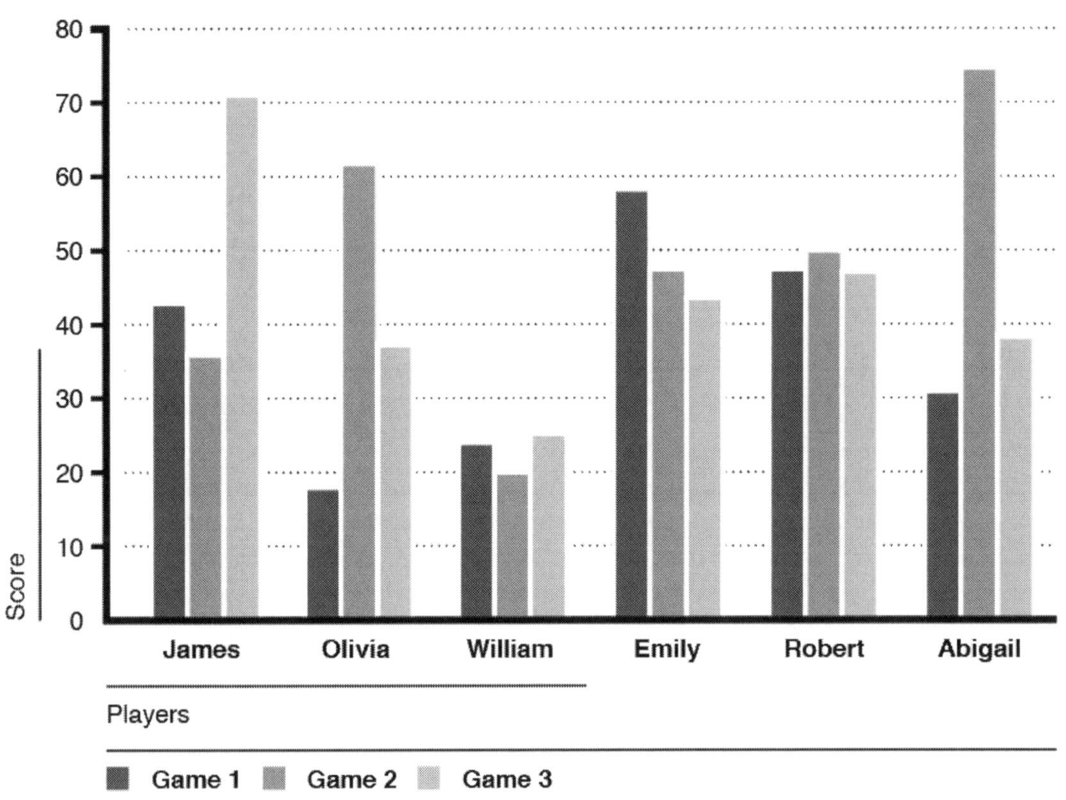

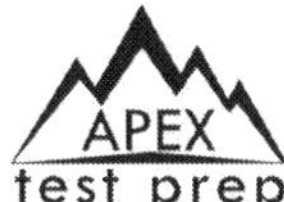

A line graph is a way to compare two variables that are plotted on opposite axes of a graph. The line indicates a continuous change as it rises or falls. The line's rate of change is known as its slope. The horizontal axis often represents a variable of time. Audiences can quickly see if an amount has grown or decreased over time. The bottom of the graph, or the x-axis, shows the units for time, such as days, hours, months, etc. If there are multiple lines, a comparison can be made between what the two lines represent. For example, the following line graph shows the change in temperature over five days. The top line represents the high, and the bottom line represents the low for each day.

Looking at the top line alone, the high decreases for a day, then increases on Wednesday. Then it decreases on Thursday and increases again on Friday. The low temperatures have a similar trend, shown in the bottom line. The range in temperatures each day can also be calculated by finding the difference between the top line and bottom line on a particular day. On Wednesday, the range was 14 degrees, from 62 to 76° F.

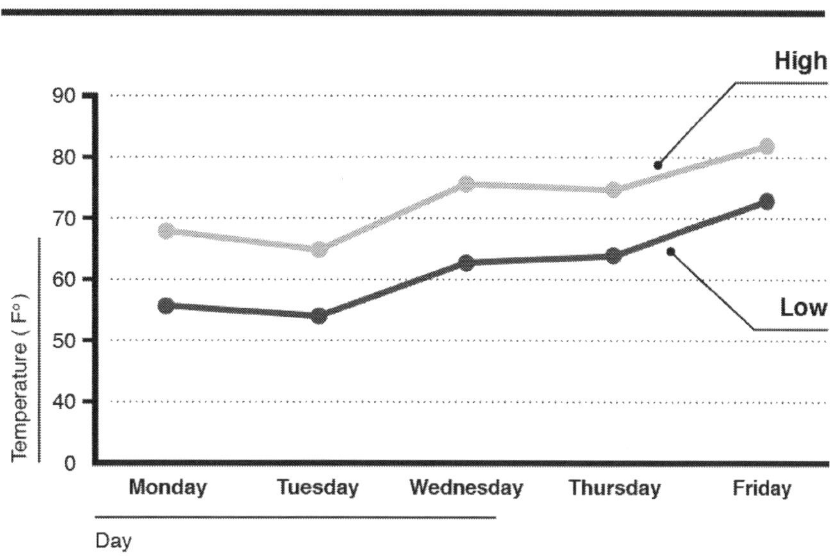

Pie charts are used to show percentages of a whole, as each category is given a piece of the pie, and together all the pieces make up a whole. They are a circular representation of data which are used to highlight numerical proportion. It is true that the arc length of each pie slice is proportional to the amount it individually represents. When a pie chart is shown, an audience can quickly make comparisons by comparing the sizes of the pieces of the pie. They can be useful for comparison between different categories. The following pie chart is a simple example of three different categories shown in comparison to each other.

Light gray represents cats, dark gray represents dogs, and the medium shade of gray represents other pets. These three equal pieces each represent just more than 33 percent, or $\frac{1}{3}$ of the whole. Values 1 and 2 may be combined to represent $\frac{2}{3}$ of the whole. In an example where the total pie represents 75,000 animals, then cats would be equal to $\frac{1}{3}$ of the total, or 25,000. Dogs would equal 25,000 and other pets also equal 25,000.

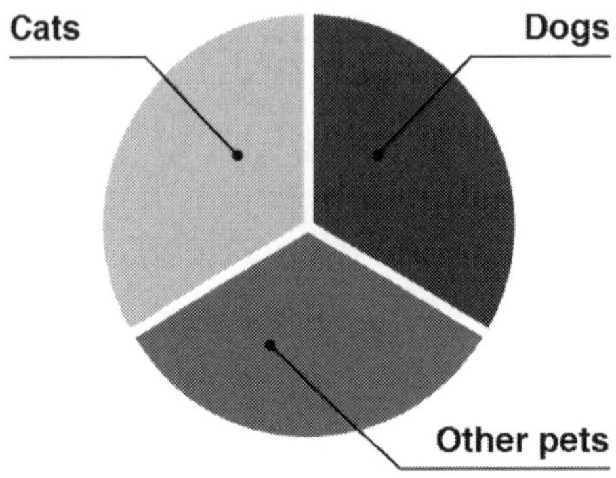

Since circles have 360 degrees, they are used to create pie charts. Because each piece of the pie is a percentage of a whole, that percentage is multiplied times 360 to get the number of degrees each piece represents. In the example above, each piece is $\frac{1}{3}$ of the whole, so each piece is equivalent to 120 degrees. Together, all three pieces add up to 360 degrees.

Stacked bar graphs, also used fairly frequently, are used when comparing multiple variables at one time. They combine some elements of both pie charts and bar graphs, using the organization of bar graphs and the proportionality aspect of pie charts. The following is an example of a stacked bar graph that represents the number of students in a band playing drums, flutes, trombones, and clarinets. Each bar graph is broken up further into girls and boys.

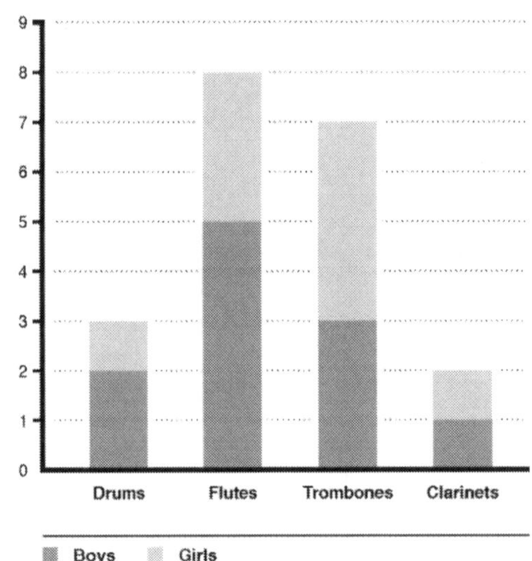

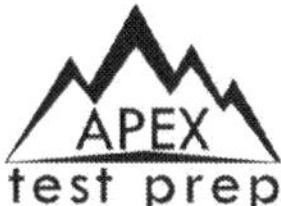

To determine how many boys play tuba, refer to the darker portion of the trombone bar, resulting in 3 students.

A **scatterplot** is another way to represent paired data. It uses Cartesian coordinates, like a line graph, meaning it has both a horizontal and vertical axis. Each data point is represented as a dot on the graph. The dots are never connected with a line. For example, the following is a scatterplot showing people's weight versus height.

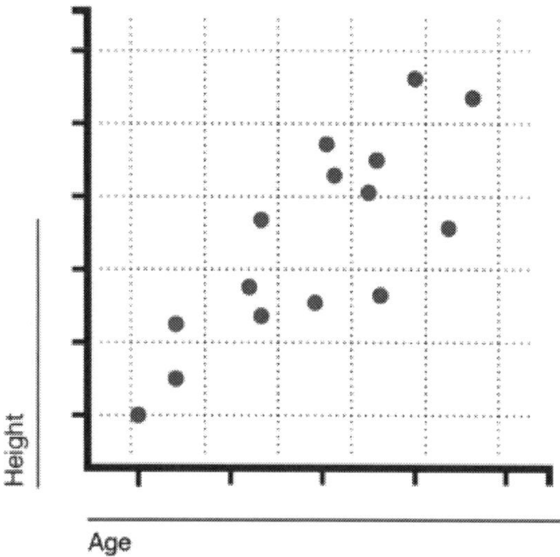

A scatterplot, also known as a **scattergram,** can be used to predict another value and to see if an association, known as a **correlation,** exists between a set of data. If the data resembles a straight line, the data is **associated.** The following is an example of a scatterplot in which the data does not seem to have an association:

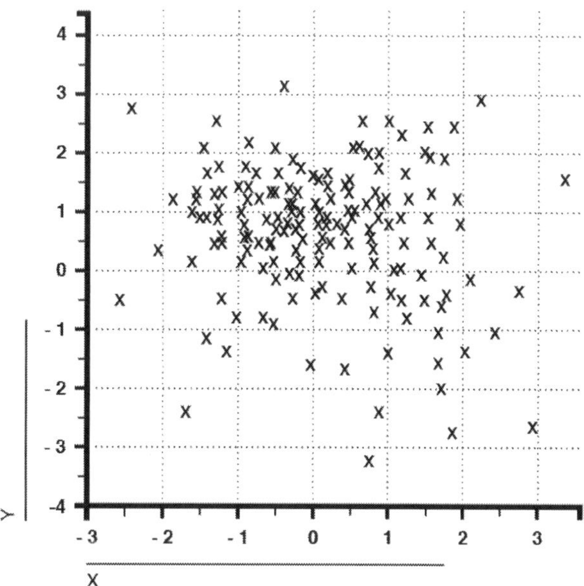

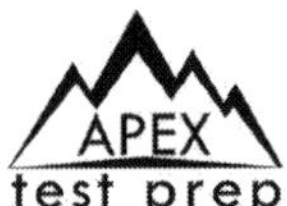

Sets of numbers and other similarly organized data can also be represented graphically. Venn diagrams are a common way to do so. A **Venn diagram** represents each set of data as a circle. The circles overlap, showing that each set of data is overlapping. A Venn diagram is also known as a **logic diagram** because it visualizes all possible logical combinations between two sets. Common elements of two sets are represented by the area of overlap. The following is an example of a Venn diagram of two sets A and B:

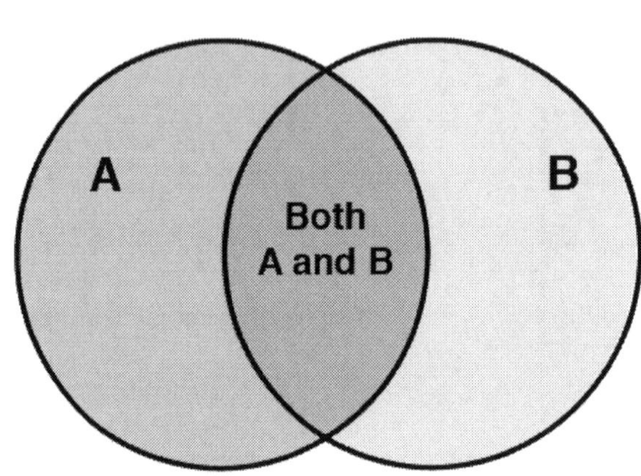

Another name for the area of overlap is the **intersection.** The intersection of A and B, $A \cap B$, contains all elements that are in both sets A and B. The **union** of A and B, $A \cup B$, contains all elements in both sets A and B. Finally, the **complement** of $A \cup B$ is equal to all elements that are not in either set A or set B. These elements are placed outside of the circles.

The following is an example of a Venn diagram representing 24 students who were surveyed about their siblings. Ten students only had a brother, seven students only had a sister, and five had both a brother and a sister. Therefore, five is the intersection, represented by the section where the circles overlap. Two students did not have a brother or a sister. Eight is therefore the complement and is placed outside of the circles.

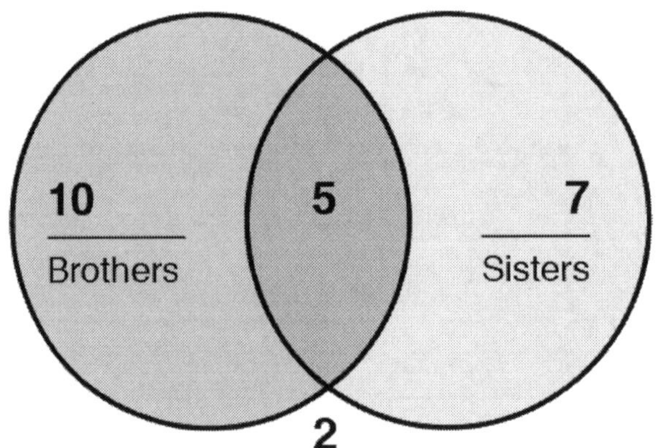

Venn diagrams can have more than two sets of data. The more circles, the more logical combinations are represented by the overlapping. The following is a Venn diagram that represents favorite colors. There were 30 students surveyed. The innermost region represents those students that have a cat, bird, and dog. Therefore, 2 students had all three. In this example, all students had at least one pet, so no one exists in the complement.

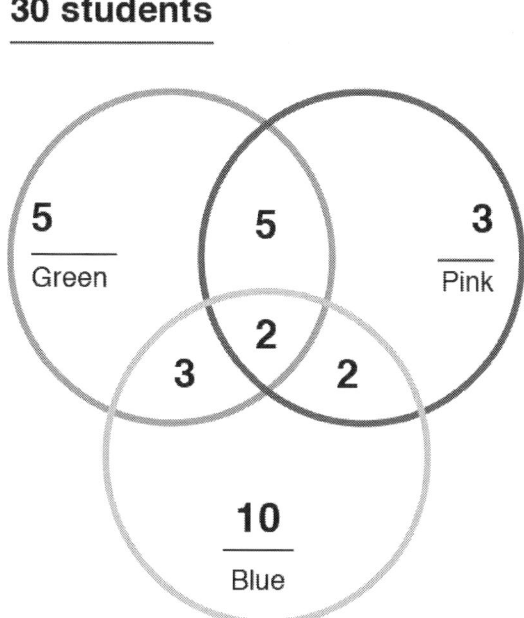

Venn diagrams are typically not drawn to scale; however, if they are, and if each circle's area is proportional to the amount of data it represents, then it is called an area-proportional Venn diagram.

Data Sets, Tables, Charts, And Graphs Using Statistics

One way information can be interpreted from tables, charts, and graphs is through statistics. The three most common calculations for a set of data are the mean, median, and mode. These three are called **measures of central tendency**, which are helpful in comparing two or more different sets of data. The **mean** refers to the average and is found by adding up all values and dividing the total by the number of values. In other words, the mean is equal to the sum of all values divided by the number of data entries. For example, if you bowled a total of 532 points in 4 bowling games, your mean score was $\frac{532}{4} = 133$ points per game. Students can apply the concept of mean to calculate what score they need on a final exam to earn a desired grade in a class.

The *median* is found by lining up values from least to greatest and choosing the middle value. If there is an even number of values, then calculate the mean of the two middle amounts to find the median. For example, the median of the set of dollar amounts \$5, \$6, \$9, \$12, and \$13 is \$9. The **median** of the set of dollar amounts \$1, \$5, \$6, \$8, \$9, \$10 is \$7, which is the mean of \$6 and \$8. The **mode** is the value that occurs the most. The mode of the data set {1, 3, 1, 5, 5, 8, 10} actually refers to two numbers: 1 and 5. In this case, the data set is bimodal because it has two modes. A data set can have no mode if no amount is repeated. Another useful statistic is range. The **range** for a set of data refers to the difference between the highest and lowest value.

In some cases, numbers in a list of data might have weights attached to them. In that case, a weighted mean can be calculated. A common application of a weighted mean is GPA. In a semester, each class is assigned a number of credit hours, its weight, and at the end of the semester each student receives a grade. To compute GPA, an A is a 4, a B is a 3, a C is a 2, a D is a 1, and an F is a 0. Consider a student that takes a 4-hour English class, a 3-hour math class, and a 4-hour history class and receives all B's. The weighted mean, GPA, is found by multiplying each grade times its weight, number of credit hours, and dividing by the total number of credit hours. Therefore, the student's GPA is:

$$\frac{3 \times 4 + 3 \times 3 + 3 \times 4}{11} = \frac{33}{11} = 3.0$$

The following bar chart shows how many students attend a cycle on each day of the week. To find the mean attendance for the week, add each day's attendance together:

$$10 + 7 + 6 + 9 + 8 + 14 + 4 = 58$$

Then divide the total by the number of days, $58 \div 7 = 8.3$. The mean attendance for the week was 8.3 people. The median attendance can be found by putting the attendance numbers in order from least to greatest: 4, 6, 7, 8, 9, 10, 14, and choosing the middle number: 8 people. This set of data has no mode because no numbers repeat. The range is 10, which is found by finding the difference between the lowest number, 4, and the highest number, 14.

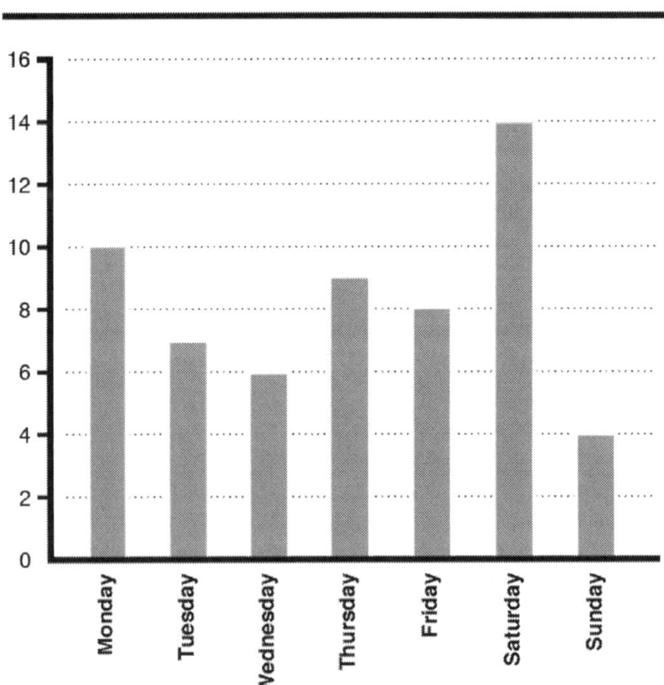

A **histogram** is a bar graph used to group data into "bins" that cover a range on the horizontal, or x-axis. Histograms consist of rectangles whose heights are equal to the frequency of a specific category. The

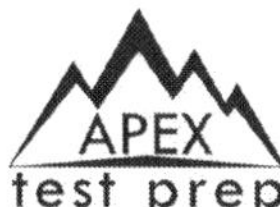

horizontal axis represents the specific categories. Because they cover a range of data, these bins have no gaps between bars, unlike the bar graph above. In a histogram showing the heights of adult golden retrievers, the bottom axis would be groups of heights, and the y-axis would be the number of dogs in each range. Evaluating this histogram would show the height of most golden retrievers as falling within a certain range. It also provides information to find the average height and range for how tall golden retrievers may grow.

The following is a histogram that represents exam grades in a given class. The horizontal axis represents ranges of the number of points scored, and the vertical axis represents the number of students. For example, approximately 33 students scored in the 60 to 70 range.

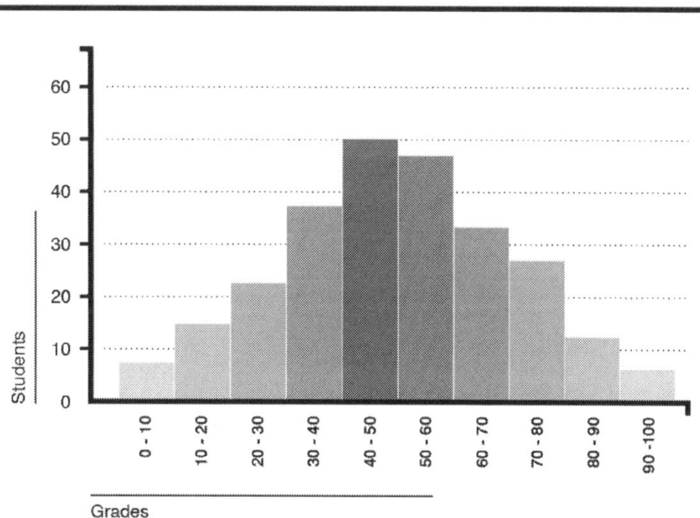

Certain measures of central tendency can be easily visualized with a histogram. If the points scored were shown with individual rectangles, the tallest rectangle would represent the mode. A bimodal set of data would have two peaks of equal height. Histograms can be classified as having data **skewed to the left, skewed to the right,** or **normally distributed**, which is also known as **bell-shaped**. These three classifications can be seen in the following chart:

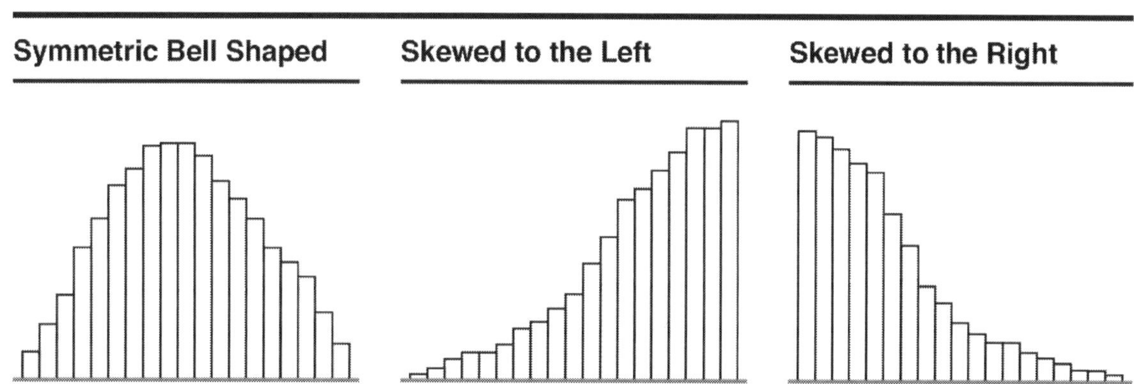

When the data is normal, the mean, median, and mode are very similar because they all represent the most typical value in the data set. In this case, the mean is typically considered the best measure of central tendency because it includes all data points. However, if the data is skewed, the mean becomes less meaningful because it is dragged in the direction of the skew. Therefore, the median becomes the best measure because it is not affected by any outliers.

The measures of central tendency and the range may also be found by evaluating information on a line graph.

In the line graph from a previous example that showed the daily high and low temperatures, the average high temperature can be found by gathering data from each day on the triangle line. The days' highs are 69, 65, 75, 74, and 81. To find the average, add them together to get 364, then divide by 5 (because there are 5 temperatures). The average high for the five days is 72.8. If 72.8 degrees is found on the graph, it will fall in the middle of all the values. The average low temperature can be found in the same way.

Given a set of data, the **correlation coefficient**, r, measures the association between all the data points. If two values are correlated, there is an association between them. However, correlation does not necessarily mean causation, or that one value causes the other. There is a common mistake made that assumes correlation implies causation. Average daily temperature and number of sunbathers are both correlated and have causation. If the temperature increases, that change in weather causes more people to want to catch some rays. However, wearing plus-size clothing and having heart disease are two variables that are correlated but do not have causation. The larger someone is, the more likely he or she is to have heart disease. However, being overweight does not cause someone to have the disease.

Relationships Between Two Variables

Independent and dependent are two types of variables that describe how they relate to each other. The **independent variable** is the variable controlled by the experimenter. It stands alone and is not changed by other parts of the experiment. This variable is normally represented by x and is found on the horizontal, or x-axis, of a graph. The **dependent variable** changes in response to the independent variable. It reacts to, or depends on, the independent variable. This variable is normally represented by y and is found on the vertical, or y-axis of the graph.

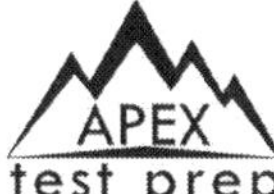

The relationship between two variables, x and y, can be seen on a scatterplot.

The following scatterplot shows the relationship between weight and height. The graph shows the weight as x and the height as y. The first dot on the left represents a person who is 45 kg and approximately 150 cm tall. The other dots correspond in the same way. As the dots move to the right and weight increases, height also increases. A line could be drawn through the middle of the dots to move from bottom left to top right. This line would indicate a **positive correlation** between the variables. If the variables had a **negative correlation**, then the dots would move from the top left to the bottom right.

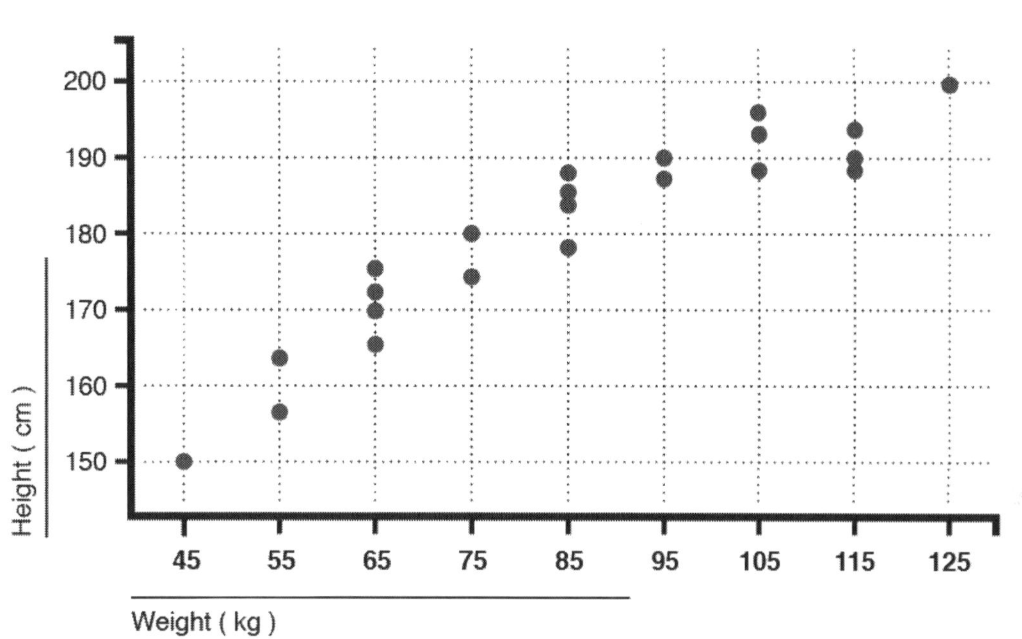

A scatterplot is useful in determining the relationship between two variables, but it is not required. Consider an example where a student scores a different grade on his math test for each week of the month. The independent variable would be the weeks of the month. The dependent variable would be the grades because they change depending on the week. If the grades trended up as the weeks passed, then the relationship between grades and time would be positive. If the grades decreased as the time passed, then the relationship would be negative. (As the number of weeks went up, the grades went down.)

The relationship between two variables can further be described as strong or weak. The relationship between age and height shows a strong positive correlation because children grow taller as they grow up. In adulthood, the relationship between age and height becomes weak, and the dots will spread out. People stop growing in adulthood, and their final heights vary depending on factors like genetics and health. The closer the dots on the graph, the stronger the relationship. As they spread apart, the relationship becomes weaker. If they are too spread out to determine a correlation up or down, then the variables are said to have no correlation.

Variables are values that change, so determining the relationship between them requires an evaluation of who changes them. If the variable changes because of a result in the experiment, then it's dependent. If the variable changes before the experiment, or is changed by the person controlling the experiment, then it's the independent variable. As they interact, one is manipulated by the other. The manipulator is the independent, and the manipulated is the dependent. Once the independent and dependent variable are determined, they can be evaluated to have a positive, negative, or no correlation.

Calculating Geometric Quantities

Perimeter and **area** are geometric quantities that describe objects' measurements. **Perimeter** is the distance around an object. The perimeter of an object can be found by adding the lengths of all sides. Perimeter may be used in problems dealing with lengths around objects such as fences or borders. It may also be used in finding missing lengths or working backwards. If the perimeter is given, but a length is missing, use subtraction to find the missing length. Given a square with side length s, the formula for perimeter is $P = 4s$. Given a rectangle with length l and width w, the formula for perimeter is $P = 2l + 2w$. The perimeter of a triangle is found by adding the three side lengths, and the perimeter of a trapezoid is found by adding the four side lengths. The units for perimeter are always the original units of length, such as meters, inches, miles, etc. When discussing a circle, the distance around the object is referred to as its circumference, not perimeter. The formula for the circumference of a circle is $C = 2\pi r$, where r represents the radius of the circle. This formula can also be written as $C = d\pi$, where d represents the diameter of the circle.

Area is the two-dimensional space covered by an object. These problems may include the area of a rectangle, a yard, or a wall to be painted. Finding the area may require a simple formula or multiple formulas used together. The units for area are square units, such as square meters, square inches, and square miles. Given a square with side length s, the formula for its area is $A = s^2$. Some other formulas for common shapes are shown below.

Shape	Formula	Graphic
Rectangle	$Area = length \times width$	width length
Triangle	$Area = \frac{1}{2} \times base \times height$	height base
Circle	$Area = \pi \times radius^2$	radius

The following formula, not as widely used as those shown above, but very important, is the area of a trapezoid:

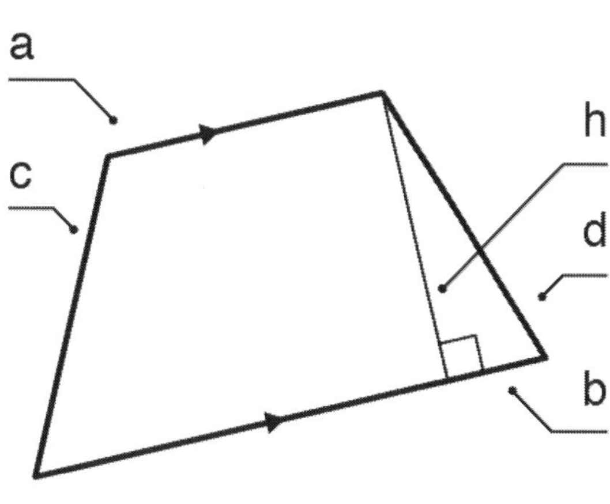

$$A = \frac{1}{2}(a + b)h$$

Geometric figures may be shown as pictures or described in words. If a rectangular playing field with dimensions 95 meters long by 50 meters wide is measured for perimeter, the distance around the field must be found. The perimeter includes two lengths and two widths to measure the entire outside of the field. This quantity can be calculated using the following equation:

$$P = 2(95) + 2(50) = 290 \text{ m}$$

The distance around the field is 290 meters.

Perimeter and area are two-dimensional descriptions; volume is three-dimensional. Volume describes the amount of space that an object occupies, but it differs from area because it has three dimensions instead of two. The units for volume are cubic units, such as cubic meters, cubic inches, and cubic millimeters. Volume can be found by using formulas for common objects such as cylinders and boxes.

To find the area of the shapes above, use the given dimensions of the shape in the formula. Complex shapes might require more than one formula. To find the area of the figure below, break the figure into two shapes. The rectangle has dimensions 11 cm by 6 cm. The triangle has dimensions 3 cm by 6 cm. Plug the dimensions into the rectangle formula: $A = 11 \times 6$. Multiplication yields an area of 66 cm^2. The triangle's area can be found using the formula:

$$A = \frac{1}{2} \times 4 \times 6$$

Multiplication yields an area of 12 cm^2. Add the two areas to find the total area area of the figure, which is 78 cm^2.

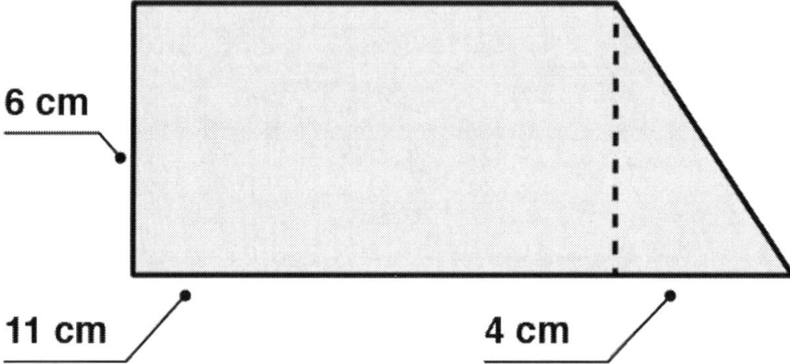

Instead of combining areas, some problems may require subtracting them, or finding the difference.

To find the area of the shaded region in the figure below, determine the area of the whole figure. Then subtract the area of the circle from the whole.

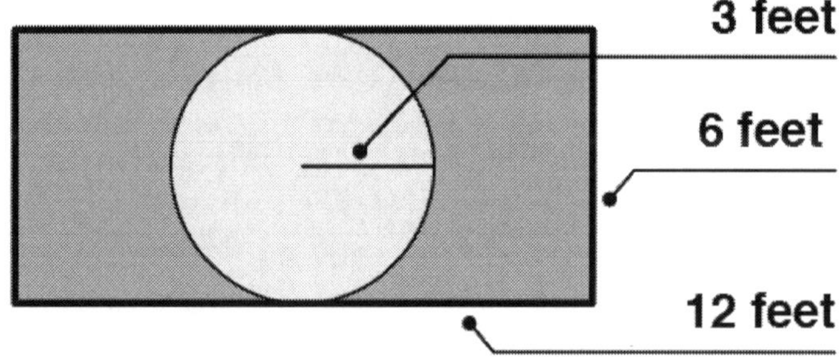

The following formula shows the area of the outside rectangle:

$$A = 12 \times 6 = 72 \text{ ft}^2$$

The area of the inside circle can be found by the following formula:

$$A = \pi(3)^2 = 9\pi = 28.3 \text{ ft}^2$$

As the shaded area is outside the circle, the area for the circle can be subtracted from the area of the rectangle to yield an area of 43.7 ft^2.

The following chart shows a diagram and formula for the volume of two objects.

Shape	Formula	Diagram
Rectangular Prism (box)	$V = length \times width \times height$	height, width, length
Cylinder	$V = \pi \times radius^2 \times height$	radius, height

Volume formulas of these two objects are derived by finding the area of the bottom two-dimensional shape, such as the circle or rectangle, and then multiplying times the height of the three-dimensional shape. Other volume formulas include the volume of a cube with side length s: $V = s^3$; the volume of a sphere with radius r: $V = \frac{4}{3}\pi r^3$; and the volume of a cone with radius r and height h:

$$V = \frac{1}{3}\pi r^2 h$$

If a soda can has a height of 5 inches and a radius on the top of 1.5 inches, the volume can be found using one of the given formulas. A soda can is a cylinder. Knowing the given dimensions, the formula can be completed as follows:

$$V = \pi(radius)^2 \times height$$

$$\pi(1.5 \text{ in})^2 \times 5 \text{ in} = 35.325 \text{ in}^3$$

Notice that the units for volume are inches cubed because it refers to the number of cubic inches required to fill the can.

With any geometric calculations, it's important to determine what dimensions are given and what quantities the problem is asking for. If a connection can be made between them, the answer can be found.

Other geometric quantities can include angles inside a triangle. The sum of the measures of any triangle's three angles is 180 degrees. Therefore, if only two angles are known, the third can be found by subtracting the sum of the two known quantities from 180. Two angles that add up to 90 degrees are known as complementary angles. For example, angles measuring 72 and 18 degrees are complementary. Finally, two angles that add up to 180 degrees are known as supplementary angles. To find the supplement of an angle, subtract the given angle from 180 degrees. For example, the supplement of an angle that is 50 degrees is $180 - 50 = 130$ degrees.

These terms involving angles can be seen in many types of word problems. For example, consider the following problem: The measure of an angle is 60 degrees less than two times the measure of its complement. What is the angle's measure? To solve this, let x be the unknown angle. Therefore, its complement is $90 - x$. The problem gives that:

$$x = 2(90 - x) - 60$$

To solve for x, distribute the 2, and collect like terms. This process results in:

$$x = 120 - 2x$$

Then, use the addition property to add $2x$ to both sides to obtain $3x = 120$. Finally, use the multiplication properties of equality to divide both sides by 3 to get $x = 40$. Therefore, the angle measures 40 degrees. Also, its complement measures 50 degrees.

Converting Unites

When working with dimensions, sometimes the given units don't match the formula, and conversions must be made. When performing operations with rational numbers, it might be helpful to round the numbers in the original problem to get a rough idea of what the answer should be. This system expands to three places above the base unit and three places below. These places correspond to prefixes that each signify a specific base of 10.

The following table shows the conversions:

kilo-	**hecto-**	**deka-**	**base**	**deci-**	**centi-**	**milli-**
1,000 times the base	100 times the base	10 times the base		1/10 times the base	1/100 times the base	1/1,000 times the base

To convert between units within the metric system, values with a base ten can be multiplied. The decimal can also be moved in the direction of the new unit by the same number of zeros on the number. For example, 3 meters is equivalent to 0.003 kilometers. The decimal moved three places (the same number of zeros for kilo-) to the left (the same direction from base to kilo-). Three meters is also equivalent to 3,000 millimeters. The decimal is moved three places to the right because the prefix milli- is three places to the right of the base unit.

The English Standard system, which is used in the United States, uses the base units of foot for length, pound for weight, and gallon for liquid volume. Conversions within the English Standard system are not as easy as those within the metric system because the former does not use a base ten model. The following table shows the conversions within this system.

Length	Weight	Capacity
1 foot (ft) = 12 inches (in) 1 yard (yd) = 3 feet 1 mile (mi) = 5,280 feet 1 mile = 1,760 yards	1 pound (lb) = 16 ounces (oz) 1 ton = 2,000 pounds	1 tablespoon (tbsp) = 3 teaspoons (tsp) 1 cup (c) = 16 tablespoons 1 cup = 8 fluid ounces (oz) 1 pint (pt) = 2 cups 1 quart (qt) = 2 pints 1 gallon (gal) = 4 quarts

When converting within the English Standard system, most calculations include a conversion to the base unit and then another to the desired unit. For example, take the following problem: $3 \text{ qt} = \_\_\_ \text{c}$. There is no straight conversion from quarts to cups, so the first conversion is from quarts to pints. There are 2 pints in 1 quart, so there are 6 pints in 3 quarts. This conversion can be solved as a proportion:

$$\frac{3 \text{ qt}}{x} = \frac{1 \text{ qt}}{2 \text{ pt}}$$

It can also be observed as a ratio 2:1, expanded to 6:3. Then the 6 pints must be converted to cups. The ratio of pints to cups is 1:2, so the expanded ratio is 6:12. For 6 pints, the measurement is 12 cups. This problem can also be set up as one set of fractions to cancel out units. It begins with the given information and cancels out matching units on top and bottom to yield the answer. Consider the following expression:

$$\frac{3 \text{ qt}}{1} \times \frac{2 \text{ pt}}{1 \text{ qt}} \times \frac{2 \text{ c}}{1 \text{ pt}}$$

It's set up so that units on the top and bottom cancel each other out:

$$\frac{3 \not{\text{qt}}}{1} \times \frac{2 \not{\text{pt}}}{1 \not{\text{qt}}} \times \frac{2 \text{ c}}{1 \not{\text{pt}}}$$

The numbers can be calculated as $3 \times 2 \times 2$ on the top and 1 on the bottom. It still yields an answer of 12 cups.

This process of setting up fractions and canceling out matching units can be used to convert between standard and metric systems. A few common equivalent conversions are $2.54 \text{ cm} = 1 \text{ in}$, $3.28 \text{ ft} = 1 \text{ m}$, and $2.205 \text{ lb} = 1 \text{ kg}$. Writing these as fractions allows them to be used in conversions. For the problem $5 \text{ meters} = \_\_\_$ ft, use the feet-to-meter conversion and start with the expression $\frac{5 \text{ m}}{1} \times \frac{3.28 \text{ ft}}{1 \text{ m}}$. The "meters" will cancel each other out, leaving "feet" as the final unit. Calculating the numbers yields 16.4 feet. This problem only required two fractions. Others may require longer expressions, but the underlying rule stays the same. When a unit in the numerator of a fraction matches a unit in the denominator, then they cancel each other out. Using this logic and the conversions given above, many units can be converted between and within the different systems.

The conversion between Fahrenheit and Celsius is found in a formula:

$$°C = (°F - 32) \times \frac{5}{9}$$

For example, to convert 78 °F to Celsius, the given temperature would be entered into the formula:

$$°C = (78 - 32) \times \frac{5}{9}$$

Solving the equation, the temperature comes out to be 25.56°C. To convert in the other direction, the formula becomes:

$$°F = °C \times \frac{9}{5} + 32$$

Remember the order of operations when calculating these conversions.

Mathematics Practice Quiz

1. What is the solution to the equation $10 - 5x + 2 = 7x + 12 - 12x$?
   a. $x = 12$
   b. No solution
   c. $x = 0$
   d. All real numbers

2. Paul took a written driving test, and he got 12 of the questions correct. If he answered 75% of the total questions correctly, how many questions were on the test?
   a. 25
   b. 16
   c. 20
   d. 18

3. The population of coyotes in the local national forest has been declining since 2000. The population can be modeled by the function $y = -(x - 2)^2 + 1600$, where y represents number of coyotes and x represents the number of years past 2000. When will there be no more coyotes?
   a. 2020
   b. 2040
   c. 2012
   d. 2042

4. The number of members of the House of Representatives varies directly with the total population in a state. If the state of New York has 19,800,000 residents and has 27 total representatives, how many should Ohio have with a population of 11,800,000?
   a. 10
   b. 16
   c. 11
   d. 5

5. The mass of the Moon is about 7.348×10^{22} kilograms and the mass of Earth is 5.972×10^{24} kilograms. How many times greater is Earth's mass than the Moon's mass?
   a. 8.127×10^1
   b. 8.127
   b. 812.7
   d. 8.127×10^{-1}

See answers on next page.

Answer Explanations

1. D: First, like terms are collected to obtain:

$$12 - 5x = -5x + 12$$

Then, if the addition principle is used to move the terms with the variable, $5x$ is added to both sides and the mathematical statement $12 = 12$ is obtained. This is always true; therefore, all real numbers satisfy the original equation.

2. B: The unknown quantity is the number of total questions on the test. Let x be equal to this unknown quantity. Therefore, $0.75x = 12$. Divide both sides by 0.75 to obtain $x = 16$.

3. D: There will be no more coyotes when the population is 0, so set y equal to 0 and solve the quadratic equation:

$$0 = -(x - 2)^2 + 1{,}600$$

Subtract 1,600 from both sides, and divide through by -1. This results in:

$$1600 = (x - 2)^2$$

Then, take the square root of both sides. This process results in the following equation:

$$\pm 40 = x - 2$$

Adding 2 to both sides results in two solutions: $x = 42$ and $x = -38$. Because the problem involves years after 2000, the only solution that makes sense is 42. Add 42 to 2000; therefore, in 2042 there will be no more coyotes.

4. B: The number of representatives varies directly with the population, so the equation necessary is $N = k \times P$, where N is number of representatives, k is the variation constant, and P is total population in millions. Plugging in the information for New York allows k to be solved for. This process gives $27 = k \times 19.8$, so $k = 1.36$. Therefore, the formula for number of representatives given total population in millions is:

$$N = 1.36 \times P$$

Plugging in $P = 11.8$ for Ohio results in $N = 16.05$, which rounds to 16 total representatives.

5. A: Division can be used to solve this problem. The division necessary is:

$$\frac{5.972 \times 10^{24}}{7.348 \times 10^{22}}$$

To compute this division, divide the constants first then use algebraic laws of exponents to divide the exponential expression.

This results in about 0.8127×10^2, which, written in scientific notation, is 8.127×10^1.

Science

Human Anatomy and Physiology

General Orientation of Human Anatomy

Levels of Organization of the Human Body

There are six levels of organization that can help describe the human body. These levels, in smallest to largest size order, are chemical, cellular, tissue, organ, organ system, and organism. The **chemical level** includes atoms and molecules, which are the smallest building blocks of matter. When atoms bind together, they form molecules, which in turn make up chemicals. All body structures are made up of these small elements. **Cells** are the smallest units of living organisms. They function independently to carry out vital functions of every organism. Cells that are similar then bind together to form tissues. **Tissues** perform specific functions by having all of the cells work together. For example, muscle tissue is made up of contractile cells that help the body move. **Organs** are made up of two or more types of tissue and perform physiological functions. **Organ systems** are made up of several organs together that work to perform a major bodily function. **Organisms** include the human body as a whole and all of its structures that perform life-sustaining functions.

There are eleven major organ systems of the human body. The **integumentary system** comprises the skin, hair, and nails, which are all on the outside of the body. It is responsible for enclosing and protecting the internal body structures. It contains many sensory receptors on its surface. The **skeletal system** comprises cartilage, bones, and joints. It supports the body and allows for movement of the body in conjunction with the **muscular system**, which is composed of skeletal muscles and tendons and also helps maintain body temperature. The **nervous system** is made up of the brain, spinal cord, and peripheral nerves. It is in charge of detecting and processing sensory information from the entire body and then sending out an appropriate response, such as taking a hand away quickly after touching something hot.

The **endocrine system** includes the pituitary gland, thyroid gland, pancreas, adrenal glands, the testes in males, and the ovaries in females. It is responsible for regulating most bodily processes and secreting hormones. The **cardiovascular system** comprises the heart and blood vessels. Together, these structures are responsible for taking nutrients and oxygen to all of the tissues in the body. This system also helps regulate body temperature. The **lymphatic system** includes the thymus, lymph nodes, spleen, and lymphatic vessels. It is in charge of returning bodily fluids to the blood and fighting off pathogens that enter the body.

The **respiratory system** includes the nasal passage, trachea, and lungs. It works to take in oxygen from the environment and deliver it to the blood and to remove carbon dioxide from the body. The **digestive system** consists of the stomach, liver, gallbladder, large intestine, and small intestine. It processes food and liquid into energy for the body and removes waste from undigested food. The **urinary system** includes the kidneys and urinary bladder. It removes and excretes waste from the blood and controls water balance within the body. The **reproductive system** in males includes the epididymis and testes and in females the mammary glands, ovaries, and uterus. Both the male and female systems produce hormones and gametes. The male system delivers its gametes to females. The female system supports an embryo until birth and then produces milk for the baby.

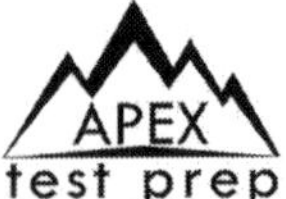

Body Cavities

Body cavities in humans are the fluid-filled spaces that contain the organs. They are located just under the skin. They provide room for the organs to adjust as the body changes position, and they contain protective membranes. Some cavities contain bones that protect the organs as well. The **dorsal cavity** is located along the posterior, or back, side of the body. It contains the brain and spinal cord in the **cranial cavity** and the **spinal cavity**, respectively, although these two subdivided cavities are continuous. The dorsal cavity contains the **meninges,** which is a multilayered membrane that runs around the brain and spinal cord and helps protect these delicate organs. The cranial cavity is the anterior portion of the dorsal cavity. In addition to the brain, it specifically contains the meninges of the brain and cerebrospinal fluid.

The spinal cavity is the posterior portion of the dorsal cavity and contains the meninges of the spinal cord and the fluid-filled spaces in between the vertebrae, in addition to the spinal cord. This portion of the dorsal cavity is the narrowest of all of the body's cavities. The **ventral cavity** is the interior space in the front of the body, anterior to the dorsal cavity. It comprises the **thoracic** and **abdominopelvic cavities**. The thoracic cavity is located within the rib cage in the chest. It encases the cardiovascular and respiratory system organs, as well as the thymus and esophagus.

It is lined by two types of membranes: the **pleura,** which is a membrane that goes around the lungs, and the **pericardium**, which is the membrane that lines the outside of the heart. The abdominopelvic cavity is located below the thoracic cavity and underneath the diaphragm. The diaphragm is a sheet of skeletal muscle that is located just beneath the lungs. This cavity contains the organs of the digestive, renal, urinary, and reproductive systems, as well as some endocrine glands. It is lined by a membrane called the **peritoneum**. It can be divided into four quadrants: right upper, right lower, left upper, and left lower.

Lateral view | **Anterior view**

Cranial cavity
Dorsal body cavity
Vertebral cavity
Thoracic cavity
Superior mediastinum
Pleural cavity
Pericardial cavity with the mediastinum
Diaphragm
Abdominal cavity
Pelvic cavity
Ventral body cavity
both thoracic and abdominopelvic cavities
Abdomino-pelvic cavity

Three Primary Body Planes

Since humans can take on many different positions, it is important to learn about the body from a standard position. Directional and regional descriptions refer to the body in a standard anatomical position, which is the body standing with lower limbs together with feet flat on the floor and facing forward, arms at the sides with palms facing forward and thumbs pointing away from the body, and head and eyes facing forward. This standard position avoids confusion when discussing the body and making comparisons between individuals.

Body planes are the hypothetical geometric planes that divide the body into different sections. There are three primary planes of the body. The **transverse plane** is a horizontal plane that separates the superior, or top, portion of the body from the inferior, or bottom, portion of the body. It is parallel to the ground and runs through the center of the body. The **sagittal plane** is a vertical plane that separates the right and left portions of the body. It runs perpendicular to the ground. The **midsagittal plane** runs through the center of the body, splitting the head into two equal parts, and all other sagittal planes are parallel to it. The **coronal plane** is a vertical plane that separates the anterior, or front, and posterior, or back, portions of the body.

The planes of the body can be used to identify the location of an individual's organs and to describe anatomical motion. The three main planes of the body create an X-Y-Z coordinate system to describe the motion in a three-dimensional manner. The planes are also helpful for describing embryologic changes and development. When a human embryo first develops, the coronal plane of the embryo is horizontal, or parallel to the ground in standard anatomical position of the mother. As the embryo develops into a fetus, its position changes within the mother, and the coronal plane becomes vertical, or perpendicular to the ground with the mother in standard anatomical position.

Medical imaging technology makes use of the body planes. Ultrasounds, CT scans, MRI scans, and PET scans allow images of the body to be seen in all three dimensions. This allows medical issues and the location of anatomical anomalies to be pinpointed within the body.

Body Planes

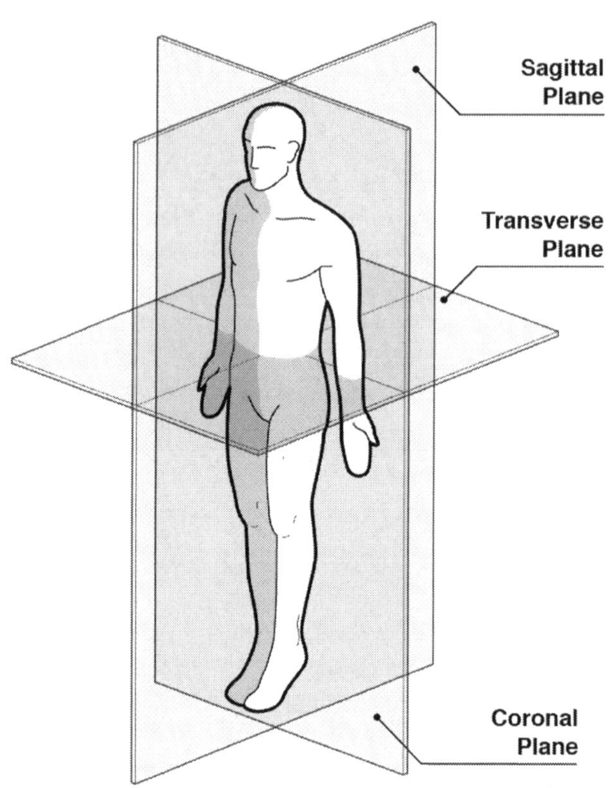

Terms of Direction

In addition to the body planes, using consistent directional terms aids in understanding the human body. It allows different structures to be compared to each other within the same body. There are two other body positions that can be studied in addition to the anatomical position. The **supine** position is when an individual is lying down, face up, in the anatomical position. The **prone** position is when an individual is lying down, face down, in the anatomical position.

There are distinct directional terms used to study the human body. The terms each have an equal and opposite term to describe the opposite side or opposing view of the body. **Anterior** means at or near the front of the body. **Posterior** means at or near the back of the body. The **midline** is the imaginary vertical line that splits the body into equal parts on the left and right. **Lateral** means farther from the midline. **Medial** means closer to the midline. **Superior** means toward the upper part of a structure or toward the head. **Inferior** means toward the lower part of a structure or away from the head. **Superficial** indicates that something is close to the surface of the body. **Deep** means away from the surface of the body. **Proximal** describes something as being near the origin of a structure, whereas **distal** describes it as being away from the origin of a structure. Most of these terms can also be used in combination. For example, a view of the front of the body from above could be called an **anterosuperior** view.

Body Regions

Body regions help separate the body into distinct anatomical compartments. The **axial** part of the body includes everything around the center of the body except the limbs. The **appendicular** part of the body comprises the appendages or limbs. The following table contains a list of body region terms and which part of the body they refer to.

Term	**Body Region**
	Axial
Head and Neck	
Cephalic	Head
Cervical	Neck
Cranial	Skull
Frontal	Forehead
Nasal	Nose
Occipital	Base of skull
Oral	Mouth
Ocular	Eyes
Thorax	
Axillary	Armpit
Costal	Ribs
Deltoid	Shoulder
Mammary	Breast
Pectoral	Chest
Scapular	Shoulder blade
Sternal	Breastbone
Vertebral	Backbone
Abdomen	
Abdominal	Abdomen
Gluteal	Buttocks
Inguinal	Bend of hip
Lumbar	Lower back
Pelvic	Area between hip bones
Perineal	Area between anus and external genitalia
Pubic	Genitals
Sacral	End of vertebral column
	Appendicular
Upper Extremity	
Antebrachial	Forearm
Antecubital	Inner elbow
Brachial	Upper arm
Carpal	Wrist
Cubital	Elbow
Digital	Fingers and toes
Manual	Hand
Palmar	Palm

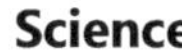

Term	Body Region
Lower Extremity	
Crural	Shin
Femoral	Thigh
Patellar	Front of knee
Pedal	Foot
Plantar	Arch of foot
Popliteal	Back of knee
Sural	Calf
Tarsal	Ankle

Abdominopelvic Regions and Quadrants

The abdominopelvic region of the body can be divided into four quadrants and nine regions. These areas are used to divide the region into smaller areas, since there are quite a few organs and structures located within the abdomen. The four quadrants are created by intersecting a sagittal plane with a transverse plane through the navel. These quadrants are often used by clinicians to pinpoint where abdominal pain is originating. It is important to note that the directional terms that are used refer to that location on the person's body and are not from the clinician's point of view. For example, when looking at a picture of the abdomen, the right upper quadrant is on the left side of the picture when the body is facing forward. The **right upper quadrant** contains the right kidney, a small portion of the stomach, the duodenum, the gallbladder, the head of the pancreas, the right portion of the liver, parts of the small intestine, and parts of the transverse and ascending colon. Pain in this region is often caused by gallbladder inflammation, liver inflammation, or stomach ulcers.

The **left upper quadrant** contains the left kidney, the left portion of the liver, part of the stomach, the spleen, the pancreas, portions of the transvers and descending colon, and parts of the small intestine. Pain in this region is often caused by abnormal rotations of the intestine and colon. The **right lower quadrant** contains the cecum, appendix, part of the small intestine, the right ureter, and the right half of the female reproductive system. Appendicitis pain is associated with this quadrant. The **left lower quadrant** contains most of the small intestine, some of the large intestine, the left ureter, and the left half of the female reproductive system. Pelvic inflammatory disease, ovarian cysts, and inflammation of the large intestine can cause pain in this region.

The nine regions of the abdomen are created by two parasagittal planes and two transverse planes centered around the navel. Once again, the directional terms associated with these regions are from the point of view of the individual's body and not the clinician's view. The nine divisions are the right hypochondriac, left hypochondriac, epigastric, right lumbar, left lumbar, umbilical, right iliac, left iliac, and hypogastric. The **perineum** is the area below the hypogastric region, at the bottom of the abdominopelvic cavity, and can sometimes be considered a tenth region. Most organs are located within two or more regions. The **right hypochondriac region** contains parts of the gallbladder, the right kidney, the small intestine, and the liver. The **left hypochondriac** region contains parts of the left kidney, the pancreas, the stomach, the spleen, and the colon.

The **epigastric region** contains the adrenal glands, most of the stomach, and parts of the liver, pancreas, duodenum, and spleen. The **right lumbar region** contains parts of the gallbladder, the left kidney, the liver, and the ascending colon. The **left lumbar region** contains parts of the descending colon, the left kidney, and the spleen. The **umbilical region** contains the navel and parts of the small intestine, both kidneys, and the transverse colon. The **right iliac region** contains the appendix, cecum, and right iliac fossa. The **left iliac region** contains parts of the descending colon, the sigmoid colon, and the left iliac fossa. The **hypogastric region** contains the organs around the pubic bone, including the bladder, the anus, organs of the reproductive system, and part of the sigmoid colon.

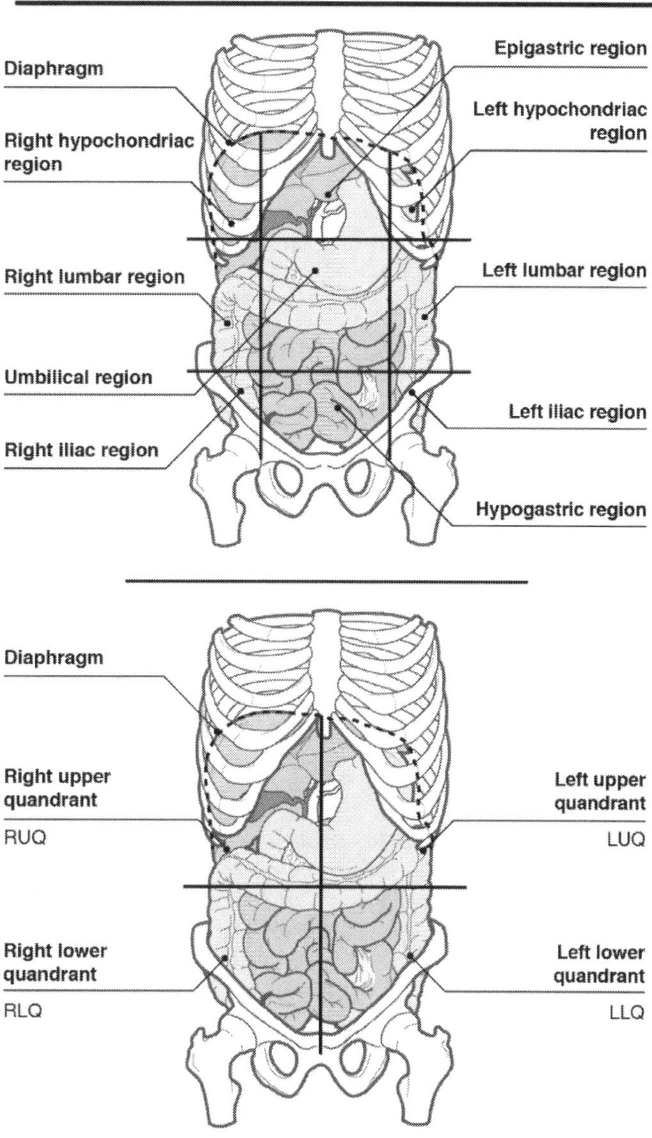

Respiratory System

The **respiratory system** is responsible for gas exchange between air and the blood, mainly via the act of breathing. It is divided into two sections: the upper respiratory system and the lower respiratory system. The **upper respiratory system** consists of the nose, the nasal cavity and sinuses, and the pharynx, while the **lower respiratory system** comprises the larynx (voice box), the trachea (windpipe), the small passageways leading to the lungs, and the lungs. The upper respiratory system is responsible for filtering, warming, and humidifying the air that gets passed to the lower respiratory system, protecting the lower respiratory system's more delicate tissue surfaces.

The human body has two lungs, each having its own distinct characteristics. The right lung is divided into three lobes (superior, middle, and inferior), and the left lung is divided into two lobes (superior and inferior). The left lung is smaller than the right lung, most likely because it shares space in the chest cavity with the heart. Together, the lungs contain approximately fifteen hundred miles of airway passages, which are the site of gas exchange during the act of breathing.

When a breath of air is inhaled, oxygen enters the nose or mouth and passes into the sinuses, which is where the temperature and humidity of the air get regulated. The air then passes into the trachea and is filtered. From there, it travels into the bronchi and reaches the lungs. Bronchi are lined with cilia and mucus that collect dust and germs along the way. Within the lungs, oxygen and carbon dioxide are exchanged between the air in the **alveoli,** a type of airway passage in the lungs, and the blood in the **pulmonary capillaries**, a type of blood vessel in the lungs. Oxygen-rich blood returns to the heart and gets pumped through the systemic circuit. Carbon dioxide-rich air is exhaled from the body.

The respiratory system has many important functions in the body. Primarily, it is responsible for **pulmonary ventilation**, or the process of breathing. During pulmonary ventilation, air is inhaled through the nasal cavity or oral cavity and then moves through the pharynx, larynx, and trachea before reaching the lungs. Air is exhaled following the same pathway. When air is inhaled, the diaphragm and external intercostal muscles contract, causing the rib cage to rise and the volume of the lungs to increase. When air is exhaled, the muscles relax, and the volume of the lungs decreases.

The respiratory system also provides a large area for gas exchange between the air and the circulating blood. During the process of external respiration, oxygen and carbon dioxide are exchanged within the lungs. Oxygen goes into the bloodstream, binds to hemoglobin in the red blood cells, and circulates through the body. Carbon dioxide moves from the deoxygenated blood into the alveoli of the lungs and is then exhaled from the body through the nose or mouth. Internal respiration is a process that allows gases to be exchanged between the circulating blood and body tissues. Arteries carry oxygenated blood throughout the body. When the oxygenated blood reaches narrow capillaries in the body tissue, the red blood cells release the oxygen.

The oxygen then diffuses through the capillary walls into the body tissues. At the same time, carbon dioxide diffuses from the body tissues into the blood of the narrow capillaries. Veins carry the deoxygenated blood back to the lungs for waste removal. Another function of the respiratory system is that it produces the sounds that the body makes for speaking and singing, as well as for nonverbal communication. The larynx is also known as the voice box. When air is exhaled, it passes through the larynx. The muscles of the larynx move the arytenoid cartilages, which then push the vocal cords together. When air passes through the larynx while the vocal cords are being pushed together, the vocal cords vibrate and create sound.

Higher-pitched sounds are made when the vocal cords are vibrating more rapidly, and lower-pitched sounds are made when the vibrations are slower. The respiratory system also helps with an individual's sense of smell. Olfactory fibers line the nasal cavity. When air enters the nose, chemicals within the air bind to the olfactory fibers. Neurons then take the olfactory signal from the nasal cavity to the olfactory area of the brain for sensory processing. In addition to these major functions, the respiratory system also protects the delicate respiratory surfaces from environmental variations and defends them against pathogens and helps regulate blood volume, blood pressure, and body fluid pH.

Respiratory System

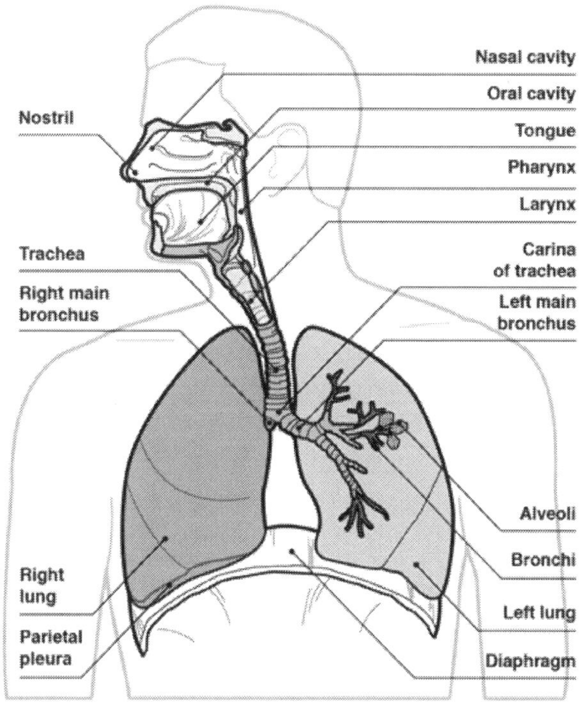

Infections of the respiratory system are common. Most upper respiratory infections are caused by viruses and include the common cold and sinusitis. Bacterial infections of the upper respiratory system are less common and include epiglottitis and croup. This part of the respiratory system gets infected by an organism entering the nasal or oral cavity and invading the mucosa that is present. The organism then begins to destroy the epithelium of the upper respiratory system. Infections of the lower respiratory system can be caused by viruses or bacteria. They include bronchitis, bronchiolitis, and pneumonia. These infections are caused by an organism entering the airway and multiplying itself in or on the epithelium in the lower respiratory system. Inflammation ensues, as well as increased mucus secretion and impaired function of the cilia lining the airways and lungs.

Cardiovascular System

The **cardiovascular system** is composed of the heart and blood vessels. It has three main functions in the human body. First, it transports nutrients, oxygen, and hormones through the blood to the body tissues and cells that need them. It also helps to remove metabolic waste, such as carbon dioxide and nitrogenous waste, through the bloodstream. Second, the cardiovascular system protects the body from attack by foreign microorganisms and toxins. The white blood cells, antibodies, and complement proteins that circulate within the blood help defend the body against these pathogens. The clotting system of the blood also helps protect the body from infection when there is blood loss following an injury. Lastly, this system helps regulate body temperature, fluid pH, and water content of the cells.

Blood Vessels

Blood circulates throughout the body in vessels called arteries, veins, and capillaries. These vessels are muscular tubes that allow gas exchange to occur. **Arteries** carry oxygen-rich blood from the heart to the other tissues of the body. **Veins** collect oxygen-depleted blood from tissues and organs and return it back to the heart. **Capillaries** are the smallest of the blood vessels and do not function individually; instead, they work together in a unit called a **capillary bed**.

Blood

Blood is an important vehicle for transport of oxygen, nutrients, and hormones throughout the body. It is composed of plasma and formed elements, which include red blood cells (RBCs), white blood cells (WBCs), and platelets. **Plasma** is the liquid matrix of the blood and contains dissolved proteins. ***RBCs*** contain **hemoglobin**, which carries oxygen through the blood. Red blood cells also transport carbon dioxide. **WBCs** are part of the immune system and help fight off diseases. **Platelets** contain enzymes and other factors that help with blood clotting.

Heart

The heart, which is the main organ of the cardiovascular system, acts as a pump and circulates blood throughout the body. Gases, nutrients, and waste are constantly exchanged between the circulating blood and interstitial fluid, keeping tissues and organs alive and healthy. The heart is located behind the sternum, on the left side, in the front of the chest. The heart wall is made up of three distinct layers. The outer layer, called the **epicardium,** is a serous membrane that is also known as the **visceral pericardium**. The middle layer is called the **myocardium** and contains connective tissue, blood vessels, and nerves within its layers of cardiac muscle tissue. The inner layer is called the **endocardium,** and is made up of a simple squamous epithelium. It includes the heart valves and is continuous with the endothelium of the attached blood vessels. The heart has four chambers: the **right atrium**, the **right ventricle,** the **left atrium,** and the **left ventricle**.

The atrium and ventricle on the same side of the heart have an opening between them that is regulated by a valve. The valve maintains blood flow in only one direction, moving from the atrium to the ventricle, and prevents backflow. The right side of the heart has a **tricuspid valve** (because it has three leaflets) between the chambers, and the left side of the heart has a **bicuspid valve** (with two leaflets) between the chambers, also called the **mitral valve**. Oxygen-poor blood from the body enters the right atrium through the superior vena cava and the inferior vena cava and is pumped into the right ventricle. The blood then enters the pulmonary trunk and flows into the pulmonary arteries, where it can become re-oxygenated. Oxygen-rich blood from the lungs then flows into the left atrium from four pulmonary veins, passes into the left ventricle, enters the aorta, and gets pumped to the rest of the body.

Cardiac Cycle

The **cardiac cycle** is the series of events that occur when the heart beats. During the cardiac cycle, blood is circulated throughout the pulmonary and systemic circuits of the body. There are two phases of the cardiac cycle—diastole and systole. During the **diastole** period, the ventricles of the heart are relaxed and are not contracting. Blood is flowing passively from the left atrium to the left ventricle and from the right atrium to the right ventricle through the atrioventricular valves. At the end of the diastole phase, both the left and right atria contract, and an additional amount of blood is pushed through to the respective ventricles. The **systole** period occurs when the left and right ventricles both contract. The aortic valve opens at the left ventricle and pushes blood through to the aorta, and the pulmonary valve opens at the right ventricle and pushes blood through to the pulmonary artery. During this phase, the atrioventricular valves are closed, and blood does not enter the ventricles from the atria.

Types of Circulation

Circulating blood carries oxygen, nutrients, and hormones throughout the body, which are vital for sustaining life. There are two types of cardiac circulation: pulmonary circulation and systemic circulation. The heart is responsible for pumping blood in both types of circulation. The **pulmonary circulatory system** carries blood between the heart and the lungs. It works in conjunction with the respiratory system to facilitate external respiration. Deoxygenated blood flows to the lungs through the vessels of the cardiovascular system to obtain oxygen and release carbon dioxide from the respiratory system. Blood that is rich with oxygen flows from the lungs back to the heart. Pulmonary circulation occurs only in the pulmonary loop. The pulmonary trunk takes the deoxygenated blood from the right ventricle to the arterioles and capillary beds of the lungs. Once the blood that is filling these spaces has been reoxygenated, it passes into the pulmonary veins and is transported to the left atrium of the heart.

The **systemic circulatory system** carries blood from the heart to the rest of the body and works in conjunction with the respiratory system to facilitate internal respiration. The oxygenated blood flows out of the heart through the vessels and reaches the body tissues, while the deoxygenated blood flows through the vessels from the body back to the heart. Unlike the pulmonary loop, the systemic loop covers the whole body. Oxygen-rich blood moves out of the left ventricle into the aorta. The aorta circulates the blood to the systemic arteries and then to the arterioles and capillary beds that are present in the body tissues, where oxygen and nutrients are released into the tissues. The deoxygenated blood then moves from the capillary beds to the venules and systemic veins. The systemic veins bring the blood back to the right atrium of the heart.

Here's a visual representation of this:

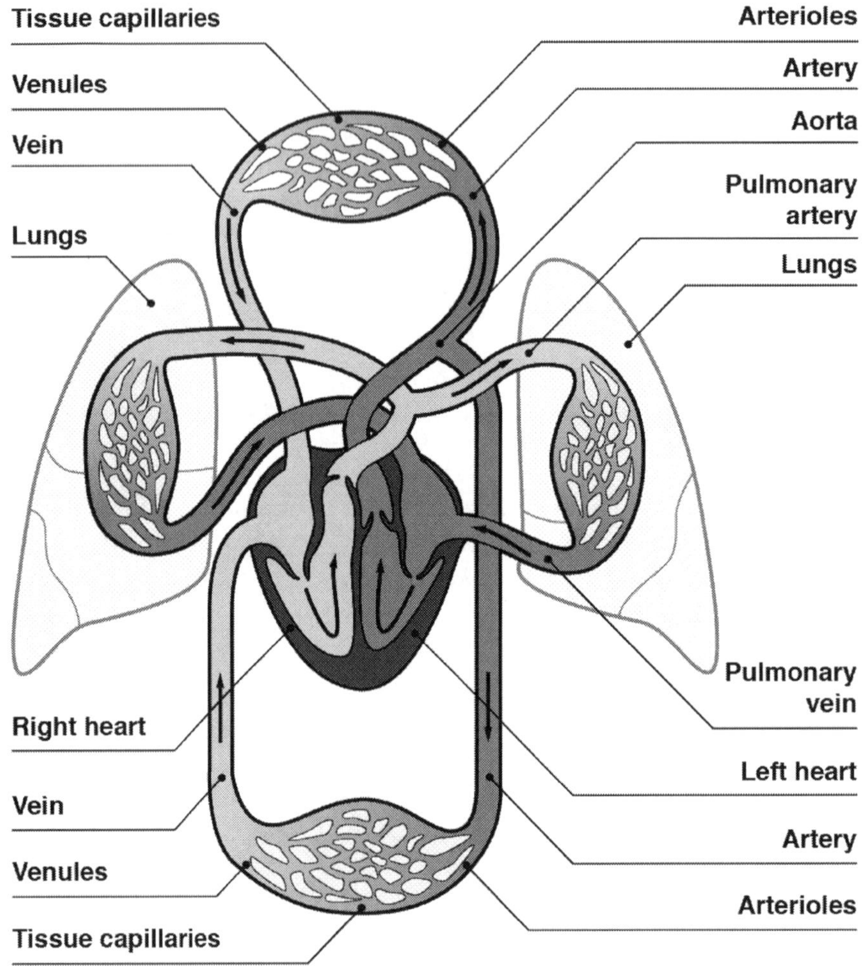

Digestive System

The **gastrointestinal system** is a group of organs that work together to fuel the body by transforming food and liquids into energy. After food is ingested, it passes through the **alimentary canal**, or **GI tract,** which comprises the mouth, pharynx, esophagus, stomach, small intestine, and large intestine. Each organ has a specific function to aid in digestion. Listed below are seven steps that incorporate the transformation of food as it travels through the gastrointestinal system.

- Ingestion: Food and liquids enter the alimentary canal through the mouth.
- Mechanical processing: Food is torn up by the teeth and swirled around by the tongue to facilitate swallowing.
- Digestion: Chemicals and enzymes break down complex molecules, such as sugars, lipids, and proteins, into smaller molecules that can be absorbed by the digestive epithelium.

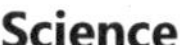

- Secretion: Most of the acids, buffers, and enzymes that aid in digestion are secreted by the accessory organs, but some are provided by the digestive tract.
- Absorption: Vitamins, electrolytes, organic molecules, and water are absorbed by the digestive epithelium and moved to the interstitial fluid of the digestive tract.
- Compaction: Indigestible materials and organic wastes are dehydrated and compacted before elimination from the body.
- Excretion: Waste products are secreted into the digestive tract.

Digestive Enzymes

Digestive enzymes are vital for breaking down food into simple molecules that can be metabolized by the body. The main digestive enzymes in humans are amylase, maltase, lactase, sucrase, lipase, and protease. These digestive enzymes are released when we eat food and can even be secreted when we smell food or anticipate eating. Amylase is readily available in one's mouth and secreted from the salivary glands. Its purpose is to break starches down into maltose immediately in the mouth. Maltase is released into the small intestines and breaks maltose into glucose. Lactose is secreted by enterocytes in the small intestines, and it breaks down lactose into glucose and galactose. Sucrase is also secreted in the small intestines, and it breaks sucrose down into fructose and glucose. Lipase is produced primarily in the pancreas, but it is also produced in the mouth and stomach. Lipase breaks down fatty acids into the sugar alcohol glycerol.

Proteases are types of digestive enzymes that break apart proteins into smaller peptides or free amino acids. There are three main proteases: pepsin, trypsin, and chymotrypsin. These proteases can break specific bonds in an amino acid chain. Pepsin is secreted in the stomach and breaks proteins apart into smaller peptides that can be broken down further in the intestines. Trypsin is secreted from the pancreas into the small intestine where it breaks peptides down further. The activity of trypsin activates the secretion of other proteases. Chymotrypsin breaks peptide chains in the small intestine into individual amino acids that can be absorbed. In addition to these, carboxypeptidase A and carboxypeptidase B are secreted by the pancreas into the small intestine, where they cleave peptide bonds to convert remaining peptides into free amino acids, which can then be transported through the intestinal wall. In addition to the enzymes, bicarbonate is an important aspect of digestion. Bicarbonate raises the pH of the stomach after the proteins in the contents being digested are denatured so the remainder of the intestinal tract is not damaged by the acidity of the stomach acid.

Mouth and Stomach

The mouth is the first point at which food and drink enter the gastrointestinal system. It is where food is chewed and torn apart by the teeth. Salivary glands in the mouth produce saliva, which is used to break down starches. The tongue also helps grip the food as it is being chewed and push it posteriorly toward the esophagus. The food and drink then move down the esophagus by the process of swallowing and into the stomach. The inferior end of the esophagus, at the stomach end, has a lower esophageal sphincter that closes off the esophagus and traps food in the stomach. The stomach stores food so that the body has time to digest large meals. It secretes enzymes and acids and also helps with mechanical processing through **peristalsis** or muscular contractions. The upper muscle of the stomach relaxes to let food in, and the lower muscle mixes the food with the digestive juices. The stomach secretes stomach acid to help break down proteins. Once digestion is completed in the stomach, the broken-down contents, called **chyme,** are passed into the small intestine.

Small Intestine

The **small intestine** is a thin tube that is approximately ten feet long and takes up most of the space in the abdominal cavity. The three structural parts of the small intestine are the duodenum, the jejunum, and the ileum. The **duodenum** is shaped like a C and receives the chyme from the stomach along with the digestive juices from the pancreas and the liver. The **jejunum** is the middle portion of the small intestine. It is the section with the most circular folds and villi to increase its surface area. The digestive products are absorbed into the bloodstream in the jejunum.

The **ileum** follows the jejunum portion of the small intestine. It mainly absorbs bile acids and vitamin B12 and passes it into the bloodstream. The ileum connects to the large intestine. The entire small intestine secretes enzymes and has folds that increase its surface area and allow for maximum absorption of nutrients from the digested food. The small intestine digestive juice along with juices from the pancreas to liver in combination with peristalsis work to complete the digestion of starches, proteins, and carbohydrates. By the time food leaves the small intestine, approximately 90 percent of the nutrients have been absorbed. These nutrients are carried to the rest of the body. The undigested and unabsorbed food particles are passed into the large intestine.

Large Intestine

The **large intestine** is a long, thick tube that is about five feet in length, also known as the **colon.** It is the final part of the gastrointestinal tract. It has five main sections. The ascending colon connects to the small intestine and runs upward along the right side of the body. It also includes the appendix. The transverse colon runs parallel to the ground from the ascending colon to the left side of the abdominal cavity. The descending colon runs downward along the left side of the body. The sigmoid colon is an S-shaped region that connects the descending colon to the rectum. The rectum is the end of the colon and is a temporary storage place for feces. The function of the large intestine is to absorb water from the digested food and transport waste to be excreted from the body. It also contains symbiotic bacteria that break down the waste products even further, allowing for any additional nutrients to be absorbed. The final waste products are converted to stool and then stored in the rectum.

Pancreas

The pancreas is a large gland that is about 6 inches long. It secretes buffers and digestive enzymes into the duodenum of the small intestine. It contains specific enzymes for each type of food molecule, such as amylases for carbohydrates, lipases for lipids, and proteases for proteins. This digestive function of the pancreas is called the exocrine role of the pancreas. The cells of the pancreas are present in clusters called **acini**. The digestive enzymes are secreted into the middle of the acini into intralobular ducts. These ducts drain into the main pancreatic duct, which then drains into the duodenum.

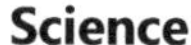

In addition to these main organs, the gastrointestinal system has a few accessory organs that help break down food without having the food or liquid pass directly through them. The liver produces and secretes **bile,** which is important for the digestion of lipids. The bile mixes with the fat in food and helps dissolve it into the water contents within the small intestine, which helps fatty foods to be digested. The liver also plays a large role in the regulation of circulating levels of carbohydrates, amino acids, and lipids in the body. Excess nutrients are removed by the liver and deficiencies are corrected with its stored nutrients. The gallbladder is responsible for storing and concentrating bile before it gets secreted into the small intestine. It recycles the bile from the small intestine so that it can be used to digest subsequent meals.

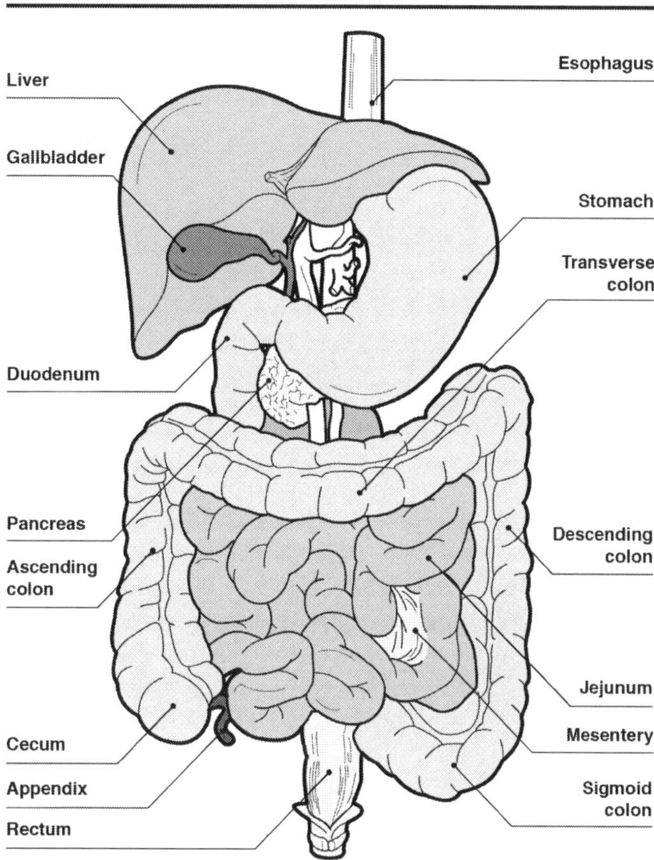

Gallbladder

As the liver secretes a greenish-yellowish fluid called bile, the gallbladder stores bile between meals. Hepatocyte cells are found in the liver and are responsible for the production of bile salts. The salts are derived from cholesterol and are the byproduct of a neutralization reaction. For example, the reaction of an alkaline substance and an acid will create the bile salts. **Bile salts** make up a major portion of bile and act as detergents (emulsifiers) that break apart lipid globules and fat. Not only do the salts help in the digestion of fats, they also allow our body to absorb fat-soluble organic molecules such as vitamins K, E, D, and A. Bile salts also remove waste products.

If there is a lack of bile salts, toxins will accumulate within our bodies, causing complications such as diarrhea and weight loss. Long term bile salt deficiency can also result in the formation of gallstones and kidney stones. Irritable bowel syndrome and Crohn's disease are the results of bile salt malabsorption. After food consumption, fats are present inside the digestive tract. Hormones then signal the gallbladder to release bile. Within the lumen of the small intestine, the bile salts will breakdown large fat globules into smaller fat globules. The surface area of the fat molecules (triglycerides) increases and allows enzymatic hydrolysis to occur readily. Lipase breaks down the smaller exposed fat droplets to monoglycerides and fatty acids. Both fatty substances then diffuse into the epithelial cells and reform into triglycerides.

Nervous System

The nervous system is made up of the central nervous system (CNS) and the peripheral nervous system (PNS). The CNS includes the brain and the spinal cord, while the PNS includes the rest of the neural tissue that is not included in the CNS. **Neurons,** or nerve cells, are the main cells responsible for transferring and processing information between the brain and other parts of the body. **Neuroglia** are cells that support the neurons by providing a framework around them and isolating them from the surrounding environment.

Neuron Form and Function

The overall purpose of a neuron is to send information as electrochemical signals using action potentials. A neuron is composed of five main components: the dendrites, the soma, the axon, the Schwann cells, and the axon terminal. The dendrites are where a neuron receives and processes a signal from the axons of neighboring neurons. The soma is the main cell body of a neuron, and it contains the nucleus of the cell. Since the nucleus and other organelles reside in the soma, it is the site of the metabolic activities of the neuron.

The axon is a long, thin structure that joins with the soma at what is known as the axon hillock. The axons is insulated with a fatty substance called myelin. The breaks between each portion of myelin, called the nodes of Ranvier, contain sodium and potassium channels. The insulation separating the ion channels enable the nerve impulse to be transmitted incredibly faster. The Schwann cells are glial cells that surround the axon of a neuron, with the purpose of forming myelin sheaths. The axon terminal is a tiny swelling at the end of an axon that stores neurotransmitters that are used in a synapse. Axon terminals are arranged near dendrites of neighboring neurons and normally are the sites where a synapse will occur.

Central Nervous System

The CNS is located within the dorsal body cavity, with the brain in the cranial cavity and the spinal cord in the spinal canal. The brain is protected by the skull, and the spinal cord is protected by the vertebrae. The brain is made up of white and gray matter. The white matter contains axons and oligodendrocytes. **Axons** are the long projection ends of neurons that are responsible for transmitting signals through the nervous system, while **oligodendrocytes** act as insulators for the axons and provide support for them. The gray matter consists of neurons and fibers that are unmyelinated. Neurons are nerve cells that receive and transmit information through electrical and chemical signals.

Glial cells and astrocytes are located in both types of tissue. Different types of glial cells have different roles in the CNS. Some are immunoprotective, while others provide a scaffolding for other types of nerve cells. **Astrocytes** provide nutrients to neurons and clear out metabolites. The spinal cord has projections within it from the PNS. This allows the information that is received from the areas of the body that the PNS reaches to be transmitted to the brain. The CNS as a whole is responsible for processing and coordinating sensory data and motor commands. It receives information from all parts of the body, processes it, and then sends out action commands in response. Some of the reactions are conscious, while others are unconscious.

Infections of the CNS include **encephalitis**, which is an inflammation of the brain, and **poliomyelitis**, which is caused by a virus and causes muscle weakness. Other developmental neurological disorders include ADHD and autism. Some diseases of the CNS can occur later in life and affect the aging brain, such as Alzheimer's disease and Parkinson's disease. Cancers that occur in the CNS can be very serious and have high mortality rates.

Brain Regions and Neurons

There are five main regions of the brain, and they have intricate processing tasks: the parietal lobe, the frontal lobe, the temporal lobe, the occipital lobe, and the cerebellum. The parietal lobe is responsible for processing touch sensation signals and proprioception, which is spatial navigation. The frontal lobe is responsible for controlling and directing motor activity and the dopamine system, which involves memory and attention. The temporal lobe is responsible for processing auditory information and language comprehension. It contains the Broca and Wernicke areas, which are vital for language comprehension and speech production. The occipital lobe contains the visual processing portions of the brain and is therefore responsible for sight and image perception.

Lastly, the cerebellum at the base of the brain is solely responsible for one's balance and coordination. The brain stem, although not a structure of the brain itself, is vital for controlling involuntary actions such as heartbeat, swallowing, and breathing. Within the central nervous system, there are two tissue types: the gray matter, which contains mainly cell bodies, and the white matter, which is made up of myelin-coated axons. The central nervous system is composed of four different types of nerve cells with unique functions: astrocytes, microglial cells, ependymal cells, and oligodendrocytes.

Peripheral Nervous System

The PNS consists of the nerves and ganglia that are located within the body outside of the brain and spinal cord. It connects the rest of the body, organs, and limbs to the CNS. Unlike the CNS, the PNS does not have any bony structures protecting it. The PNS is responsible for relaying sensory information and motor commands between the CNS and peripheral tissues and systems. It has two subdivisions, known as the afferent, or sensory, and efferent, or motor, divisions. The **afferent division** relays sensory information to the CNS and supplies information from the skin and joints about the body's sensation and balance. It carries information away from the stimulus back to the brain.

The afferent division provides the brain with sensory information about things such as taste, smell, and vision. It also monitors organs, vessels, and glands for changes in activity and can alert the brain to send out appropriate responses for bringing the body back to homeostasis. The **efferent division** transmits motor commands to muscles and glands. It sends information from the CNS to the organs and muscles to provide appropriate responses to sensations. The electrical responses from the neurons are initiated in the CNS, but the axons terminate in the organs that are part of the PNS. The efferent division consists of the **autonomic nervous system (ANS),** which regulates activity of smooth muscle, cardiac muscle, and glands, and allows the brain to control heart rate, blood pressure, and body temperature, and the **somatic nervous system (SNS),** which controls skeletal muscle contractions and allows the brain to control body movement.

Diseases of the PNS can affect single nerves or the whole system. Single nerve damage, or **mononeuropathy,** can occur when a nerve gets compressed due to trauma or a tumor. It can also be damaged as a result of being trapped under another part of the body that is increasing in size, such as in carpal tunnel syndrome. These diseases can cause pain and numbness at the affected area.

Autonomic Nervous System

The **autonomic nervous system** is made up of pathways that extend from the CNS to the organs, muscles, and glands of the body. The pathway is made up of two separate neurons. The first neuron has a cell body that is located within the CNS, for example, within the spinal cord. The axon of that first neuron synapses with the cell body of the second neuron. Part of the second neuron innervates the organ, muscle, or gland that the pathway is responsible for.

The autonomic nervous system consists of the sympathetic nervous system and the parasympathetic nervous system. The **sympathetic nervous system** is activated when mentally stressful or physically dangerous situations are faced, also known as "fight or flight" situations. Neurotransmitters are released that increase heart rate and blood flow in critical areas, such as the muscles, and decrease activity for nonessential functions, such as digestion. This system is activated unconsciously. The **parasympathetic system** has some voluntary control. It releases neurotransmitters that allow the body to function in a restful state. Heart rate and other sympathetic responses are often decreased when the parasympathetic system is activated.

Somatic Nervous System and the Reflex Arc

The **somatic nervous system** is considered the voluntary part of the PNS. It comprises motor neurons whose axons innervate skeletal muscle. However, nerve cells and muscle cells do not come into direct contact with each other. Instead, the neurotransmitter acetylcholine transfers the signal between the nerve cell and muscle cell. These junctions are called **neuromuscular junctions**. When the muscle cell receives the signal from the nerve cell, it causes the muscle to contract.

Although most muscle contractions are voluntary, reflexes are a type of muscle contraction that is involuntary. A **reflex** is an instantaneous movement that occurs in response to a stimulus and is controlled by a neural pathway called a **reflex arc.** The reflex arc carries the sensory information from the receptor to the spinal cord and then carries the response back to the muscles. Many sensory neurons synapse in the spinal cord so that reflex actions can occur faster, without waiting for the signal to travel to the brain and back. For somatic reflexes, stimuli activate somatic receptors in the skin, muscles, and tendons. Then, afferent nerve fibers carry signals from the receptors to the spinal cord or brain stem. The signal reaches an integrating center, which is where the neurons synapse within the spinal cord or brain stem. Efferent nerve fibers then carry motor nerve signals to the muscles, and the muscles carry out the response.

Muscular System

Muscular System

There are approximately seven hundred muscles in the body. They are attached to the bones of the skeletal system and make up half of the body's weight. There are three types of muscle tissue in the body: skeletal muscle, smooth muscle, and cardiac muscle. An important characteristic of all types of muscle is that they are **excitable,** which means that they respond to electrical stimuli.

Skeletal Muscles

Skeletal muscle tissue is a voluntary, striated muscle tissue, which means that the contractile fibers of the tissue are aligned parallel so that they appear to form stripes when viewed under a microscope. Most skeletal muscle are attached to bones by intermediary tendons. Tendons are bundles of collagen fibers. When nerve cells release acetylcholine at the neuromuscular junction, skeletal muscle contracts. The skeletal muscle tissue then pulls on the bones of the skeleton and causes body movement.

Smooth Muscles

Smooth muscle tissue is an involuntary nonstriated muscle tissue. It has greater elasticity than striated muscle but still maintains its contractile ability. Smooth muscle tissue can be of the single-unit variety or the multi-unit variety. Most smooth muscle tissues are single unit where the cells all act in unison and the whole muscle contracts or relaxes. Single-unit smooth muscle lines the blood vessels, urinary tract, and digestive tract. It helps to move fluids and solids along the digestive tract, allows for expansion of the urinary bladder as it fills and helps move blood through the vessels. Multi-unit smooth muscle is found in the iris of the eye, large elastic arteries, and the trachea.

Cardiac Muscles

Cardiac muscle tissue is an involuntary striated muscle that is only found in the walls of the heart. The cells that make up the tissue contract together to pump blood through the veins and arteries. This tissue has high contractility and extreme endurance, since it pumps for an individual's entire lifetime without any rest. Each cardiac muscle cell has finger-like projections, called **intercalated disks**, at each end that overlap with the same projections on neighboring cells. The intercalated disks form tight junctions between the cells so that they do not separate as the heart beats and so that electrochemical signals are passed from cell to cell quickly and efficiently.

Muscle Control

To initiate the muscular contractions that cause movement, an excitation (stimulus) from a nerve cell travels to the muscle fibers. This nerve cell is referred to as a ***motor neuron*** and can be responsible for movement for up to several hundred muscle fibers. The ***motor unit*** is the term used for the motor neuron and the skeletal muscle fibers that specific neuron innervates. The ***axon*** is at proximal end of the motor neuron. The portion between the axonal terminals and the muscle fibers is called the neuromuscular junction and once the signal jumps from the motor neuron to the muscle fibers, the muscle will now contract, causing movement. Each muscle fiber is only innervated by one motor neuron, though each motor neuron can have anywhere from several to several thousand skeletal muscle fibers associated with it.

Reproductive System

The **reproductive system** is responsible for producing, storing, nourishing, and transporting functional reproductive cells, or **gametes**, in the human body. It includes the reproductive organs, also known as **gonads,** the reproductive tract, the accessory glands and organs that secrete fluids into the reproductive tract, and the **perineal structures**, which are the external genitalia. The human male and female reproductive systems are very different from each other.

The primary objective of the male reproductive system is to facilitate fertilization of a female's egg to produce offspring. Male hormones, such as testosterone, are produced and secreted as part of the male reproductive system. The hormones and functions of the male reproductive system also play a major role in determining all of the secondary sex characteristics of males, such as deeper voices, muscle development, and body hair distribution.

The male gonads are called **testes.** The testes secrete androgens, mainly testosterone, and produce and store one-half billion **sperms cells**, which are the male gametes, each day. An **androgen** is a steroid hormone that controls the development and maintenance of male characteristics. Once the sperm are mature, they move through a duct system where they are mixed with additional fluids that are secreted by accessory glands, forming a mixture called **semen.** The sperm cells in semen are responsible for fertilization of the female gametes to produce offspring. The male reproductive system has a few accessory organs as well, which are located inside the body. The **prostate gland** and the **seminal vesicles** provide additional fluid that serves as nourishment to the sperm during ejaculation. The **vas deferens** is responsible for transportation of sperm to the urethra. The **bulbourethral glands** produce a lubricating fluid for the urethra that also neutralizes the residual acidity left behind by urine.

The female reproductive system has several functions; however, its primary functions are creating and sustaining eggs, growing embryos, and giving birth to offspring. Just as in the male reproductive system, the female reproductive system is an important aspect of producing and regulating the female-specific hormones, such as estrogen. The regulation of the sex hormones done by the female reproductive system determine the secondary sex characteristics and stimulate the ability to lactate to feed children.

The female gonads are called **ovaries.** Ovaries generally produce one immature gamete, or **oocyte,** per month. The ovaries are also responsible for secreting the hormones estrogen and progesterone. When the oocyte is released from the ovary, it travels along the uterine tubes, or **Fallopian tubes**, and then into the **uterus.** The uterus opens into the vagina. When sperm cells enter the vagina, they swim through the uterus. If they fertilize the oocyte, they do so in the Fallopian tubes. The resulting zygote travels down the tube and implants into the uterine wall. The uterus protects and nourishes the developing embryo for nine months until it is ready for the outside environment.

If the oocyte is not fertilized, it is released in the uterine, or menstrual, cycle. The **menstrual cycle** usually occurs monthly and involves the shedding of the functional part of the uterine lining. **Mammary glands** are a specialized accessory organ of the female reproductive system. The mammary glands are located in the breast tissue of females. During pregnancy, the glands begin to grow as the cells proliferate in preparation for lactation. After pregnancy, the cells begin to secrete nutrient-filled milk, which is transferred into a duct system and out through the nipple for nourishment of the baby.

The endocrine system is composed of various glands that produce hormones. Many of these endocrine glands are integral parts of the reproductive system. They are responsible for producing sex hormones that regulate the reproductive system and produce the secondary sex characteristics, such as facial hair and deepened voice in males and breast development and widened hips in females. Specifically within females, ovaries are considered endocrine glands due to the fact that they produce reproductive regulatory hormones like progesterone and estrogen. Estrogen and progesterone in turn are pivotal in maintaining normal reproductive development and ensuring a female's ability to successfully produce offspring.

Integumentary System

The **integumentary system** protects the body from damage from the outside. It consists of skin and its appendages, including hair, nails, and sweat glands. This system functions as a cushion, a waterproof layer, a temperature regulator, and a protectant of the deeper tissues within the body. It also excretes waste from the body. The skin is the largest organ of the human body, consisting of two layers called the epidermis and the dermis. The **epidermis** can be classified as thick or thin. Most of the body is covered with thin skin but areas such as the palm of the hands are covered with thick skin. The epidermis is

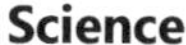

responsible for synthesizing vitamin D when exposed to UV rays. Vitamin D is essential to the body for the processes of calcium and phosphorus absorption, which maintain healthy bones. The **dermis** lies under the epidermis and consists of a superficial papillary layer and a deeper reticular layer. The **papillary layer** is made up of loose connective tissue and contains capillaries and the axons of sensory neurons. The **reticular layer** is a meshwork of tightly packed irregular connective tissue and contains blood vessels, hair follicles, nerves, sweat glands, and sebaceous glands.

The three major functions of skin are protection, regulation, and sensation. Skin acts as a barrier and protects the body from mechanical impacts, variations in temperature, microorganisms, and chemicals. It regulates body temperature, peripheral circulation, and fluid balance by secreting sweat. It also contains a large network of nerve cells that relay changes in the external environment to the body.

Hair provides many functions for the human body. It provides sensation, protects against heat loss, and filters air that is taken in through the nose. Nails provide a hard layer of protection over soft skin. Sweat glands and sebaceous glands are two important exocrine glands found in the skin. **Sweat glands** regulate temperature and remove bodily waste by secreting water, nitrogenous waste, and sodium salts to the surface of the body. **Sebaceous glands** secrete **sebum,** which is an oily mixture of lipids and proteins. Sebum protects the skin from water loss and bacterial and fungal infections.

The integumentary system also plays a vital role in maintaining homeostasis. Homeostasis is the regulation of the body to maintain proper body functions. The skin specifically is one of the most important elements in maintaining homeostasis. The skin regulates temperature through sweating, contains temperature sensors that induce shivering, and allows absorption of certain materials. All of these functions facilitate proper temperature, water balance, and vitamin and mineral regulation.

Epithelial Tissues and Skin Cells

The majority of epithelial tissues are layers of cells that cover the surfaces of the body and line all the organs. A majority of the epithelial tissue exposed to the outside environment is the skin; however, some epithelial tissues exposed to the outside environment are not skin, such as in the airways, the reproductive and urinary systems, and the digestive tract. There are three different epithelial cell shapes: the columnar epithelium, the cuboidal epithelium, and the squamous epithelium. These different cell shapes can be arranged as a single layer referred to as **simple**. Multiple layers are referred to as **stratified** and an arrangement that appears to be stratified but is actually a single layer is called **pseudostratified**. The pseudostratified epithelium can form cilia, so it is commonly found in locations with cilia, like the airways. Additionally, a type known as transitional epithelium is composed of layers of different epithelial cell shapes with the purpose of being flexible and stretchy.

Transitional epithelium is found in structures like bladders and ureters. Simple columnar epithelium is a single row of tall cells and is found in absorptive areas, like the intestines, and areas where secretion occurs often, like the stomach. Simple cuboidal epithelium is a single layer of cube-shaped cells that are important in secretion and absorption. They are commonly found in the kidneys, pancreas, and other similar organs. Simple squamous epithelium cells are a flat single layer that is found in thin tissues where passive diffusion occurs, such as capillaries. Stratified epithelia are mainly utilized for protection of structures since they are durable. Therefore, stratified epithelium is abundant throughout the entire body. Some epithelial cells can become **keratinized**, meaning they contain the tough protein keratin. Keratinization makes cells stronger and more waterproof, and therefore it is abundant in skin. The skin is composed of five layers of cells. From outside to the inside, they are the stratum corneum, stratum lucidum, stratum granulosum, stratum spinosum, and the stratum basale.

Endocrine System

The **endocrine system** is made up of ductless tissues and glands, and is responsible for hormone secretion into either the blood or the interstitial fluid of the human body. **Hormones** are chemical substances that change the metabolic activity of tissues and organs. **Interstitial fluid** is the solution that surrounds tissue cells within the body. This system works closely with the nervous system to regulate the physiological activities of the other systems of the body in order to maintain homeostasis. While the nervous system provides quick, short-term responses to stimuli, the endocrine system acts by releasing hormones into the bloodstream, which then are distributed to the whole body. The response is slow but long lasting, ranging from a few hours to even a few weeks. While regular metabolic reactions are controlled by enzymes, hormones can change the type, activity, or quantity of the enzymes involved in the reaction. They can regulate development and growth, digestive metabolism, mood, and body temperature, among many other things. Often very small amounts of a hormone will lead to large changes in the body.

There are eight major glands in the endocrine system, each with its own specific function. They are described below.

- **Hypothalamus:** This gland is a part of the brain. It connects the nervous system to the endocrine system via the pituitary gland and plays an important role in regulating endocrine organs.
- **Pituitary gland:** This pea-sized gland is found at the bottom of the hypothalamus. It releases hormones that regulate growth, blood pressure, certain functions of the reproductive sex organs, and pain relief, among other things. It also plays an important role in regulating the function of other endocrine glands.
- **Thyroid gland:** This gland releases hormones that are important for metabolism, growth and development, temperature regulation, and brain development during infancy and childhood. Thyroid hormones also monitor the amount of circulating calcium in the body.
- **Parathyroid glands:** These are four pea-sized glands located on the posterior surface of the thyroid. The main hormone that is secreted is called parathyroid hormone (PTH) and helps with the thyroid's regulation of calcium in the body.
- **Thymus gland:** This gland is located in the chest cavity, embedded in connective tissue. It produces several hormones that are important for development and maintenance of normal immunological defenses.
- **Adrenal glands:** One adrenal gland is attached to the top of each kidney. Its major function is to aid in the management of stress.
- **Pancreas:** This gland produces hormones that regulate blood sugar levels in the body.
- **Pineal gland:** The pineal gland secretes the hormone **melatonin**, which can slow the maturation of sperm, oocytes, and reproductive organs. Melatonin also regulates the body's circadian rhythm, which is the natural awake-asleep cycles.

Feedback Loops: Positive and Negative Feedback

All the mechanisms of the body, like blood pressure, temperature, and nutrient control, need ways to maintain the balance of homeostasis. All aspects of the body have optimal ranges, and feedback loops are how these optimal ranges are maintained. There are two forms of feedback loops: positive feedback loops and negative feedback loops. Positive feedback amplifies the output of a system and is considered a self-reinforcing response to an input. Positive feedback loops work by a receptor sensing a small variation from what is normal and then outputting in a magnified way. A common example of a positive feedback loop in physiology is the formation of blood clots. When there is a cut that results in the loss of blood, blood pressure at the site of the cut is decreased. This fluctuation in blood pressure stimulates the release of blood clotting factors, which initiate the process of clotting blood. When clotting begins, its effect is detected and then further amplified until no more variation is detected, which is when the cut is completely sealed.

Generally speaking, negative feedback loops occur when a product of a reaction results in a decrease in the reaction. In this case, the response in negative feedback loops is opposite of the output of the event which triggered it. The baroreflex, which is the regulation of blood pressure, is a good example of a negative feedback loop. A sufficiently high blood pressure is required to successfully circulate the entirety of the body, but if it is too high it can be damaging. Baroreceptors, which are pressure sensors, in the carotid artery and the aortic arch detect alterations in blood pressure past what is within the standard range. When variations are detected, the baroreceptors send signals to the brain, then the brain signals the heart to alter heart rate. When blood pressure is detected as too high, the heart is signaled to decrease heart rate, and when blood pressure is too low, heart rate increases. Since the result is opposite of the stimulus, this is considered a negative feedback loop.

Failed feedback loops result in faulty homeostasis that is detrimental to one's health. A common example of a nonfunctioning feedback loop is seen in diabetics. In diabetic individuals, beta cells do not release insulin when there is a rise in glucose levels in blood. This results in blood glucose being concentrated above the range of homeostasis. Chronically elevated glucose levels in the blood cause countless health issues over time.

Endocrine System: Hormones and Their Sources

Function of Endocrine System: Specific Chemical Control at Cell, Tissue, and Organ Level

The endocrine system is responsible for maintaining homeostasis of the body. Endocrine glands release hormones to elicit a response or change in specific target cells. Hormones are regulated by a feedback system that will either increase or reduce the effect of the hormone. For example, blood glucose levels are regulated by the hormone insulin in a negative feedback system. Insulin is produced by the pancreas, an endocrine organ. When insulin circulates in the blood, it lowers blood glucose levels. The pancreas senses the lower blood glucose levels and stops producing insulin. Childbirth is an example of a positive feedback system. The pituitary gland releases the hormone oxytocin when the baby pushes on the muscles of the cervix. Oxytocin causes uterine muscles to contract and further dilation of the cervix. As the cervix continues to be dilated, more oxytocin is released. The feedback cycle ends with the birth of the child.

Definitions of Endocrine Gland, Hormone

Endocrine glands are ductless glands that secrete hormones into the circulatory system. Hormones are chemicals that are produced by a tissue or organ with the goal of inducing a response or change from target cells. The hormones that are secreted can reach target cells that are both near and far from the endocrine gland.

Major Endocrine Glands: Names, Locations, Products

The major endocrine glands are the hypothalamus, the pituitary gland, the thyroid, the parathyroid glands, the adrenal glands, the pancreas, the gonads, and the pineal gland. The table below provides detailed information about each gland:

Name	**Location**	**Products**
Hypothalamus	Undersurface of the brain	Neurohormones
Pituitary gland	Bottom of hypothalamus	Follicle-stimulating hormone (FSH), luteinizing hormone (LH), anti-diuretic hormone, growth hormone, oxytocin, prolactin
Thyroid	Front of neck	Thyroxin
Parathyroid glands	Posterior surface of the thyroid	Parathyroid hormone
Adrenal glands	Chest cavity	Adrenaline, aldosterone, cortisol
Pancreas	Behind the stomach	Insulin, glucagon
Gonads	Pelvis	Ovaries: estrogen, progesterone; testes: testosterone
Pineal gland	Center of the brain	Melatonin

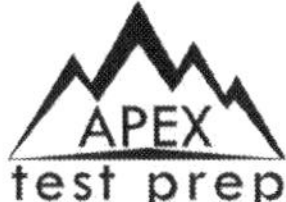

Major Types of Hormones

Hormones can be either amino acid–based hormones or steroids. Amino acid–based hormones are water soluble and derived from individual amino acids or polypeptides or proteins. Steroid hormones are lipids and are not water soluble; therefore, they are not soluble in the blood. The following figure illustrates the major hormone types:

Hormone Class	Components	Example(s)
Amine Hormone	Amino acids with modified groups (e.g. norepinephrine's carboxyl group is replaced with a benzene ring)	Norepinephrine OH, NH_2, HO, OH
Peptide Hormone	Short chains of linked amino acids	Oxytocin Gly, Leu, Pro, Cys, Asp, Cys, Glu, Tyr, Ile
Protein Hormone	Long chains of linked amino acids	Human Growth Hormone
Steroid Hormones	Derived from the lipid cholesterol	Testosterone: H_3C, OH, H_3C, O Progesterone: CH_3, C=O, H_3C, H_3C, O

Neuroendocrinology: Relation Between Neurons and Hormonal Systems

The endocrine and nervous systems both respond to changes in the internal and external environments. Neurons and hormones are both used to communicate the changes within the body. Neurons rapidly respond to stimuli through electrochemical signals. Hormones respond much slower to changes. The brain processes the change and then signals the endocrine gland to produce a hormone. The hormone then has to travel through the circulatory system to induce a response from the target cells.

Endocrine System: Mechanisms of Hormone Action

Cellular Mechanisms of Hormone Action

When hormones reach their target cell, water-soluble hormones bind to membrane receptors, but steroid hormones cross the plasma membrane and bind to an internal receptor. Signal transduction is the process by which the hormone gets converted to an intracellular response. The water-soluble hormones cause a conformational change in the receptor molecule, which then activates a second messenger. The second messenger activates the target protein, which initiates the cellular response. The steroid hormones bind to an internal receptor, and then the receptor-steroid complex moves into the nucleus where it binds directly to the cell's DNA and regulates gene expression.

Transport of Hormones: Blood Supply

Amino acid–based hormones are hydrophilic and travel through the blood stream individually until they can bind to the membrane receptors of their target cells. Non–water-soluble hormones, such as steroids, must bind to a plasma protein while traveling through the blood.

Specificity of Hormones: Target Tissue

Because hormones travel through the blood, they must be highly specific for their target tissue. The cells of the target tissue have specific receptors that only accept binding of that hormone. If the hormones were not highly specific, they would elicit changes from many different cells on their way to their target tissue.

Integration With Nervous System: Feedback Control

Several endocrine glands are linked to the nervous system. The hypothalamus and posterior pituitary glands are examples of glands that have nerve tissue that helps regulate the function of the gland. The nerve tissue sends signals to the brain, and the brain can regulate the secretion of endocrine hormones through the blood.

Regulation by Second Messengers

When hormones bind to receptors on the cell surface, the receptor-hormone complex activates a second messenger on the inside of the cell, such as calcium ions or cyclic adenosine monophosphate (AMP). These second messengers can activate an enzyme, open an ion channel, or initiate the transcription of a gene.

Hormone Secretion and Function

Aldosterone

Aldosterone is a steroid hormone produced by the adrenal cortex of the adrenal gland. Aldosterone is derived from corticosterone, which is derived from cholesterol. It is a hydroxycorticosteroid hormone that is vital in maintaining proper blood pressure and concentrations of electrolytes in the blood. Secretion of aldosterone occurs when blood pressure decreases. Upon secretion, aldosterone functions by increasing the permeability of sodium ions through membranes of the collecting ducts in the nephrons. This results in an increased blood volume, which causes blood pressure to increase as well. Aldosterone is released when baroreceptors detect low blood volume or pressure. Aldosterone is regulated by the renin angiotensin system, which is activated by low blood volume or blood pressure.

Corticosteroids

Corticosteroids, more commonly known as steroids, are a class of hormone. They are produced by the adrenal cortex in humans and often synthesized in a lab for use as medication. Glucocorticoids and mineralocorticoids are the two main divisions of *corticosteroids*. They have many functions and are involved in regulating many physiological processes, such as immune response, stress response, and inflammation. Some common corticosteroids are cortisol, cortisone, and aldosterone. Medicinally, the main use of corticosteroids is to control inflammation and pain.

Antidiuretic Hormone (Vasopressin)

Antidiuretic hormone, also known as arginine vasopressin, is a hormone that has two main functions. The first is to increase the amount of water in circulation by allowing filtrate to be reabsorbed into the bloodstream in the nephrons. Its other function is to constrict arterioles, which in turn increases blood pressure. Antidiuretic hormone is produced by the hypothalamus in the brain, then it is stored in the pituitary gland until it is needed. Secretion of antidiuretic hormone increases blood pressure through the constriction of blood vessels. In addition, it reduces concentrations of electrolytes by increasing the amount of water reabsorbed in the kidneys. Antidiuretic hormone is activated by high particle concentration in the blood or reduced blood pressure.

Oxytocin

Oxytocin is a type of peptide hormone that is synthesized in the hypothalamus. It is stored in the posterior pituitary gland, from where it is then secreted when needed. It is mainly released into one's bloodstream during childbirth or sexual activity. In childbirth, oxytocin stimulates uterine contractions. In addition, it plays a role in milk production after childbirth. Oxytocin is also involved in emotions and behaviors like trust, empathy, and relationship-forming. Isolated oxytocin is used as a medicine in childbirth to induce labor sooner, increase the speed of labor, and decrease the amount of bleeding.

Adrenocorticotropic Hormone

Adrenocorticotropic hormone, abbreviated as ACTH, is a tropic polypeptide hormone. It is synthesized and secreted by the anterior pituitary gland. ACTH's physiological function is to stimulate and increase the production of cortisol. It is produced mostly in times of biological stress. Since it stimulates the production of cortisol, it is very important in the regulation of one's circadian rhythm. Deficiency of ACTH is indicative of many health issues. In addition, a chronic overexpression of ACTH can be indicative of health issues, such as Cushing's syndrome. The synthesis and release of adrenocorticotropic hormone are regulated by corticotropin-releasing hormone.

Growth Hormone

Also known as somatotropin or HGH, growth hormone is a single-chain polypeptide that is composed of 191 amino acids with a globular shape. Growth hormone has many important functions such as stimulating cell reproduction, growth, and regeneration. It is mostly important for the growth of children but is still prevalent in adults. Growth hormone is often used as a medicinal treatment for growth disorders in children and growth hormone deficiency in adults. It is produced in, stored in, and secreted from the anterior pituitary gland by somatotropic cells. Release of growth hormone is regulated by the hypothalamus.

Luteinizing Hormone

Luteinizing hormone is a glycoprotein hormone that is synthesized by gonadotropic cells in the anterior pituitary gland. Luteinizing hormone functions differently in females and males. In females, rises in levels of luteinizing hormone initiate ovulation as well as promoting formation of the corpus luteum. In males, it stimulates production of testosterone by the leading cells. It is a heterodimeric glycoprotein composed of multiple alpha and beta subunits. Production of luteinizing hormone in the gonadotropic cells is regulated by gonadotropin releasing hormone. Monitoring levels of luteinizing hormone, alongside other hormones important to reproduction, can provide insight into an individual's reproductive health. The synthesis of luteinizing hormone is regulated by gonadotropin-releasing hormone.

Follicle-Stimulating Hormone

Follicle stimulating hormone (FSH) is a type of glycoprotein polypeptide hormone, and it is synthesized by the gonadotropic cells in the pituitary gland. Its main purpose is to regulate the development of reproductive systems. In addition, FSH is also involved in regulating growth and pubertal maturation. FSH works together with luteinizing hormone to regulate the reproductive system. In males, it regulates the production of sperm. In females, FSH assists in controlling menstrual cycles and egg growth. Secretion of FSH is regulated by both positive and negative feedback mechanisms that involve the pituitary gland, the reproductive organs, and other hormones.

Prolactin

Prolactin, also referred to as lactotropin, is another polypeptide hormone; it is secreted by lactotrophs in the pituitary gland. The most important role of prolactin is to stimulate the production of milk. When breastfeeding, a female's levels of prolactin are high and their levels of estrogen are low. Prolactin exists in men at low levels, and when levels are high in men, many health issues can occur. Dopamine, a hormone synthesized by the hypothalamus, is one element of the regulation of prolactin production. The main regulator of prolactin is the varying levels of estrogens.

Thyroid-Stimulating Hormone

Thyroid-stimulating hormone (TSH), or thyrotropin, is a glycoprotein hormone that is produced by the thyrotrope cells in the pituitary gland. The function of TSH, as its name suggests, is to stimulate the thyroid gland to make thyroxine and triiodothyronine. Triiodothyronine then stimulates metabolism in the body. TSH is present in one's body throughout one's life, but is most concentrated in times of development, quick growth, and stress. It is regulated by production of thyrotropin-releasing hormone by the hypothalamus. Levels of TSH can be measured to test for proper thyroid function. Certain synthetic pharmaceuticals that resemble TSH are used to adjust endocrine functions of thyroid cells, as well as aid in the diagnosis of thyroid cancer.

Renin

Renin, also referred to as angiotensinogenase, is an aspartic protease enzyme. It is produced by kidneys and is considered a main hormone used in regulating blood pressure and other bodily functions. Renin activates the renin-angiotensin system by cleaving angiotensinogen into angiotensin I, which is then converted into angiotensin II, which in turn increases blood pressure. Therefore, indirectly, the function of renin is to regulate blood pressure. When renin is overly active, it can lead to vasoconstriction and hypertension. A common treatment for hypertension is the use of renin inhibitors

Angiotensin

Angiotensin, like renin, is a vital aspect of the renin-angiotensin system. Angiotensin is an oligopeptide and is formed when renin cleaves angiotensinogen. As it is part of the renin-angiotensin system, it is vital in regulating blood pressure. In addition, another function of angiotensin is to stimulate the adrenal cortex to release aldosterone. There are four types of angiotensin with a wide variety of additional functions, such as regulating lipogenesis and lipolysis, acting as a vasoconstrictor, and regulating salt reabsorption. The amount of angiotensin synthesized is regulated by the amount of renin released by the kidneys.

Erythropoietin

Erythropoietin (EPO) is produced by the kidneys as a response to cellular hypoxia, which is when cells are deprived of oxygen. It is a glycoprotein cytokine, and its main function is to stimulate erythropoiesis, which is the synthesis of red blood cells in the red bone marrow. Red blood cell turnover happens continuously, so EPO is constantly secreted at low levels in healthy individuals. It is heavily secreted when one is anemic or hypoxic. EPO is mainly produced by interstitial cells in the renal cortex, and it is additionally made in the liver and the pericytes in the brain. It is believed that EPO is regulated by feedback mechanisms involving measurement of blood oxygen and iron.

Glucagon

Glucagon is a very well-known peptide hormone that is made by the alpha cells of the pancreas. The purpose of glucagon is to raise one's blood sugar by converting glycogen into glucose and releasing it into the blood. In addition to elevating blood sugar, glucagon can decrease the synthesis of fatty acids

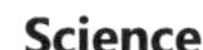

and stimulate lipolysis. Glucagon is regulated by the concentration of sugar in the blood. Alpha cells constantly output their signals to produce glucagon when blood sugar is low, and they are inhibited when blood sugar is elevated.

Insulin

Insulin is the opposite of glucagon in function and is secreted when blood sugar is elevated above the body's normal concentrations. It is also a peptide hormone, but it is made by the beta cells in the pancreatic islets. It is regulated by the beta cells, which secrete insulin into the blood stream when they detect high concentrations of glucose in the blood. Additionally, insulin production is regulated by a variety of hormones including melatonin, leptin, and growth hormone. For diabetic individuals, insulin is harvested from cow and pig pancreases to be used as a medication.

Androgens

Androgens are a class of hormones that are produced by adrenal glands, the testes in males, and the ovaries in females. Androgens are more prevalent in males, and the major androgen in males is testosterone. The ovaries and adrenal glands in females produce fewer androgens than the testes in males. The functions of androgens include acting as weak steroids, forming testes, and aiding sperm cell formation. Adrenal androgens are regulated by different hormones, such as angiotensin II, corticotropin releasing hormone, and adrenocorticotropic hormone. Testicular androgen secretion is regulated by follicle stimulating hormone and luteinizing hormone.

Testosterone

Testosterone is a key anabolic steroid, a sex hormone in males, and it is classified as an androgen. It is important in the development of the prostate and testes. It is produced by the Leydig cells of the testes in men and the ovaries in women, as well as being produced in small amounts by the adrenal glands in men and women. The production of testosterone is regulated by a process known as the hypothalamic-pituitary-testicular axis. When levels of testosterone are low, the hypothalamus secretes gonadotropin-releasing hormone, which signals the pituitary gland to release follicle stimulating hormone and luteinizing hormone. These hormones then trigger the production of testosterone.

Estrogens

Estrogens are a class of sex hormones important to female physiology. Although estrogens are most important in females, they exist in males as well. Estrone, estradiol, and estriol are the three main estrogens. The primary function of estrogens is to develop and regulate the female reproductive system. Similar to androgens, estrogens are regulated, and their synthesis is stimulated by follicle stimulating hormone, which is stimulated by gonadotropin releasing hormone from the hypothalamus. Estrogens are commonly used as medications for menopause, birth control, and feminizing therapies.

Progestogens

Progestogens are another class of steroid hormones, and their function is to activate progesterone receptors. They are the third type of sex hormone, along with estrogens and androgens. The main progestogen hormone is progesterone. Progesterone is mainly known as a female hormone, as it is vital for pregnancies to occur. However, progesterone is in males at low levels, as it is utilized in production of testosterone and other hormones. Progestogens are stimulated when there is a surge in luteinizing hormone. Like estrogens, there are many pharmaceutical uses for progestogens such as menopausal and transgender hormone therapies.

Parathyroid Hormone

Parathyroid hormone, as its name suggests, is secreted by the parathyroid glands, specifically their chief cells. It is a peptide hormone whose primary function is to regulate calcium concentrations and their specific effects on the intestines, kidneys, and bones. The secretion of parathyroid hormone is determined by calcium concentrations through negative feedback. It is secreted when decreased concentrations of serum calcium are detected by the chief cells. Excessive amounts of parathyroid hormone, known as hyperparathyroidism, may lead to many health issues, such as kidney stones and bone disease.

Thyroid Hormone

There are two main thyroid hormones, triiodothyronine and thyroxine, which play important roles in regulating skin, hair and nail growth, energy, and body weight. Thyroid hormones are regulated by feedback loops that involve the hypothalamus, thyroid gland, and pituitary gland. The difference between the two main thyroid hormones is that triiodothyronine is the active form of thyroxine. Having high concentrations of thyroid hormone in one's bloodstream is known as thyrotoxicosis, and it can be indicative of issues like a tumor, thyroid inflammation, or Graves' disease.

Epinephrine

Epinephrine, more commonly referred to as adrenaline, is a hormone classified as a catecholamine that is also considered a neurotransmitter. As a hormone, it has influence on many parts of the body, and as a neurotransmitter it helps neurons communicate in the brain. It is mainly produced by the adrenal glands, but it is also produced by neurons in the medulla oblongata in small amounts. The most important functions of epinephrine are to induce the fight-or-flight response, regulate the activity of the heart, and signal adjustments in blood sugar concentrations. Epinephrine production is regulated by the adrenal medulla of the adrenal gland. It is secreted as a response to stress and certain imbalances in one's body.

Norepinephrine

Norepinephrine, or noradrenaline, like epinephrine, is classified as a catecholamine and is a stress hormone and neurotransmitter. The main function of norepinephrine is to increase the heart rate in response to stressful events. This has the secondary effects of increasing blood pressure, increasing blood sugar, and stimulating the breakdown of fats. Norepinephrine is regulated in the same manner as epinephrine. The adrenal medulla recognizes stress signals and physiological imbalances, and then the adrenal medulla secretes norepinephrine.

Melatonin

Melatonin is an endogenous hormone that is heavily involved in controlling the sleep-wake cycle. Melatonin is released from the pineal gland in the brain when one is exposed to low-light environments. It is a derivative of tryptophan, and its exact mechanism is not entirely known. Melatonin production begins when one is near falling asleep, is highest in the middle of the night, and drops off significantly before one wakes up. The cyclical production of melatonin is opposite of the production of cortisol, a stress hormone which stimulates wakefulness. It can be made synthetically and is often taken as an oral supplement to induce or improve sleep.

Growth Hormone-Releasing Hormone

Growth hormone releasing hormone (GHRH), or somatocrinin, is a peptide hormone that is produced from the hypothalamus in the arcuate nucleus. GHRH first occurs in humans during gestation, and its function is to stimulate the production and eventual secretion of growth hormone. Upon release by the arcuate neurons, it travels to the anterior pituitary gland, where it stimulates the secretion of growth hormone. As growth hormone is needed for growth and regulating the metabolism, GHRH is necessary for these as well. Another function of GHRH is to support slow-wave sleep.

Thyrotropin-Releasing Hormone

Thyrotropin-releasing hormone (TRH) is classified as a hypophysiotropic hormone, meaning that it is a trophic hormone that acts on the anterior lobe of the pituitary gland. TRH is produced by neurons in the hypothalamus and its function is to trigger the release of prolactin and thyroid-stimulating hormone from the pituitary gland. There are some clinical uses of TRH, such as treatment for spinocerebellar degeneration. Concentrations of thyrotropin regulates the production of thyrotropin releasing hormone. When there are high concentrations of thyrotropin, TRH production is inhibited.

Gonadotropin-Releasing Hormone

Gonadotropin-releasing hormone (GnRH) is a releasing hormone synthesized in the arcuate nucleus of the hypothalamus. Additionally, it is considered a neurohormone since it is produced from a neural cell. It is responsible for triggering the secretion of the gonadotropin hormones, follicle-stimulating hormone, and luteinizing hormone from the anterior lobe of the pituitary gland. Concentration and activity of GnRH is believed to influence sexual behaviors. Since GnRH is produced from specific neurons, it is regulated by a wide variety of sensory neurons.

Corticotropin-Releasing Hormone

Corticotropin-releasing hormone (CRH), also known as corticoliberin, is a releasing hormone that is vital in the regulation of the hypothalamic-pituitary-adrenal axis (HPA-axis), which is responsible for responding to stress. CRH stimulates the pituitary gland to synthesize and release adrenocorticotropic hormone, which in turn triggers the secretion of cortisol from the adrenal glands. Stressful events directly stimulate the production and release of CRH when the neural signals of stress converge at the HPA-axis.

Urinary System

The **urinary system** encompasses all the organs of the urinary system. In both the male and female bodies, the urinary system is made up of the kidneys, ureters, urinary bladder, and the urethra. It is the main system responsible for getting rid of the organic waste products, as well as excess water and electrolytes that are generated by the other systems of the body. Regulation of the water and electrolytes also contributes to the maintenance of blood pH.

Under normal circumstances, humans have two functioning **kidneys.** They are the main organs that are responsible for filtering waste products out of the blood and transferring them to urine. Every day, the kidneys filter approximately 120 to 150 quarts of blood and produce one to two quarts of urine. The kidneys are made up of millions of tiny filtering units called **nephrons.** Nephrons have two parts: a **glomerulus,** which is the filter, and a **tubule.** As blood enters the kidneys, the glomerulus allows for fluid and waste products to pass through it and enter the tubule.

Blood cells and large molecules, such as proteins, do not pass through and remain in the blood. The filtered fluid and waste then pass through the tubule, where any final essential minerals can be sent back to the bloodstream. The final product at the end of the tubule is called **urine.** The urine travels through the **ureters** into the **urinary bladder**, which is a hollow, elastic muscular organ. As more and more urine enters the urinary bladder, its walls stretch and become thinner so that there is no significant difference in internal pressure. The urinary bladder stores the urine until the body is ready for urination, at which time its muscles contract and force the urine through the urethra and out of the body.

Nephron Form and Function

There are approximately one million nephrons in a kidney; they have the main function of removing waste and excessive dissolved substances from the blood while preserving as much water as possible. When entering a nephron, fluid from blood passes from the glomerulus, a small cluster of blood vessels, into a structure of the nephron known as the Bowman's capsule. From the Bowman's capsule, the filtrate passes into the first of three portions of the renal tubule, the proximal convoluted tubule (PCT). The majority of reabsorption occurs in this region. In the PCT, the nephron removes amino acids, water, glucose, a large portion of salts, and vitamins from the filtrate.

The solutes that are released into the surrounding tissue return to the blood stream via capillaries known as the vasa recta. Additionally, ammonia, urea, potassium ions, and hydrogen ions are added to the filtrate at the PCT. Next, the filtrate enters the loop of Henle, where more water and salts are removed, and urea is added to the filtrate. From the loop of Henle, the filtrate enters the distal convoluted tubule (DCT). The DCT responds to aldosterone and adjusts how much sodium is removed from the filtrate to be reabsorbed into the bloodstream. Lastly, the filtrate passes from the renal tubule into the collecting duct. In the collecting duct, the final concentration of urine is determined by the presence of aldosterone and antidiuretic hormone. These hormones adjust the water permeability of the collecting duct. From the collecting ducts, the urine eventually drains into the ureter.

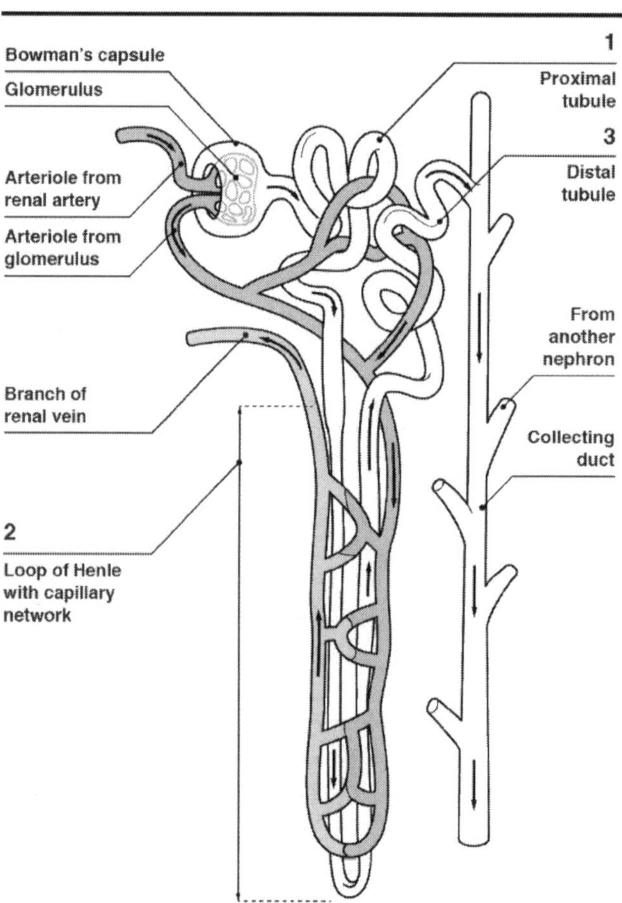

Immune System

The **immune system** comprises cells, tissues, and organs that work together to protect the body. They recognize millions of different microorganisms, such as parasites, bacteria, and fungi, and viruses that can invade and infect the body. When an attack on the body is sensed, immune cells are activated and communicate with each other through an elaborate network. They begin to produce chemicals and recruit other cells to defend the body at the infection site. It is important for the body's immune system to be able to distinguish between pathogens, such as viruses and microorganisms, and the body's own healthy tissue, so that the body does not attack itself. There are two types of immune systems that work to defend the body against infection: the innate system and the adaptive system.

Innate Immune System

The **innate immune system** is triggered when pattern recognition receptors recognize components of microorganisms that are the same among many different varieties, or when damaged or stressed cells send out help signals. It is always primed and ready to fight infections. This system works in a nonspecific way, which means that it works without having a memory of the pathogens it defended against previously and does not provide long-lasting immunity for the body. It does critical work in the first few hours and days of exposure to a pathogen to fight off infection by producing general immune responses, such as by producing inflammation and activating the complement cascade. During inflammation, immune cells that are already present in the injured tissue are activated, and chemicals stimulate inflammation of the tissue to create a physical barrier against the infection. The complement system is a cascade of events that the immune systems starts to help antibodies fight off pathogens. The proteins that are produced first recruit inflammatory cells and then tag the pathogens for destruction by coating them with opsonin. The proteins also put holes in the pathogen's plasma membrane and, lastly, help rid the body of the neutralized invader.

Mechanical, chemical, and surface barriers all function as part of the innate immune system. Mechanical barriers are the first line of defense against pathogens. Both skin and the respiratory tract are examples of mechanical barriers that provide initial protection against infection. The epithelial layer of the skin is an impermeable physical barrier that wards off many infections. When the epithelium sheds, or goes through desquamation, any microbes that are attached to the skin are removed as well. The top layers of skin are also avascular and lack a blood supply, so the environment is not ideal for survival of microbes. The respiratory tract uses a mucociliary escalator to protect against infection. Pathogens get caught in the sticky mucus that lines the respiratory tract and are moved upward toward the throat. If a mechanical barrier is passed and the pathogen enters the body, chemical barriers are activated.

These barriers include cells that have a secondary purpose of fighting off infections. For example, the gastric acid and proteases found in the stomach act as chemical barriers against pathogens that are ingested. They create unfriendly and toxic environments for bacteria to colonize. The group of proteins called **interferons** helps inhibit the replication of viruses. Biological barriers can also help prevent infection. The bacteria that is naturally found in the gastrointestinal tract acts as a biological barrier by creating competition for nutrients and space against pathogenic bacteria. The eyes have a flushing reflex to push out pathogens that may cause infection. Tears are produced by the tear ducts and collect the microbes to be released along with them from the eye.

Adaptive Immune System

The **adaptive immune system** creates a memory of the pathogen that it fought against previously so that the body can respond again in an efficient manner the next time the pathogen is encountered. When **antigens**, or allergens, such as pollen, are encountered, specific antibodies are secreted to inactivate the antigen and protect the body. The response of the adaptive immune system can take several days, which is much longer than the immediate response of the innate immune system. It uses fewer types of cells to produce its immune response compared to the innate immune system as well. The adaptive immune system provides the body with a long-lasting defense mechanism and protection against recurrent infections. Vaccines use the memory of the adaptive immune system to protect individuals against diseases they have never experienced. When vaccines are administered, an active, weakened, or attenuated virus is injected into the body, which mimics the active virus. The adaptive immune system then starts an immune response and creates a memory of the antigens associated with that disease along with the antibodies to fight them off.

Stem cells are the cells that the rest of the cells in an organism come from. With all the different types of cells in the body, stem cells have varying degrees in their ability to change, or differentiate, into other cells. The ability to differentiate into other cells is called **cell potency**. Cells capable of turning into many other cells are referred to as **pluripotent**, while other stem cells with more restricted ability to change are called **multipotent**. A cell only capable of changing into one other type of cell may similarly be called **unipotent**.

Lymphocytes are the specialized cells that are a part of the adaptive immune system. **B cells** and **T cells** are different types of lymphocytes that are derived from multipotent hematopoietic stem cells and that recognize specific target pathogens. B cells are formed in the bone marrow and then move into the lymphatic system and circulate through the body. These cells are called **naive B cells**. Naive B cells express millions of antibodies on their surfaces as well as a B-cell receptor (BCR). The BCR helps with antigen binding, internalization, and processing. It allows the B cell to then initiate signaling pathways and communicate with other immune cells. When a naive B cell encounters an antigen that fits one of its surface antibodies, it begins to mature and differentiates into a memory B cell or a plasma cell. **Memory B cells** retain their surface-bound antibodies. **Plasma cells**, on the other hand, secrete their antibodies instead of keeping them attached to the cell membrane. The freely circulating antibodies can then identify pathogens that are circulating throughout the body.

T cells are also produced inside the bone marrow—the spongy tissue found inside the bone. The T cells migrate to the thymus where they mature and start to express T-cell receptors (TCRs) as well as one of two other types of receptors—CD4 or CD8. These receptors help T cells identify antigens that are bound to specific receptors on antigen-presenting cells, such as macrophages and dendritic cells. CD4 and CD8 bind to the receptor-antigen complex on these cells, which activates the T cells to produce an immune response. After maturation, the three types of T cells that are produced are helper T cells, cytotoxic T cells, and T regulatory cells. **Helper T cells** express CD4 and help activate B cells, cytotoxic T cells, and other immune cells. **Cytotoxic T cells** express CD8 and remove pathogens and infected host cells. **T regulatory cells** express CD4 and help distinguish between molecules that belong to the individual and foreign molecules.

Helper T Cells

Helper T cells can initiate an adaptive immunity to a foreign substance by activating a humoral and cell-mediated immune response. A **humoral immune response** occurs in the lymph and blood, and causes antibodies to remove pathogens and toxins in body fluids. In a **cell-mediated response**, differentiated

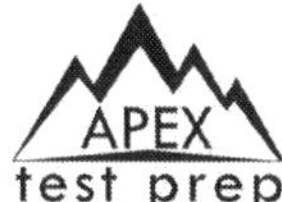

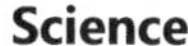

cytotoxic T cells will destroy infected host cells that present specific antigens. Two requirements are needed for the helper T cells to activate. First, a foreign molecule must be able to bind to the antigen receptor (TCR) on the Helper T cell. Second, that antigen needs to be available on the surface of an **antigen-presenting cell**. B cells, macrophages, and dendritic cells are examples of antigen-presenting cells. The following figure shows how a dendritic cell activates a helper T cell.

In the first stage, the dendritic antigen-presenting cell engulfs a pathogen and breaks it down. At the surface of the dendritic cell is a Class II major histocompatibility complex (MHC) molecule that displays a fragment of the antigen. With the help of an accessory protein (CD4), the helper T cell binds to the MHC complex with its antigen receptor. In the second stage, the dendritic cell produces cytokines, which stimulates the helper T cell to secrete its own set of cytokines. In the last stage, the release of cytokines by the helper T cells results in **self-proliferation**—the production of helper T cell clones. These clones secrete more cytokines that activate B cells and cytotoxic T cells.

The activation of B cells, a humoral immune response, can lead to the secretion of antibodies, as shown in the next figure. First, a dendritic antigen-presenting cell engulfs and breaks apart the pathogen. A class II MHC molecule from the dendritic antigen-presenting cell forms a complex with an antigen fragment of the destroyed pathogen. The helper T cell's TCR antigen receptor binds to the complex. The helper T cell activates and detaches from the complex of the dendritic cell. Next, the activated helper T cell contains receptors specific to the class II MHC complex on the B cell. This complex presents an antigen to the helper T cell, which results in direct cell contact between the helper T cell and B cell. Lastly, specific receptors on the helper T cell bind to the MHC complex on the B cell and causes the helper T cell secretes a set of cytokines. As a result, the B cell proliferates into specialized antibody-secreting plasma cells and memory B cells. The antibodies that are presented are specific to the same antigen that initiated B cell activation.

Malfunctions of the Immune System

An **immunodeficiency** occurs when the body cannot respond to a pathogen because a component of the immune system is inactive. This can be caused by a genetic mutation or by behavior. For example, smoking paralyzes the mucociliary escalator of the respiratory tract, disabling a critical part of the body's innate immune system. If the immune system is not functioning properly, the body may attack its own self and develop an autoimmune disorder. When the body cannot distinguish between itself and foreign pathogens, the immune system becomes overactive and the body attacks itself unnecessarily. To diagnose an autoimmune disease, it is important to identify which antibodies an individual's body is producing and then determine which of those antibodies is attacking the individual itself. Autoantibody tests look for specific antibodies within an individual's tissues; antinuclear antibody tests are specific autoantibody tests that look for antibodies that attack the nuclei of cells; complete blood count tests count the number of red and white cells in the blood, which reveals if the body is actively fighting an infection; and C-reactive protein tests determine whether there is inflammation occurring throughout the body.

Diseases such as type I diabetes and rheumatoid arthritis are autoimmune disorders. The pancreas contains cells that produce insulin to regulate blood sugar levels. In type I diabetes, auto-aggressive T cells infiltrate the pancreas and destroy the insulin-producing beta cells population. Without the insulin-producing cells, the body cannot regulate blood sugar levels on its own and requires external sources of insulin to maintain healthy levels. Rheumatoid arthritis occurs when the body's immune system attacks the joint linings of its own body. This causes inflammation and damage in healthy tissue around the joints, leading to pain and immobility.

Lymphatic System

The lymphatic system is a type of circulatory system that is composed of valved one-way vessels that progressively become larger as they near the center of the body. In the lymphatic system, B-cells develop and multiply, making the lymphatic system vital for one's immune system. The lymphatic system is composed of five major components: lymphatic vessels, lymph nodes, the tonsils/adenoids, the spleen, and the thymus. Lymphatic vessels collect and then transport a fluid known as lymph away from tissues and toward larger collecting ducts. The lymph nodes are small structures throughout the network of lymphatic vessels that filter the lymph.

Lymph nodes contain white blood cells and are vital in preventing infections and diseases. Lymph nodes swell when one is sick because they are making an increased number of immune cells to fight infection. The tonsils and adenoids trap bacteria in the mouth and nasal cavity to prevent infections; however, they are not entirely necessary, as many people have them surgically removed to improve impaired breathing. The spleen contains lymphocytes, controls the levels of all types of blood cells, and filters the blood of old and damaged red blood cells. Lastly, the thymus is where white blood cells and T lymphocytes are made.

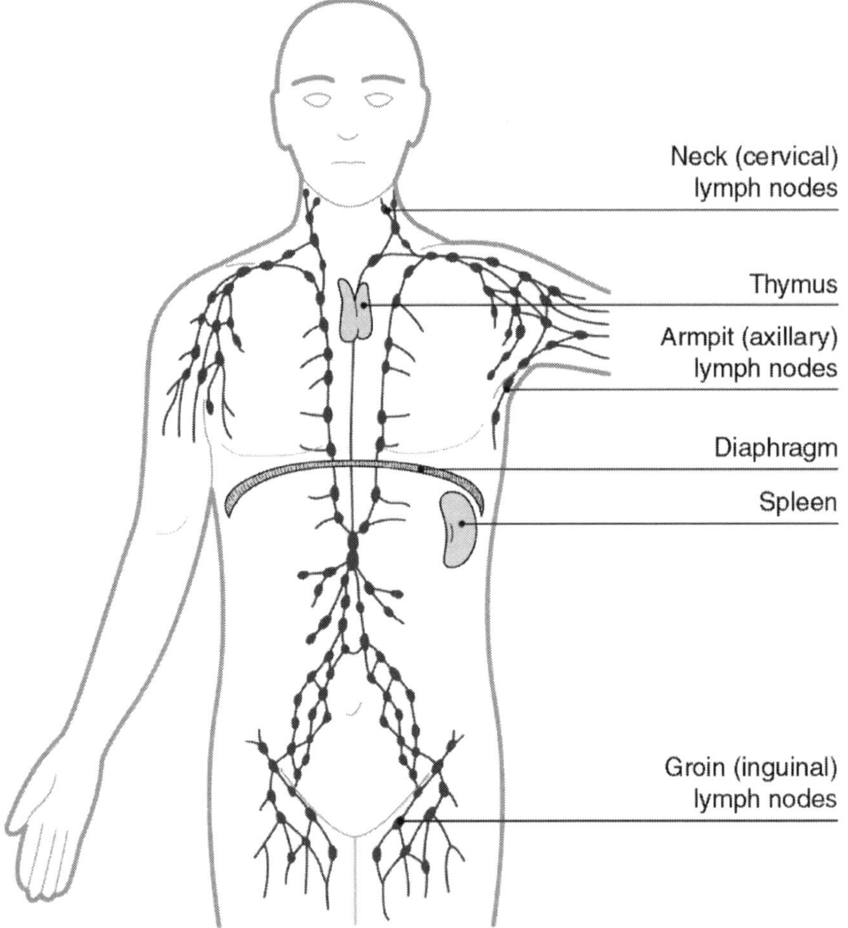

Skeletal System

The adult **skeletal system** consists of the 206 bones that make up the skeleton, as well as the cartilage, ligaments, and other connective tissues that stabilize them. Babies are born with roughly three hundred bones, some of which fuse together during growth. Bone is made up of collagen fibers and calcium salts.

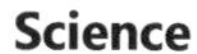

The calcium salts are strong but brittle, and the collagen fibers are weak but flexible, so the combination makes bone very resistant to shattering.

Axial Skeleton

The **axial skeleton** comprises the bones found in the head, trunk of the body, and vertebrae—a total of eighty bones. It is the central core of the body and is responsible for connecting the pelvis to the rest of the body. The axial skeleton can be divided into the following five parts:

1. The **skull bones** are made up of the cranium and the facial bones. While the skeleton gets frailer with age, the skull remains strong to protect the brain. The cranium is formed from eight flat bones that fit together without spaces in between. These meeting points are called **sutures.** The brain is held in a space inside the cranium called the **cranial vault**. The lower front part of the skull is formed by fourteen facial bones. Together with the cranium, the facial bones form spaces to hold the eyes, internal ear, nose, and mouth.

2. There are three **middle ear ossicles** in each ear, called the **malleus, incus,** and **stapes**, respectively, positioned between the eardrum and inner ear. They are among the smallest bones found in the human body. These bones transmit sounds from the air to the fluid-filled cochlea, and without them, individuals suffer from hearing loss.

3. The **hyoid bone** is a horseshoe-shaped bone located in the anterior midline of the neck. It is held in place by muscles and is only distantly articulated to other bones. It aids in swallowing and movement of the tongue.

4. The **rib cage** includes the **sternum,** or breastbone, and twelve pairs of **ribs.** The ribs each have one flat end and one rounded end, similar to a crescent shape. The flat ends of the upper seven ribs come together at the sternum, while their rounded ends are attached at joints to the vertebrae. The eighth, ninth, and tenth pairs of ribs connect to the ribs above with noncostal cartilage. The last two sets of ribs are floating ribs and do not attach to any other structure. The rib cage protects the heart and lungs.

5. The adult **vertebral column** comprises twenty-four vertebrae, the sacrum, and the coccyx. The **sacrum** is formed from five fused vertebrae, and the **coccyx** is formed from three to five fused vertebrae, so the vertebral column is thought to have thirty-three bones total. The seven cervical vertebrae are the uppermost vertebrae and connect the cranium. Below the cervical vertebrae are twelve thoracic vertebrae, followed by five lumbar vertebrae.

Appendicular Skeleton

The appendicular skeleton comprises 126 bones that support the body's appendages. It helps with movement of the body as well as with manipulation of external objects and interactions with the environment. It is divided into the following four parts:

1. The pectoral girdles include four bones, which are the right and left clavicle and two scapula bones. The scapulae help keep the shoulders in place.

2. The upper limbs comprise the arms and the hands. The arms each consist of three bones. The humerus is in the upper part of the arm, and the ulna and radius are below the elbow, making up the forearm. The arm bones provide attachment points for muscles that allow for movement of the arms and wrist. Each hand has twenty-seven bones.

3. The pelvis comprises two coxal bones that provide an attachment point for the lower limbs and the axial skeleton.

4. The lower limbs comprise the legs, ankles, and feet. The legs are each made up of four bones. The femur is located in the thigh. The patella covers the knee. The tibia and fibula are in the lower leg below the knee. These bones have muscles attached to them that allow for movement of the leg. The foot and ankle of each leg have twenty-six bones total.

Functions of the Skeletal System

One of the major functions of the skeletal system is to provide structural support for the entire body. It provides a framework for the soft tissues and organs to attach to. The skeletal system also provides a reserve of important nutrients, such as calcium and lipids. Normal concentrations of calcium and phosphate in body fluids are partly maintained by the calcium salts stored in bone. Lipids that are stored in yellow bone marrow can be used as a source of energy. Yellow bone marrow also produces some white blood cells. Red bone marrow produces red blood cells, most white blood cells, and platelets that circulate in the blood. Certain groups of bones form protective barriers around delicate organs. The ribs, for example, protect the heart and lungs, the skull encloses the brain, and the vertebrae cover the spinal cord.

The skeletal system has several functions, which include maintaining the shape of the body, supporting its weight, protecting the vital organs, and attaching to muscles to facilitate movement. When the skeletal and muscular system function together, it is referred to as the musculoskeletal system. The most important aspect of the musculoskeletal system is that it supports and stabilizes the body and allows movement to occur. Movement is made possible through muscles attaching to bones then contracting to pull the bones in a specific direction. In addition to this, the musculoskeletal system assists in homeostasis by regulating minerals like calcium and producing antibodies within the bone marrow.

Compact and Spongy Bone

There are two types of bone: compact and spongy. **Compact bone** is dense with a matrix filled with organic substances and inorganic salts. There are only tiny spaces left between these materials for the **osteocytes**, or bone cells, to fit into. **Spongy bone**, in contrast to compact bone, is lightweight and porous. It has a branching network of parallel lamellae called **trabeculae**. Although spongy bone forms an open framework inside the compact bone, it is still quite strong. Different bones have different ratios of compact to spongy bone depending on their function. The outside of the bone is covered by a **periosteum**, which has four major functions. It isolates and protects bones from the surrounding tissue, provides a place for attachment of the circulatory and nervous system structures, participates in growth and repair of the bone, and attaches the bone to the deep fascia. An **endosteum** is found inside the bone; it covers the trabeculae of the spongy bone and lines the inner surfaces of the central canals.

Biology

Cell Structure, Function, and Organization

Biology is the study of life and the most basic unit of life is the cell—the smallest individual thing containing the necessary components to be considered alive. All organisms are made up of one or more cells, and the characteristics of the cells are determined by these components.

Nucleus

Compartmentalization, Storage of Genetic Information

The nucleus is the command center of the cell. The genetic information of the cell is stored within the chromosomes in the nucleus.

Nucleolus: Location and Function

Within the nucleus resides the nucleolus, which is the site of rRNA synthesis and ribosome assembly.

Nuclear Envelope, Nuclear Pores

The nucleus is surrounded by two phospholipid bilayer membranes, known as the **nuclear envelope.** Certain areas of the two membranes are fused together to form protein-gated nuclear pores, which allow for the transport of material in and out of the nucleus.

Mitochondria

Site of ATP Production

Mitochondria are the energy-creating organelles of the cell. They convert glucose into ATP that is ready to be used by the cell.

Inner and Outer Membrane Structure

Mitochondria are surrounded by an outer membrane, an inner membrane space, and an inner membrane that has many folds and is held in a viscous matrix. Whereas the outer membrane has many protein channels that allow substances to enter the organelle, the inner membrane is impermeable except through very specific transporters.

Self-Replication

Mitochondria self-replicate by splitting through fission.

Lysosomes: Membrane-Bound Vesicles Containing Hydrolytic Enzymes

Lysosomes are membrane-bound vesicles that contain hydrolytic digestive enzymes for breaking down cell waste. They fuse with vesicles that enter the cell through phagocytosis and use their enzymes on those contents. They are also involved in apoptosis, and when a cell dies, the digestive enzymes within the lysosome break down other cell components.

Endoplasmic Reticulum

The endoplasmic reticulum (ER) is a network of membranes and fluid-filled flattened sacs that run throughout the cytoplasm, connecting the plasma membrane of the cell to the nuclear membrane.

Rough and Smooth Components

Rough ER has ribosomes attached to its membrane and is a site of protein synthesis within the cell. Smooth ER does not have ribosomes attached and is the site of lipid and steroid synthesis as well as carbohydrate metabolism.

Rough Endoplasmic Reticulum Site of Ribosomes

Ribosomes can be found on the outer (cytoplasmic) surface of the rough ER and are considered membrane bound. These ribosomes are responsible for translation of mRNA into polypeptide chains, which is the essential mechanism of protein synthesis. Proteins synthesized by rough ER are targeted for transport to specific final destinations.

Membrane Structure
The membrane structure of rough ER extends continuously from the outer membrane of the cell's nuclear membrane. This proximity to the nucleus allows the ER special control over the cell's protein processing.

Role in Membrane Biosynthesis
Smooth ER is responsible for the synthesis of lipids, particularly cholesterol and phospholipids, which are the essential components of cellular membranes.

Role in Biosynthesis of Secreted Proteins
Proteins destined for secretion outside of the cell begin with their synthesis in ribosomes on rough ER and then are sent to the Golgi apparatus. From there, the proteins are packaged into vesicles and transported to the cell membrane for secretion.

Golgi Apparatus: General Structure and Role in Packaging and Secretion

The Golgi apparatus is also a network of flattened, fluid-filled sacs. They receive the proteins and lipids that are synthesized by the ER through transport vesicles; modify them, such as through glycosylation or phosphorylation; and then send them to their final destination in secretory vesicles that join the plasma membrane and release the contents to the extracellular space.

Peroxisomes: Organelles That Collect Peroxides

Peroxisomes are vesicles similar to lysosomes but contain different enzymes. Peroxisomes contain enzymes that require oxygen and are crucial for the breakdown of hydrogen peroxide, a toxic byproduct of metabolic reactions, into oxygen and water.

Cytoskeleton

General Function in Cell Support and Movement

The cytoskeleton gives eukaryotic cells shape and structure. It comprises three types of protein: actin filaments, intermediate filaments, and microtubules. It also has an important role in transporting substances within a cell, cell movement, and cell adhesion.

Microfilaments: Composition and Role in Cleavage and Contractility

Microfilaments comprise two thin threads of actin that twist around each other. They are responsible for the formation of a cleavage furrow during cell division, which is the indentation of the cell surface during the final stage of division. The actin fibers give microfilaments tensile strength, making them responsible for the contraction of muscle cells.

Microtubules: Composition and Role in Support and Transport

Microtubules are hollow tubes of the protein tubulin. They are found in the cytoplasm, where they provide support for the cell structure, and can be lengthened and shortened with the addition or subtraction of tubulin dimers, which gives them the ability to push and pull materials through the cytoplasm. Microtubules play an important role in the transport of organelles and intracellular materials.

Intermediate Filaments, Role in Support

Intermediate filaments are larger than microfilaments but smaller than microtubules. They work with both to provide a cytoskeletal matrix within the nucleus and to form a structural matrix in the cytoplasm.

Composition and Function of Cilia and Flagella

Cilia are made up of short clusters of microtubules. They are found on the outside of the cell membrane, and their motility can transport mucus across the membrane or cause the cell to move itself. **Flagella** are made up of long bundles of microtubules that project outward from the cell membrane. They propel larger molecules or organisms, such as spermatozoa or single-cells protists, through the liquid extracellular environment.

Centrioles, Microtubule Organizing Centers

Centrioles are cylindrical organelles, similar in structure to cilia and flagella, that occur in pairs. They are found in the centrosomes of animal cells. Centrosomes are microtubule rings that organize the microtubules within the cell.

Human Tissues

There are four primary types of **tissue** found in the human body: epithelial, connective, muscle, and neural. Each tissue type has specific characteristics that enable organs and organ systems to function properly. **Epithelial tissue** includes epithelia and glands. **Epithelia** are the layers of cells that cover exposed surfaces and line internal cavities and passageways. The cells are laid out in sheets and have tight cell bonds between them. The three main cell shapes in epithelia are squamous, which appear flattened; cuboidal, which appear as cubes; and columnar, which appear as tall columns. The cell layers can be described as simple, which is when the cells are in one row; stratified, which is when there are multiple rows of cells with only one of the layers connected to the basement membrane and the other layers strongly connected to each other; or pseudostratified, which is when cells are in one row but the nuclei of the cells appear stratified and are not in line with each other.

Epithelia do not contain blood vessels and can often regenerate quickly to replace dead and damaged cells. Since they are avascular, they receive nutrition from the substances that diffuse through the blood vessels of the underlying connective tissue. **Glands** are structures that are made up of epithelial tissue and are involved in secretion of fluids. They synthesize substances, such as hormones, and then release them into the bloodstream, into inner-body cavities, or onto the surface of the body. Epithelial tissue has five main functions: (1) to protect underlying tissue from toxins and physical trauma, (2) to absorb substances in the digestive tract lining, (3) to regulate and excrete chemicals between body cavities and underlying tissue surfaces, (4) to secrete hormones into the blood vascular system, and (5) to detect sensations.

Connective tissue fills internal spaces and is never exposed to the outside of the body. It provides structural support for the body and stores energy. This type of tissue is also a protective barrier for delicate organs and for the body against microorganisms. Connective tissue is made up of cells, ground substance, and fibers. The cells are surrounded by extracellular fluid. The ground substance is a viscous substance that is clear and colorless and contains glycosaminoglycans and proteoglycans to keep the collagen fibers within the intercellular spaces. The fibers can be collagenous, which bind bones to other tissues; elastic, which allow organs to stretch and return to their original form; or reticular, which form a scaffolding for other cells. Connective tissue can be described as loose or dense based on how many cells are present and how tightly the fibers are woven together in the tissue.

Muscle tissue has characteristics that make it specialized for contraction, which is the force that produces movement in the body. It also helps the body maintain posture and is responsible for controlling body temperature. Three types of muscle tissue are found in the human body: skeletal, smooth, and cardiac. **Skeletal muscle** contracts voluntarily according to impulses of the central nervous system. It helps support the body and maintain its posture. It also carries out movements of the body. Smooth and cardiac

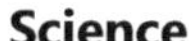

muscle tissue contract involuntarily. They work without conscious thought or impulse to regulate bodily functions. **Smooth muscle** is found in blood vessels and hollow organs, such as the urinary bladder. **Cardiac muscle** is found solely in the heart.

Neural tissue conducts electrical impulses, which help send information and instructions throughout the body. Most of it is concentrated in the brain and spinal cord. Neural tissue comprises neurons and neuroglia. The **neurons** receive and transmit impulses, while the **neuroglia** provide nutrients to the neuron and help pass the impulses from the neurons through the tissue.

Cell Structure and Function

Although there are trillions of cells in the human body, there are only two hundred different types of cells. The **cell** is the basic functional unit of all living organisms. Humans are made up of eukaryotic cells, which means that the cells contain their DNA in a nucleus that is bound by a membrane, and the cells contain organelles. Organelles are membrane-enclosed structures that each have a specific function. The outside of each cell is surrounded by a phospholipid bilayer membrane, which means that it is a two-layer membrane made up of a chain of phospholipid molecules. Phospholipids have a hydrophobic tail and a hydrophilic head, so the tails of the two layers face each other on the inside, and the hydrophilic heads face the extracellular and internal cellular environments.

Molecules can pass through the membrane in a regulated manner. The nucleus of the cell also has a membrane around it to protect the delicate and important DNA inside. The DNA of each cell contains important genetic information from the parent cells and to be passed down to daughter cells. Each organelle contributes a different function to the cell. The endoplasmic reticulum is a network of membranous sacs and tubes that are responsible for packaging and transporting proteins into vesicles to move them out of the cell. The flagella are clusters of microtubules that stick out of the plasma membrane and help the cell move around. The peroxisome contains enzymes that are involved in the cell's metabolic functions. The mitochondrion is the most important cell organelle, as it is responsible for generating the cell's ATP by aerobic cellular respiration. Lysosomes are responsible for digestion of macromolecules. The Golgi apparatus is responsible for composition, modification, organization, and secretion of cell products. Ribosomes make up a complex that manufactures proteins within the cell.

Cellular Respiration

In simple terms, cellular respiration is the cellular process of breaking up sugars to create energy in the form of **adenosine 5′-triphosphate** (**ATP**). Cellular respiration consists of three main stages: glycolysis, the citric acid or Krebs cycle, and the electron transport chain. Glycolysis is the first step of cellular respiration. It is where glucose is progressively broken down in the cytosol of the cell. Through glycolysis, one molecule of glucose produces two molecules of ATP, two molecules of NADH, and two molecules of pyruvate. Since glycolysis is done in the cytoplasm, without the need to enter an organelle, it is a rapid process. The next step, the citric acid cycle, is a series of energy molecule producing reactions in the matrix of the mitochondria, in which pyruvate is converted to acetyl-CoA, combined with oxaloacetate to form citrate, and then broken down into oxaloacetate again, where it can cycle through again.

The two pyruvates produced from glycolysis result in four CO_2, six NADH, six protons, two $FADH_2$, and two ATP through the citric acid cycle. The final main step of cellular respiration is the **electron transport chain** (**ETC**). The primary purpose of the ETC is to carry electrons from the NADH and $FADH_2$ electron carriers through a series of proteins embedded in the inner mitochondrial membrane to pump protons from the matrix to the intermembrane space of the mitochondria. The protons pumped into the intermembrane space create a proton gradient known as the **proton-motive force** which allows protons to flow back into the mitochondrial matrix through the ATP synthase motor. The proton flow through ATP synthase allows it to mechanically combine ADP and a phosphate to make ATP.

The final net equation of cellular respiration is:

$$1 \text{ glucose} + 6\ O_2 \rightarrow 6\ CO_2 + 6\ H_2O + 38 \text{ ATP} + \text{heat}$$

Plants also produce their energy through these steps; however, since plants do not consume glucose, they make it themselves through light-driven photosynthesis before cellular respiration.

The net chemical equation for photosynthesis is:

$$6\ CO_2 + 6\ H_2O \rightarrow 1 \text{ glucose} + 6\ O_2$$

Mitosis and Meiosis

Mitosis

Mitosis is a process that cells use to reproduce exact copies of themselves. It helps organisms to grow themselves and their population. Single-celled organisms can only use mitosis to reproduce (this is considered asexual reproduction). Multicellular organisms use mitosis to reproduce all cells except for their germ cells, which are reproduced by meiosis. Mitosis is a five-stage process that divides the genetic material in the nucleus of the cells. The first stage, *prophase*, is when the mitotic spindles begin to form. The spindles comprise centrosomes and microtubules. The microtubules lengthen and the centromeres move towards opposite ends of the cell. Two identical chromosomes join together. Next, during *prometaphase*, the chromosome pairs develop a kinetochore, which is a specialized protein that joins them together, and become further condensed. The nuclear envelope starts to break down.

In *metaphase*, the microtubules stretch across the cell and the centrosomes have reached opposite ends of the cell. The chromosomes align in the middle of the cell, along the metaphase plate, which is a plane that runs exactly between the two centrosomes. As mitosis begins to reach completion, during the penultimate stage of *anaphase*, the chromosome pairs break apart, forming two fully developed, independent chromosomes. One set of chromosomes moves to each end of the cell. The cell elongates while the microtubules shorten towards opposite ends of the cell.

Telophase is the final stage of mitosis. Two nuclei form at each end of the cell and a nuclear envelope begins to form around each nucleus. The chromosomes become less condensed and the microtubules are broken down. The cytoplasm is divided by a process called *cytokinesis*, which marks the end of mitosis.

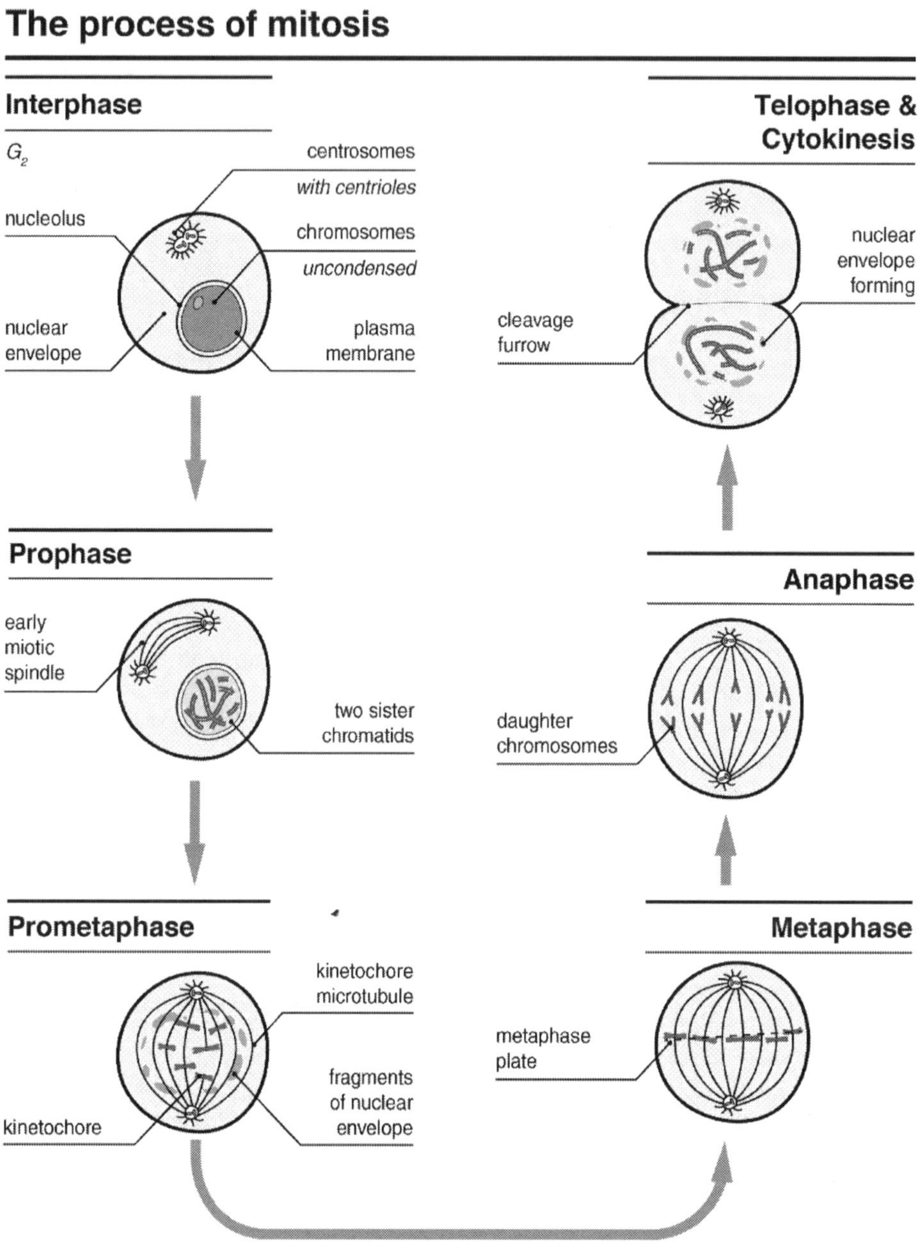

The process of mitosis

Interphase

G_2

centrosomes *with centrioles*

nucleolus

chromosomes *uncondensed*

nuclear envelope

plasma membrane

Prophase

early miotic spindle

two sister chromatids

Prometaphase

kinetochore microtubule

fragments of nuclear envelope

kinetochore

Metaphase

metaphase plate

Anaphase

daughter chromosomes

Telophase & Cytokinesis

nuclear envelope forming

cleavage furrow

Meiosis

Unlike mitosis, **meiosis** produces daughter cells that are not identical to the parent cells. In addition, the parent cell is diploid and the daughter cells are haploid, which means that the parent cell has twice as many chromosomes as the daughter cells it produces. At the end of meiosis, four daughter cells are produced, whereas in mitosis, two daughter cells are produced. Meiosis follows the same stages as mitosis; however, they occur twice—once during meiosis I and again during meiosis II.

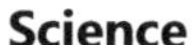

The parent cell has two sets of chromosomes, set A and set B. One set comes from the germ cell from each parent, which in the case of humans, is the sperm and the egg. During prophase I, each chromosome set duplicates itself exactly and then pairs up with its identical chromosome so that they are matched up along their entire lengths. A protein structure called the synaptonemal complex holds the pairs together. Between prophase I and metaphase I, a process called *crossing over* occurs. This is when the genes on the chromosomes are traded between each other, producing chromosomes that are no longer identical to the parent chromosomes. The synaptonemal complex helps with the exchange of genes during this process. The areas where the paired chromosomes are linked together during crossing over, called chiasmata, can be visualized under a microscope.

Chiasmata are responsible for holding the new remixed chromosomes together after the synaptonemal complex breaks down. Once crossing over is complete, the mitotic spindles take hold of the chromosomes and move them towards the center of the cell. The two homologues of the same chromosome pairs attach to spindles that are attached to opposite poles of the cell. In anaphase I, the homologues are pulled apart in opposite directions and in telophase I, the chromosomes have reached the opposite poles. The parent cell then splits into two cells. Next, in meiosis II, the intermediate daughter cells divide again. The chromosomes are not duplicated, however. During this stage, the chromosome pairs are separated from each other into four haploid cells, each with one set of chromosomes.

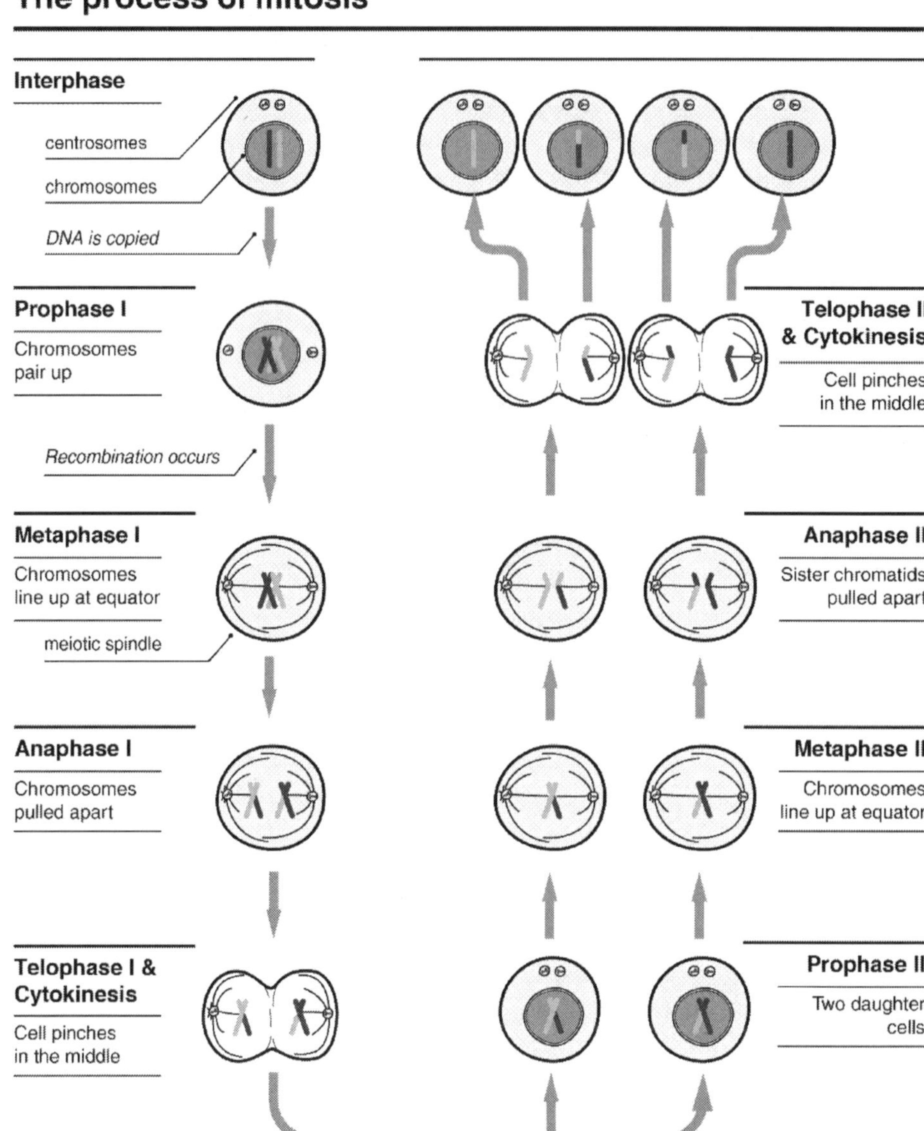

Genetic Material and The Structure of Proteins

Chromosomes

A **chromosome** is a molecule of DNA that contains the genetic material of an organism, located in the nucleus of the cell. It is a threadlike structure made up of genes that is coiled tightly around proteins called **histones**. DNA is negatively charged and histones are positively charged, so DNA is easily wrapped around the histones to support the more fragile form of the chromosome. The Chromosomes are too small to even be seen under a microscope when a cell is not dividing. However, when a cell is undergoing division, the DNA making up the chromosomes becomes much more tightly packed and microscopically visible. During cell division, each chromosome makes an exact copy of itself that it is attached to at a constriction point called the **centromere**. The double chromosome structure, called **sister chromatids**, has an X shape, with one set of the chromosome's arms being longer than the other. In other words, the centromere is located closer to one end of the chromosome than the other. The shorter part of the chromosome sticking out from the centromere is called the **p-arm,** and the longer arm is called the **q-arm**.

For genetic information to be conserved from one generation to the next, chromosomes must be replicated and divided within the parent cell before being passed on to the daughter cell. Humans have twenty-three pairs of chromosomes. Twenty-two pairs are **autosomes,** or body chromosomes that contain most of the genetic hereditary information, and one pair is an **allosome,** or sex chromosome. Some genetic traits are sex-linked, so those genes are located on the allosome. Chromosomes are divided in humans during the process of meiosis.

Meiosis is a special type of cell division in which a parent cell produces four daughter cells, each with half the number of chromosomes as the parent cell. As a precursor to meiosis, each chromosome replicates itself to form a sister chromatid. When a sperm cell meets an egg cell, each brings with it twenty-three sister chromatids. When meiosis starts, the homologous chromosomes pair up and undergo a crossing-over event where they can switch gene alleles. The remixed sister chromatids move toward the center of the cell along spindles and then are pulled to opposite poles and divided into two cells. These two cells divide again, breaking up the sister chromatids, and leaving each of the four cells with one set of chromosomes.

Nucleic acids are macromolecules that are abundant in all forms of life. Deoxyribonucleic acid (DNA) is a double-stranded helical structure containing specific sequences of nitrogenous bases that encode information for producing specific proteins. Ribonucleic acid (RNA) is a single stranded structure of bases, copied from DNA during the process of transcription, which carries the information encoded by DNA. RNA interacts with ribosomes to create proteins from the information in the DNA.

The vast majority of DNA is composed of sequences that do not contain protein-coding regions and have other purposes, such as controlling the activity of the regions that code proteins. The actual segments of DNA that do encode specific proteins are known as genes. Genes are the fundamental units of heredity that determine traits passed on to offspring. Strands of DNA are further organized into structures known as chromosomes to reduce the amount of space in a cell occupied by DNA and to aid in the regulation of gene expression. A chromosome is composed of one strand of DNA wrapped around simple proteins known as histones.

Genes

Genes are made up of DNA and are the basic functional unit of heredity. They can be as short as a few hundred DNA base pairs in length to over 2 million DNA base pairs long. Humans have between 20,000 and 25,000 genes on their twenty-three pairs of chromosomes. Each chromosome contains two **alleles,** or variations, of each gene—one inherited from each parent. Genes contain information about a specific trait that was inherited from one of the individual's parents. They provide instructions for making proteins to express that specific trait. Generally, one allele of a gene has a more dominant **phenotype,** or physical characteristic, than the other. This means that when both variations are present on a gene, the dominant variation or phenotype would always be expressed over the recessive phenotype. Since the dominant phenotype is always expressed when present, the recessive phenotype is only expressed when the gene only contains two recessive phenotype alleles.

Although this is the case for almost all genes, some gene alleles have either codominance or incomplete dominance expression. With codominance, if both alleles are present, they are equally expressed in the phenotype. For example, certain cows can have red hair with two red hair alleles and white hair with two white hair alleles. However, when one of each allele is present, these cows have a mix of red and white hair on their bodies, not pink hair. Incomplete dominance occurs when two different alleles on a gene produce a third phenotype. For example, in certain types of flowers, two red alleles produce red flowers, and two white alleles produce white flowers. One of each allele produces pink flowers, a completely different color of flower.

Gene Mutations

Sometimes when genes are replicated, a permanent alteration in the DNA sequence occurs, and a gene mutation is formed. Mutations can be small and affect a single DNA base pair or be large and affect multiple genes in a chromosome. They can either be **hereditary,** which means they were present in the parent cell as well, or **acquired,** which means the mutation occurred at some point during cell replication within that individual's lifetime. Acquired mutations do not get passed on to subsequent generations. Most mutations are rare and occur in very small portions of the population. When the genetic alteration occurs in more than 1 percent of the population, it is called a **polymorphism.** Polymorphisms cause many of the variations seen in normal populations, such as hair and eye color, and do not affect a person's health. However, some polymorphisms put an individual at greater risk of developing some diseases.

Genetic mutations can alter an amino acid sequence produced in a variety of ways. There are several different forms of mutations that can occur. Base substitutions occur when one nucleotide is swapped for an incorrect one during replication. In this case, since only one base is incorrect, typically only one amino acid in a sequence would be incorrect (missense mutation). Sometimes the incorrect base will still code for the same amino acid and not affect its sequence (silent mutation); yet in some cases, the incorrect base could end the amino acid synthesis (nonsense mutation). Mutations may result in insertion or deletion of a base. This mutation results in a frameshift that alters the entire sequence of codons, resulting in a completely different amino acid chain.

Histones

In eukaryotic cells, DNA and proteins make up a complex called **chromatin**. The function of chromatin is to pack long DNA molecules into compact, dense structures. **Histones** make up a significant portion of chromatin and are involved in gene regulation. The first level of DNA packing in chromatin is carried out by histones, which act as spools for DNA. For example, these proteins act to anchor and bind DNA such that DNA wraps around the histone to form a nucleosome.

The **nucleosome** is the basic structural unit for the packaging of DNA and results in a 'beads-on-a-string' nucleosome array called **euchromatin**. Within a human diploid cell, about 1.8 meters of DNA is wound on the histones. The mass of DNA is nearly equal to the total weight of histone within chromatin. The size of each histone is approximately 100 amino acids. Almost twenty percent of the histone's amino acids consist of positively charged amino acids, such as lysine or arginine. Due to the negatively charged phosphate backbone within DNA, it allows the positively charged segments of the histone to bind to DNA tightly. There are four types of histones that are vital in DNA packing, namely, Histones H2A, H2B, H3, and H4. However, a fifth type of histone called H1/H5 linker histone is involved in a later stage of packing. These histones can wrap into 30-nanometer fibers composed of several compact nucleosome arrays called **heterochromatin**. These nanometer-sized fibers can undergo a higher-level of DNA supercoiling to produce the metaphase chromosome.

DNA

DNA is the material that carries all of the hereditary information about an individual. It is present in every cell of the human body. DNA is a double-stranded molecule that coils up into a helical structure. Each strand is made from a sequence of four chemical bases, which are adenine, guanine, cytosine, and thymine. Each base pairs with only one of the four other bases when it is linked to the second strand—adenine with thymine and guanine with cytosine. The order of the base pairs and length of the strand determine what type of information is being coded. It varies for each gene that it makes up.

DNA Replication

An important characteristic of DNA is its ability to replicate itself. Each strand of the double-stranded DNA structure serves as a template for creating an exact replica of the DNA molecule. When cells divide, they require an exact copy of the DNA for the new cell. During DNA replication, the helical molecule is untwisted, and the strands are separated at one end. Specific replication proteins attach to each separated strand and begin forming new strands with matching base pairs for each of the strands. While some of the DNA molecule is untwisted, the remainder becomes increasingly twisted in response. Topoisomerase enzymes help relieve the strain of the excess twisting by breaking, untwisting, and rejoining the DNA strands. Once the replication proteins have copied the strands from one end to the other, two new DNA molecules are formed. Each DNA molecule is made from one original base pair strand and one newly synthesized base pair strand joined together.

Transcription

Transfer RNA (tRNA); Ribosomal RNA (rRNA)

tRNA is a folded RNA molecule that transports amino acids from the cytoplasm to the ribosomes where translation occurs. It is the physical link between mRNA and the amino acids that build a protein. Ribosomal RNA (rRNA) comprises the structural part of ribosomes. rRNA moves along the mRNA and then binds tRNA and other molecules that help with the organization of amino acids to assemble the protein.

Mechanism of Transcription

Transcription is a three-part process. **Initiation** occurs at the **promoter site** of DNA, which is a specific sequence of bases that resides on the strand of DNA before the actual DNA sequence. Next, **elongation** occurs. The DNA strands are uncoiled, and the template strand, or **antisense strand**, is read in the 3' to 5' direction. An RNA transcript that is complementary to the template strand is elongated from the template strand. Lastly, **termination** occurs when the RNA polymerase that was generating the RNA transcript reaches a termination sequence on the DNA template strand.

mRNA Processing in Eukaryotes, Introns, and Exons

Eukaryotes have an RNA processing step that occurs after transcription but before translation. Genes from DNA include exons and introns. **Exons** are the parts of the sequence that code for a functional part of the final protein product post-translation. **Introns** are sequences found in between exons that do not code for a part of the final product. Introns are transcribed from DNA to RNA, but before the RNA is translated into a protein, the introns are removed in a process called splicing.

Ribozymes, Spliceosomes, Small Nuclear Ribonucleoproteins (snRNPs), and Small Nuclear RNAs (snRNAs)

A ribozyme is an enzyme made of RNA instead of protein. Small nuclear ribonucleoproteins (snRNPs) help to splice transcribed RNA and are formed from small nuclear RNAs (snRNAs) that are combined with other proteins. snRNPs combine with other proteins to form spliceosomes, which remove the introns and join the ends of the remaining exons in the RNA molecule.

Functional and Evolutionary Importance of Introns
Although introns are noncoding sections of currently produced proteins, there are theories that during evolution, they were used to produce new genes by producing multiple types of mRNA during the translation process.

Translation

Roles of mRNA, tRNA, and rRNA
During translation, mRNA is decoded within a ribosome to figure out which amino acids are needed to form the protein. tRNA carries the appropriate amino acids from the cytoplasm of a cell to the ribosome and links them to the mRNA. rRNA reads the order of the amino acids and links them together to form the final protein product.

Role of Structure of Ribosomes
The subunits of the ribosome surround the mRNA strand from both sides. They attract the tRNA molecules that are attached to amino acids to the site of translation. The ribosomes decode the mRNA sequence and then form the new protein.

Initiation and Termination Cofactors
Initiation factors help to bring all parts of the translational process together to start the formation of the protein. They attach the 5' end of the mRNA, the ribosomal subunits, and the tRNA with the correct amino acid together. When the stop codon is encountered by the ribosome, termination factors bind to the ribosome instead of another tRNA molecule, and protein synthesis is completed.

Posttranslational Modification of Proteins
Different functional groups can attach to proteins after translation to increase the functionality of the protein, including methylation, acetylation, phosphorylation, and glycosylation. The groups can be added to the end of the protein or to an amino acid side chain. These additions can regulate activity, localization, and interaction with other cellular molecules. They can also help with protein folding and increase stability of the molecule.

Mendel's Laws of Inheritance

Gregor Mendel was a monk who came up with one of the first models of inheritance in the 1860s. He is often referred to as the father of genetics. At the time, his theories were largely criticized because biologists did not believe that these ideas could be generally applicable and could also not apply to different species. They were later rediscovered in the early 1900s and given more credence by a group of European scientists. Mendel's original ideas have since been combined with other theories of inheritance to develop the ideas that are studied today.

Between 1856 and 1863, Gregor Mendel experimented with about five thousand pea plants that had different color flowers in his garden to test his theories of inheritance. He crossed purebred white flower and purple flower pea plants and found that the results were not a blend of the two flowers; they were instead all purple flowers. When he then fertilized this second generation of purple flowers with itself, both white flowers and purple flowers were produced, in a ratio of one to three. Although he used different terms at the time, he proposed that the color trait for the flowers was regulated by a gene, which he called a **factor,** and that there were two alleles, which he called **forms,** for each gene. For each gene, one allele was inherited from each parent. The results of these experiments allowed him to come up with his **Principles of Heredity**.

There are two main laws that Mendel developed after seeing the results of his experiments. The first law is the **Law of Segregation**, which states that each trait has two versions that can be inherited. In the parent cells, the allele pairs of each gene separate, or segregate, randomly during gamete production. Each gamete then carries only one allele with it for reproduction. During the process of reproduction, the gamete from each parent contributes its single allele to the daughter cell. The second law is the **Law of Independent Assortment,** which states that the alleles for different traits are not linked to one another and are inherited independently. It emphasizes that if a daughter cell selects allele A for gene 1, it does not also automatically select allele A for gene 2. The allele for gene 2 is selected in a separate, random manner.

Mendel theorized one more law, called the **Law of Dominance**, which has to do with the expression of a genotype but not with the inheritance of a trait. When he crossed the purple flower and white flower pea plants, he realized that the purple flowers were expressed at a greater ratio than the white flower pea plants. He hypothesized that certain gene alleles had a stronger outcome on the phenotype that was expressed. If a gene had two of the same allele, the phenotype associated with that allele was expressed. If a gene had two different alleles, the phenotype was determined by the dominant allele, and the other allele, the recessive allele, had no effect on the phenotype.

Genotype and Phenotype

A genotype is the genetic code that determines the specific traits that an organism will express. It is the specific genetic information of heredity that is passed from parent organisms into an offspring. One's genotype takes the form of the various genes found within their DNA. On the other hand, a phenotype is the visible traits that are a result of an organism's genotype and its exposure to certain environmental factors that can alter it. While the genotype of an organism is inherited by parents, the phenotype is not necessarily inherited. Different organisms with the same phenotype may not always have the same genotype.

Dominant and Recessive Traits

Dominant traits are traits that are more likely to be expressed when their dominant allele is passed on to offspring. Recessive traits are essentially the opposite of dominant traits. For example, if an organism were to receive one dominant allele and one recessive allele from their parents for a specific trait, the dominant trait associated with the dominant allele will be expressed. Additionally, if offspring were to inherit the dominant allele from both parents, the dominant trait will occur. The only way for a recessive trait to occur is if offspring receives both recessive alleles for the trait and no dominant allele.

Organisms contain a set number of paired chromosomes. Typically, within humans, there are 46 chromosomes in every cell. 22 pairs of autosomes and 1 pair of sex chromosomes. One of each pair is passed from each parent to makeup the chromosomes of the offspring. Alleles are variations of a specific gene on a chromosome. Both chromosomes inherited from the parents have the same genes, yet they may have different alleles of each gene. The different alleles inherited from parents together make the unique genotype of the offspring.

Genetic Variation from Gene Mutations

Meiosis is the process of individual sex cells dividing to produce sperm or eggs. During meiosis, a single germ cell divides twice to produce four haploid cells, meaning that they contain half the number of chromosomes as the parent cell. Through this division of cells, new combinations of chromosomes appear in the four resulting daughter cells. The separation allows single chromosomes from one parent to combine with the single chromosomes of the other parent's gamete to produce unique offspring. This separation of genetic material followed by recombination with the other parent is what allows genetic variation of the offspring.

Predicting Traits with Punnett Squares

First utilized by Reginald Punnett, Punnett squares are diagrams that can be employed to predict the genotypes of offspring through breeding. The Punnett square is used to visualize mendelian inheritance. For example, if one were to use a Punnett square to determine the genotype of an offspring from a parent with homozygous recessive alleles and a parent with homozygous dominant alleles, it would show that there is a 100% chance that the offspring will have heterozygous genes. If the parents both had heterozygous alleles, the offspring would have a 25% chance of being homozygous dominant, a 25% chance of being homozygous recessive, and a 50% chance of being heterozygous.

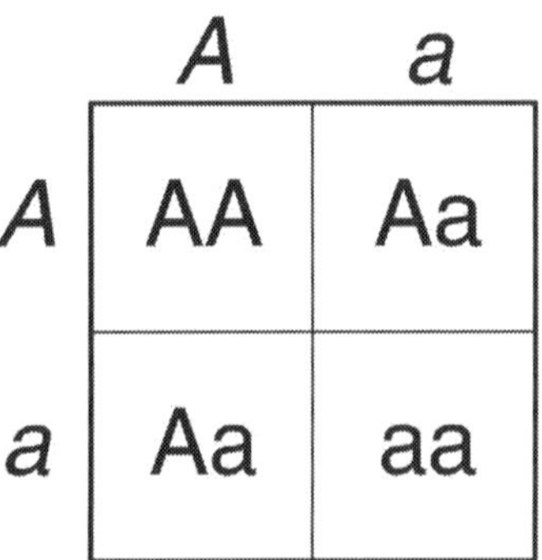

Basic Macromolecules in A Biological System

There are six major elements found in most biological molecules: carbon, hydrogen, oxygen, nitrogen, sulfur, and phosphorus. These elements link together to make up the basic macromolecules of the biological system, which are lipids, carbohydrates, nucleic acids, and proteins. Most of these molecules use carbon as their backbone because of its ability to bond four different atoms. Each type of macromolecule has a specific structure and important function for living organisms.

Lipids

Lipids are made up of hydrocarbon chains, which are large molecules with hydrogen atoms attached to a long carbon backbone. These biological molecules are characterized as hydrophobic because their structure does not allow them to form bonds with water. When mixed together, the water molecules bond to each other and exclude the lipids. There are three main types of lipids: triglycerides, phospholipids, and steroids.

Triglycerides are made up of one glycerol molecule attached to three fatty acid molecules. **Glycerols** are three-carbon atom chains with one hydroxyl group attached to each carbon atom. **Fatty acids** are hydrocarbon chains with a backbone of sixteen to eighteen carbon atoms and a double-bonded oxygen molecule. Triglycerides have three main functions for living organisms. They are a source of energy when carbohydrates are not available, they help with absorption of certain vitamins, and they help insulate the body and maintain normal core temperature.

Phospholipid molecules have two fatty acid molecules bonded to one glycerol molecule, with the glycerol molecules having a phosphate group attached to it. The phosphate group has an overall negative charge, which makes that end of the molecule **hydrophilic,** meaning that it can bond with water molecules. Since the fatty acid tails of phospholipids are hydrophobic, these molecules are left with the unique characteristic of having different affinities on each of their ends. When mixed with water, phospholipids create **bilayers,** which are double rows of molecules with the hydrophobic ends on the inside facing each other and the hydrophilic ends on the outside, shielding the hydrophobic ends from the water molecules. Cells are protected by phospholipid bilayer cell membranes. This allows them to mix with aqueous solutions while also protecting their inner contents.

Steroids have a more complex structure than the other types of lipids. They are made up of four fused carbon rings. Different types of steroids are defined by the different chemical groups that attach to the carbon rings. Steroids are often mixed into phospholipid bilayers to help maintain the structure of the cell membrane and aid in cell signaling from these positions. They are also essential for regulation of metabolism and immune responses, among other biological processes.

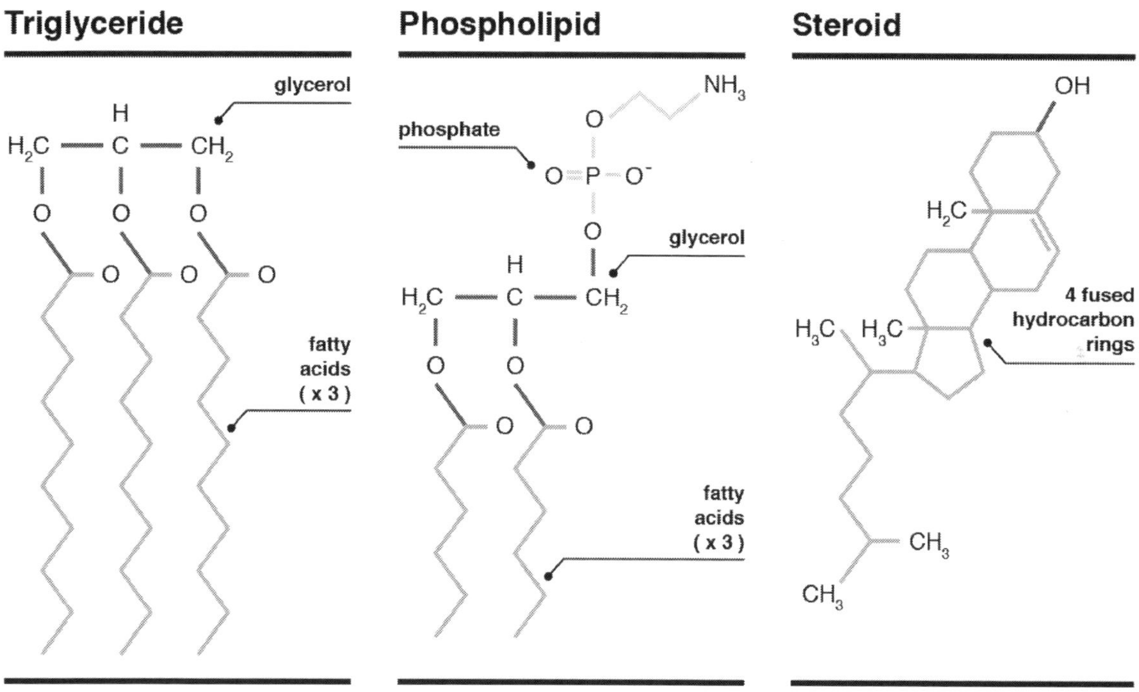

Triglyceride | **Phospholipid** | **Steroid**

glycerol
fatty acids (x 3)
phosphate
glycerol
fatty acids (x 3)
4 fused hydrocarbon rings

Lipid metabolism involves the breakdown and storage of fats for energy consumption, and the synthesis of fats for specific functions or structures. Lipids are first broken down during digestion. During this phase, they are broken down into triglycerides by various lipase enzymes. After digestion, they are eventually absorbed into the bloodstream within the small intestines. From this point they can be stored by the body as adipose tissue or continue into lipid catabolism in the mitochondria, where fatty acids are broken down into acetyl CoA while creating the energy molecules NADH and $FADH_2$. Acetyl CoA and fatty acids can be utilized within the endoplasmic reticulum to synthesize a wide variety of lipids in the body as well. These processes are membrane lipid, triglyceride, fatty acid, and cholesterol biosynthesis.

Carbohydrates

Carbohydrates are made up of sugar molecules. **Monomers** are small molecules, and **polymers** are larger molecules that consist of repeating monomers. The smallest sugar molecule, or monosaccharide, has the chemical formula of CH_2O. Monosaccharides can be made up of one of these small molecules or a multiple of this formula (such as $C_2H_4O_2$). **Polysaccharides** consist of repeating monosaccharides in lengths of a few hundred to a few thousand linked together.

Monosaccharides are broken down by living organisms to extract energy from the sugar molecules for immediate consumption. Glucose is a common monosaccharide used by the body as a primary energy source and which can be metabolized immediately. The more complex structure of polysaccharides allows them to have a more long-term use. They can be stored and broken down later for energy. Glycogen is a molecule that consists of 1700 to 600,000 glucose units linked together. It is not soluble in water and can be stored for long periods of time. If necessary, the glycogen molecule can be broken up into single glucose molecules in order to provide energy for the body. Polysaccharides also form structurally strong materials, such as chitin, which makes up the exoskeleton of many insects, and cellulose, which is the material that surrounds plant cells.

Carbohydrates are broken down much faster than the other molecules, as it occurs outside of organelles in the cytosol. Initially upon consumption, digestive enzymes break carbohydrates down into simple sugars, which are all broken down into glucose. Glucose can then be stored for later use in the liver as glycogen or broken down through the process of glycolysis. Glycolysis occurs in the cytoplasm of every cell, breaking down glucose into pyruvate that can be used in the citric acid cycle, all while producing the energy molecules ATP and NADH. Although larger carbohydrates are not synthesized by the human body, glucose can be created from non-carbohydrate macromolecules through the process of gluconeogenesis.

Nucleic Acids

Nucleotides are made up of a five-carbon sugar molecule with a nitrogen-containing base and one or more phosphate groups attached to it. **Nucleic acids** are polymers of nucleotides, or polynucleotides. There are two main types of nucleic acids: deoxyribonucleic acid (DNA) and ribonucleic acid (RNA). **DNA** is a double strand of nucleotides that are linked together and folded into a helical structure. Each strand is made up of four nucleotides, or bases: adenine, thymine, cytosine, and guanine. The adenine bases only pair with thymine on the opposite strand, and the cytosine bases only pair with guanine on the opposite strand. It is the links between these base pairs that create the helical structure of double-stranded DNA. DNA is in charge of long-term storage of genetic information that can be passed on to subsequent generations. It also contains instructions for constructing other components of the cell. **RNA,** on the other hand, is a single-stranded structure of nucleotides that is responsible for directing the construction of proteins within the cell. RNA is made up of three of the same nucleotides as DNA, but instead of thymine, adenine pairs with the base uracil.

Through digestion, various protease and peptidase enzymes break down ingested proteins into individual amino acids that can be absorbed by the small intestines and eventually be used for protein anabolism. The synthesis of proteins begins during the transcription of DNA, where mRNA strands are produced from genes on the DNA. From there, ribosomes bind to mRNA and work with tRNA to create a chain of amino acids from the 3-base-long segments of mRNA known as codons. Each codon determines what amino acid will be added to the growing peptide chain next. Once the polypeptide is created, it undergoes post-translational modifications, such as methylation, phosphorylation, and disulfide bond formation. Finally, the modified polypeptide can then be folded into its final protein structure.

Proteins

Proteins are made from a set of twenty amino acids that are linked together linearly, without branching. The amino acids have peptide bonds between them and form polypeptides. These polypeptide molecules coil up, either individually or as multiple molecules linked together, and form larger biological molecules, which are called proteins. Proteins have four distinct layers of structure. The primary structure consists of the sequence of amino acids. The secondary structure consists of the folds and coils formed by the hydrogen bonding that occurs between the atoms of the polypeptide backbone. The tertiary structure consists of the shape of the molecule, which comes from the interactions of the side chains that are linked to the polypeptide backbone. Lastly, the quaternary structure consists of the overall shape that the protein takes on when it is made up of two or more polypeptide chains. Proteins have many vital roles in living organisms. They help maintain and repair body tissue, provide a source of energy, form antibodies to aid the immune system, and are a large component in transporting molecules within the body, among many other functions.

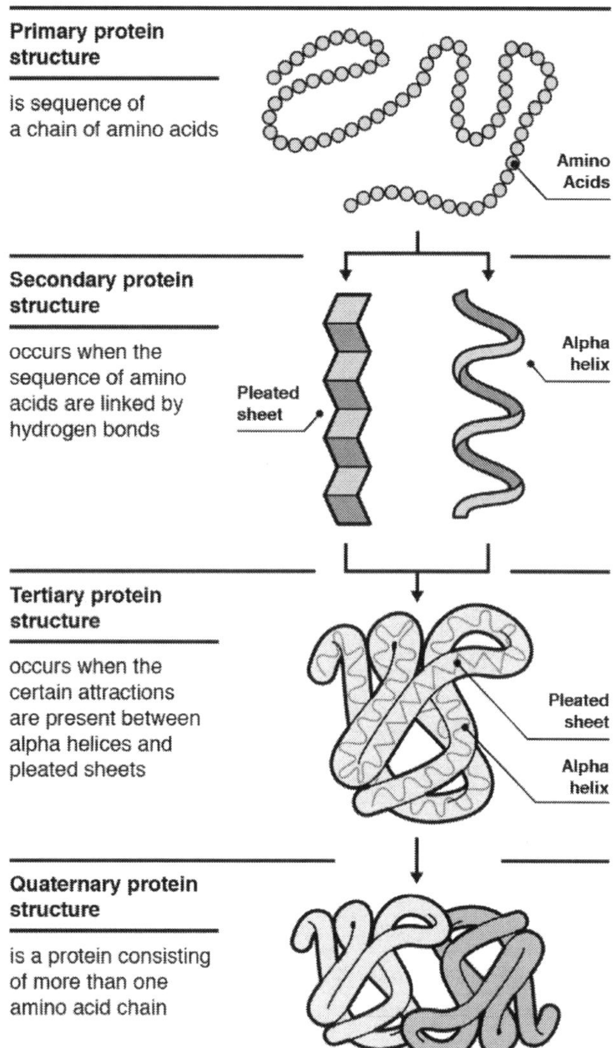

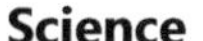

The nucleic acids DNA and RNA are constantly broken down and replaced in cells. DNA is broken down into nucleotides, nucleosides, then eventually bases through the use of several catabolic enzymes. The catabolism of purines and pyrimidines utilize different pathways of enzymes since they have different structures. Bases can be salvaged in the synthesis of new nucleic acid; however, they can be broken down further into uric acid for excretion. The nucleotides used in DNA and RNA can be synthesized through two different pathways, one for purines and the other for pyrimidines. Both processes require phosphoribosyl pyrophosphate to add the ribose and phosphate to a base and create a nucleotide. To become DNA, the ribose of the nucleotide is reduced to make deoxyribose.

Role of Micro-Organisms in Disease

Microorganisms are any living organism that requires a microscope for humans to view. Although we cannot see them, microorganisms exist in every environment on earth, and within our bodies there are ten times more microorganisms than human cells. Microorganisms can be a single cell or a colony of cells. They are separated into the major groups of bacteria, archaea, viruses, algae, fungi, and protozoa. Many microorganisms work in symbiosis with other organisms, such as gut microbes within a human digestive tract, yet many can be considered pathogenic and hazardous to the health of other organisms.

Pathogens are types of organisms that may cause disease in a host organism. The main groups of pathogens are viruses, bacteria, protozoans, fungi, and animals. Pathogenic viruses infect host cells and utilize the cellular mechanisms of the host to replicate within the cell by inserting its genetic information in the host's DNA. Pathogenic bacteria are types of bacteria that reproduce quickly within a host and release a toxin that can damage the host, making them sick. Pathogenic protozoa are single celled and eukaryotic organisms that are much larger than bacteria and contain a nucleus and cellular structures. Protozoan infections are considered parasitic infections. An example of a protozoan pathogen is malaria. Pathogenic fungi are more relevant to plants, but they may infect humans as well. They may produce toxins and carcinogens. For example, Aspergillus produces aflatoxin and is known to contaminate foods like nuts. Aflatoxin can cause allergic diseases and severe symptoms in individuals with nut allergies. Certain pathogens may be carried by other animals, which are referred to as vectors. An example of this would be bird flu, swine flu, or any of the various pathogenic protozoa, viruses, and bacteria that ticks transmit.

Microbial Causes of Disease

Overall, a disease is a condition that is detrimental to one's health and proper body functions and infects cells, tissues, and organs. Disease can be either classified as infectious or non-infectious. Infectious diseases are said to be communicable because they can spread from the host to other people. Communicable diseases can infect healthy individuals and are caused by pathogens. Non-infectious diseases do not spread from the host to others, staying only in the infected individual. Non-infectious diseases are caused by pathogens as well, but many times there are other causes for an individual to be infected, such as old age, immunodeficiency, or poor diet.

Microbes can infect humans in many different ways. The most common ways infections begin are from pathogens being ingested with food, entering the body through an open wound, or through the eyes, nose, mouth, or urogenital openings. The most common diseases in the world are caused by a variety of different microbe infection mechanisms. For example, the Hepatitis B virus, which infects over a quarter of the world's population, is spread through bodily fluids of one infected individual to another. Malaria infects humans when the single celled malaria parasite is injected into their bloodstream when they are bit by an infected mosquito. On the other hand, pathogenic Escherichia coli typically infects humans when it is ingested in contaminated food. Lastly, influenza infections occur when the flu virus is passed through the air as an aerosol or droplets from an infected individual into the mouth or nose of another person.

Microscopy

There are several different types of microscopes that are created to visualize items at various magnifications and resolutions. There are a couple variations on light microscopes: the simple microscope, compound microscope, stereo microscope, and confocal microscope. Light microscopes typically cannot resolve anything smaller than bacteria unless lasers are utilized. Beyond light microscopes, there are electron microscopes that employ a beam of electrons as the source of illumination. Scanning electron microscopes reflect the electrons off of a sample's surface to determine its surface topography. Transmission electron microscopes require that samples be sliced with an ultramicrotome, then the electron beam passes through the sample to allow its internal components to be viewed.

Chemistry

Basic Atomic Structure

Atoms are the smallest units of all matter and make up all chemical elements. They each have three parts: protons, neutrons, and electrons.

Measurable Properties of Atoms

Although atoms are very small in size, they have many properties that can be quantitatively measured. The **atomic mass** of an atom is equal to the sum of the protons and neutrons in the atom. The **ionization energy** of an atom is the amount of energy that is needed to remove one electron from an individual atom. The greater the ionization energy, the harder it is to remove the electron, meaning the greater the bond between the electron and that atom's nucleus. Ionization energies are always positive because atoms require extra energy to let go of an atom.

On the other hand, **electron affinity** is the change in energy that occurs when an electron is added to an individual atom. Electron affinity is always negative because atoms release energy when an electron is added. The **effective nuclear charge** of an atom is noted as $\mathbf{Z_{eff}}$ and accounts for the attraction of electrons to the nucleus of an atom as well as the repulsion of electrons to other neighboring electrons in the same atom. The **covalent radius** of an atom is the radius of an atom when it is bonded to another atom. It is equal to one-half the distance between the two atomic nuclei. The **van der Waal's radius** is the radius of an atom when it is only colliding with another atom in solution or as a gas and is not bonding to the other atom.

The Periodic Table and Periodicity

Periodic Table

The **periodic table** is a chart that describes all the known elements. Currently, there are 118 elements listed on the periodic table. Each element has its own cell on the table. Within the cell, the element's abbreviation is written in the center, with its full name written directly below. The atomic number is recorded in the top left corner, and the atomic mass is recorded at the bottom center of the cell in atomic mass units, or **amus.** The first ninety-four elements are naturally occurring, whereas the last twenty-four can only be made in laboratory environments.

The rows of the table are called **periods,** and the columns are called **groups.** Elements with similar properties are grouped together. The periodic table can be divided and described in many ways according to similarities of the grouped elements. When it is divided into blocks, each block is named in accordance with the subshell in which the final electron sits. The blocks of the periodic table are labelled by letters according to quantum numbers, or s, p, d, and f. The s-block is the leftmost block, and contains groups 1 and 2 on the periodic table, plus helium, which is formally in group 18. The p-block is the rightmost, and covers groups 13 to 18. Next is the d-block, containing the transition metals, ranging from group 3 to 12. The last is the f-block which contains the lanthanides and actinides.

The f-block is formally between the s- and d-blocks in the long periodic table, in periods 6 and 7. The elements are also classified according to their physical and chemical properties, which include alkali metals, alkaline earth metals, transition metals, basic metals, semimetals, nonmetals, halogens, noble gases, lanthanides, and actinides. If the periodic table is divided according to shared physical and chemical properties, the elements are often classified as metals, metalloids, and nonmetals.

Periodicity

Periodicity refers to the trends that are seen in the periodic table among the elements. It is a fundamental aspect of how the elements are arranged within the table. These trends allow scientists to learn the properties of families of elements together instead of learning about each element only individually. They also elucidate the relationships among the elements. There are many important characteristics that can be seen by examining the periodicity of the table, such as ionization energy, electron affinity, length of atomic radius, and metallic characteristics. Moving from left to right and from bottom to top on the periodic table, elements have increasing ionization energy and electron affinity. Moving in the opposite directions, from top to bottom and from right to left, the elements have increasing length of atomic radii. Moving from the bottom left corner to the top right corner, the elements have increasing nonmetallic properties, and moving in the opposite direction from the top right corner to the bottom left corner, the elements have increasing metallic properties.

Protons

Protons are found in the nucleus of an atom and have a positive electric charge. At least one proton is found in the nucleus of all atoms. Protons have a mass of about one atomic mass unit. The number of protons in an element is referred to as the element's atomic number. Each element has a unique number of protons and therefore its own unique atomic number. Hydrogen ions are unique in that they only contain one proton and do not contain any electrons. Since they are free protons, they have a very short lifespan and immediately become attracted to any free electrons in the environment. In a solution with water, they bind to a water molecule, H_2O, and turn it into H_3O^+.

Neutrons

Neutrons are also found in the nucleus of atoms. These subatomic particles have a neutral charge, meaning that they do not have a positive or negative electric charge. Their mass is slightly larger than that of a proton. Together with protons, they are referred to as the nucleons of an atom. Interestingly, although neutrons are not affected by electric fields because of their neutral charge, they are affected by magnetic fields and are said to have magnetic moments.

Electrons

Electrons have a negative charge and are the smallest of the subatomic particles. They are located outside the nucleus in orbitals, which are shells that surround the nucleus. If an atom has an overall neutral charge, it has an equal number of electrons and protons. If it has more protons than electrons or vice versa, it becomes an **ion.** When there are more protons than electrons, the atom is a positively charged

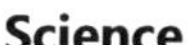
ion, or **cation**. When there are more electrons than protons, the atom is a negatively charged ion, or **anion**.

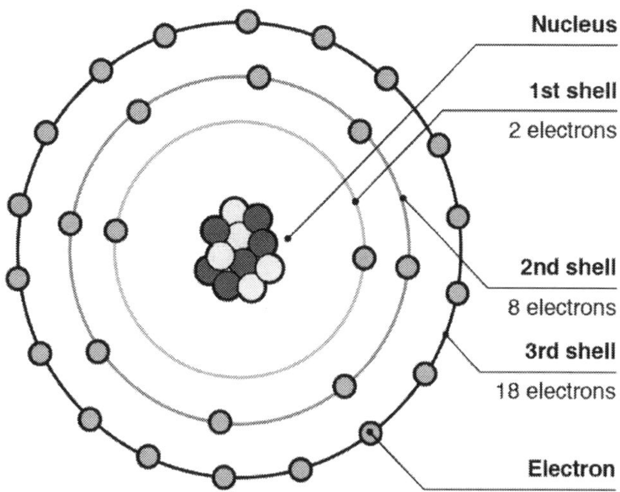

The location of electrons within an atom is more complicated than the locations of protons and neutrons. Within the orbitals, electrons are always moving. They can spin very fast and move upward, downward, and sideways. There are many different levels of orbitals around the atomic nucleus, and each orbital has a different capacity for electrons. The electrons in the orbitals closest to the nucleus are more tightly bound to the nucleus of the atom. There are three main characteristics that describe each orbital. The first is the **principle quantum number**, which describes the size of the orbital. The second is the **angular momentum quantum number**, which describes the shape of the orbital. The third is the **magnetic quantum number**, which describes the orientation of the orbital in space.

Chemical Bonds Between Atoms

Chemical bonds are formed from attractions between atoms that then create chemical compounds or molecules. The bonds can be strong or weak depending on how the bond is formed. A stable compound formed with the total energy of the molecular unit is lower than that of the atoms separately. There are many different types of chemical bonds that can form between atoms, including covalent bonds, ionic bonds, metallic bonds, and hydrogen bonds.

Biologically Significant Bonds

There are three main types of bonds that are abundant in all life: covalent bonds, ionic bonds, and hydrogen bonds. There are many other unique and important chemical bonds in a biological context, such as glycosidic, phosphodiester, phosphoanhydride, peptide, and disulfide bonds. Glycosidic bonds are the main bonds that link carbohydrates together, and carbohydrates are a major component of cell's plasma membranes; therefore, glycosidic bonds are necessary for life. Phosphodiester bonds are the bonds that make up the backbones of DNA and RNA. Phosphodiester bonds form when two hydroxyl groups in phosphoric acid react with a hydroxyl group of a different molecule, forming the double ester bond.

Phosphoanhydride bonds are the bonds that link together inorganic phosphates in the nucleoside triphosphates ATP and GTP. Since ATP and GTP are energy-carrying molecules that fuel our bodies, the phosphodiester bond is one of the most important bonds for the existence of life. Peptide bonds are formed between the carboxyl group and amino group of two amino acids to form polypeptides. Lastly, disulfide bonds form between two cysteine residues when a sulfide anion of one sulfhydryl group acts as a nucleophile and attacks the side chain of the other cysteine, creating the bond. A disulfide bond's purpose is to stabilize a protein's structure. When the disulfide bonds in a folded protein are broken, the protein loses its structural stability and denatures. In addition to these bonds, hydrogen bonding is also an important aspect of biology. Hydrogen bonds are necessary for proper protein folding, DNA structure, the formation of antibodies, and the process of chelation, which is the formation of a ring around a metal cation.

Physical Properties and Changes of Matter

Changes in States of Matter

The universe is composed completely of matter. **Matter** is any material or object that takes up space and has a mass. Although there is an endless variety of items found in the universe, there are only about one hundred elements, or individual substances, that make up all matter. These elements are different types of atoms and are the smallest units that anything can be broken down into. Different elements can link together to form compounds, or molecules. Hydrogen and oxygen are two examples of elements, and when they bond together, they form water molecules. Matter can be found in three different states: gas, liquid, or solid.

Gases

Gases have three main distinct properties. The first is that they are easy to compress. When a gas is compressed, the space between the molecules decreases, and the frequency of collisions between them increases. The second property is that they do not have a fixed volume or shape. They expand to fill large containers or compress down to fit into smaller containers. When they are in large containers, the gas molecules can float around at high speeds and collide with each other, which allows them to fill the entire container uniformly.

Therefore, the volume of a gas is generally equal to the volume of its container. The third distinct property of a gas is that it occupies more space than the liquid or solid from which it was formed. One gram of solid CO_2, also known as dry ice, has a volume of 0.641 milliliters. The same amount of CO_2 in a gaseous state has a volume of 556 milliliters. Steam engines use water in this capacity to do work. When water boils inside the steam engine, it becomes steam, or water vapor. As the steam increases in volume and escapes its container, it is used to make the engine run.

Liquids

A liquid is an intermediate state between gases and solids. It has an exact volume due to the attraction of its molecules to each other and molds to the shape of the part of the container that it is in. Although liquid molecules are closer together than gas molecules, they still move quickly within the container they are in. Liquids cannot be compressed, but their molecules slide over each other easily when poured out of a container. The attraction between liquid molecules, known as **cohesion,** also causes liquids to have surface tension. They stick together and form a thin skin of particles with an extra strong bond between them. As long as these bonds remain undisturbed, the surface becomes quite strong and can even support the weight of an insect such as a water skipper. Another property of liquids is **adhesion,** which is when different types of particles are attracted to each other. When liquids are in a container, they are drawn up above the surface level of the liquid around the edges. The liquid molecules that are in contact with the container are pulled up by their extra attraction to the particles of the container.

Solids

Unlike gases and liquids, solids have a definitive shape. They are similar to liquids in that they also have a definitive volume and cannot be compressed. The molecules are packed together tightly, which does not allow for movement within the substance. There are two types of solids: crystalline and amorphous. **Crystalline solids** have atoms or molecules arranged in a specific order or symmetrical pattern throughout the entire solid. This symmetry makes all of the bonds within the crystal of equal strength, and when they are broken apart, the pieces have straight edges. Minerals are all crystalline solids. **Amorphous solids**, on the other hand, do not have repeating structures or symmetry. Their components are heterogeneous, so they often melt gradually over a range of temperatures. They do not break evenly and often have curved edges. Examples of amorphous solids are glass, rubber, and most plastics.

Matter can change between a gas, liquid, and solid. When these changes occur, the change is physical and does not affect the chemical properties or makeup of the substance. Environmental changes, such as temperature or pressure changes, can cause one state of matter to convert to another state of matter. For example, in very hot temperatures, solids can melt and become a liquid, such as when ice melts into liquid water, or sublimate and become a gas, such as when dry ice becomes gaseous carbon dioxide. Liquids can evaporate and become a gas, such as when liquid water turns into water vapor. In very cold temperatures, gases can depose and become a solid, such as when water vapor becomes icy frost on a windshield, or condense and become a liquid, such as when water vapor becomes dew on grass. Liquids can freeze and become a solid, such as when liquid water freezes and becomes ice.

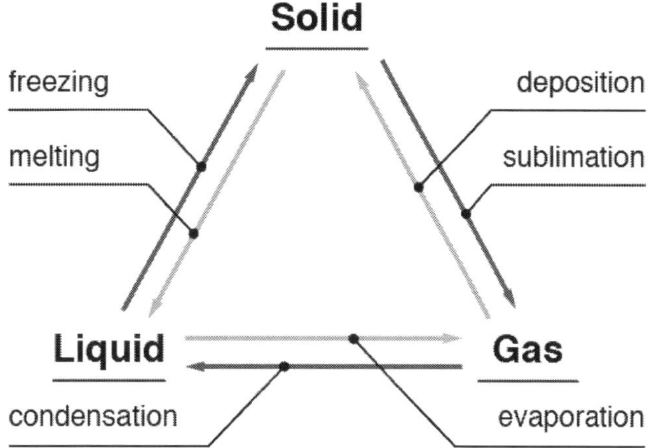

Definition of Density

The density (represented as rho, ρ, or simply D) of a substance is:

$$\rho = \frac{m}{V}$$

The units of mass (m) are in grams, and for solids, the units of the volume (V) are centimeters cubed (cm^3). For solutes or liquids, the volume is given in units of liters (L) or milliliters (mL). For water, one milliliter (mL) is also equal to one centimeter cube (cm^3) or 1.00 grams. If a sugar cube has a mass of 2.0 grams and an edge that measures 1 cm in length, then the density is:

$$\rho = \frac{2.0\text{ g}}{(1.0\text{ cm})^3} = 2.0\text{ g/cm}^3$$

Characteristic Properties of Molecules

There are two basic types of properties that can help characterize substances: physical and chemical. **Physical properties** can be detected without changing the substance's identity or composition. If a substance is subject to a physical change, its appearance changes, but its composition does not change at all. Common physical properties include color, odor, density, and hardness. Physical properties can also be classified as extensive or intensive. Extensive physical properties depend on the amount of substance that is present. These include characteristics such as mass and volume. Intensive properties do not depend on how much of the substance is present and remain the same regardless of quantity. These include characteristics such as density and color.

Chemical properties are characteristics of a substance that describe how it can be changed into a different chemical substance. A substance's composition is changed when it undergoes a chemical change. Chemical properties are measured and observed only as the substance is undergoing a change to become a different substance. Some examples of chemical properties are flammability, reactivity, toxicity, and ability to oxidize. These properties are detected by making changes to the substance's external environment and seeing how it reacts to the changes. An iron shovel that is left outside can become rusty. Rusting occurs when iron changes to iron oxide. While iron is very hard and a shiny silver color, iron oxide is flaky and a reddish-brown color. **Reactivity** is the ability of a substance to combine chemically with another substance. While some substances are very reactive, others are not reactive at all. For example, potassium is very reactive with water, and even a small amount causes an explosive reaction. Helium, on the other hand, does not react with any other substance.

It is often important to quantify the properties that are observed in a substance. Quantitative measurements are associated with a number, and it is imperative to include a unit of measure with each of those measurements. Without the unit of measure, the number may be meaningless. If the weight of a substance is noted as 100 without a unit of measure, it is unknown whether the substance is equivalent to 100 of something very light, such as milligram measurements, or 100 of something very heavy, such as kilogram measurements. There are many other quantitative measurements of matter that can be taken, including length, time, and temperature, among many others. Contrastingly, there are many properties that are not associated with a number; these properties can be measured qualitatively. The measurements of qualitative properties use a person's senses to observe and describe the characteristics. Since the descriptions are developed by individual persons, they can be very subjective. These properties can include odor, color, and texture, among many others. They can also include comparisons between two substances without using a number; for example, one substance may have a stronger odor or be lighter in color than another substance.

Chemical Reactions

A chemical reaction is a process that involves a change in the molecular arrangement of a substance. Generally, one set of chemical substances, called the reactants, is rearranged into a different set of chemical substances, called the products, by the breaking and re-forming of bonds between atoms. In a

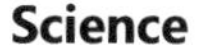

chemical reaction, it is important to realize that no new atoms or molecules are introduced. The products are formed solely from the atoms and molecules that are present in the reactants. These can involve a change in state of matter as well. Making glass, burning fuel, and brewing beer are all examples of chemical reactions.

Valence Electrons and Reactivity

Valence electrons are the electrons located on the outermost edge of an atom. Being that they are on the outside and not buried beneath other layers of electrons, valence electrons are what will interact with other atoms. The valence shell of electrons on an atom has a set number of electrons it can contain. If the valence shell is full, as it is in noble gasses, it is stable and unlikely to react with other atoms. When a valence shell of electrons is not full, it is much more likely to react with other atoms as it attempts to reach a full stable valence shell.

Covalent Bonds

An important characteristic of electrons is their ability to form covalent bonds with other atoms to form molecules. A covalent bond is a chemical bond that forms when two atoms share the same pair or pairs of electrons. There is a stable balance of attraction and repulsion between the two atoms. When these bonds are formed, energy is released because the electrons become more spatially distributed instead of being pulled toward the individual atom's nucleus. There are several different types of covalent bonds. **Sigma bonds** are the strongest type of covalent bond and involve the head-on overlapping of electron orbitals from two different atoms. **Pi bonds** are a little weaker and involve the lateral overlapping of certain orbitals. While single bonds between atoms, such as between carbon and hydrogen, are generally sigma bonds, double bonds, such as when carbon is double-bonded to an oxygen atom, are usually one sigma bond and one pi bond.

Covalent bonds can also be classified as nonpolar or polar. **Nonpolar covalent bonds** are formed when two atoms share their electrons equally, creating a very small difference of electronegativity between the atoms. Compounds that are formed with nonpolar covalent bonds do not mix well with water and other polar solvents and are much more soluble in nonpolar solvents. **Polar covalent bonds** are formed when electrons are not evenly shared between the atoms. Therefore, the electrons are pulled closer to one atom than the other, giving the molecule ionic properties and an imbalance of charge. The electronegative difference between the atoms is greater when polar bonds are formed compared to nonpolar bonds.

Coordinate covalent bonds, or **dipolar bonds**, are formed when the two shared electrons of the molecule come from the same atom. The electrons from one atom are shared with an empty orbital on the other atom, making one atom the electron pair donor and the other atom the electron pair acceptor. The electrons are shared approximately equally when these bonds are created.

Ionic Bonds

When ionic bonds are formed, instead of sharing a pair of electrons, the electrons are transferred from one atom to another, creating two ions. One of the ions is left with a positive charge, and the other one is left with a negative charge. This results in a large difference in electronegativity between the ions. The ionic bonds result from the attraction between the oppositely charged ions. However, the same two ions are not always paired with each other. Each ion is surrounded by ions with the opposite charge but are constantly moving around. Ionic bonds commonly form in metal salts. Metals have few electrons in their outermost orbitals, and by losing those electrons, they become more stable. By taking these electrons away from the metallic atoms, nonmetals can fill their valence shells and also become more stable. For example, when sodium atoms and chloride atoms combine to form sodium chloride, the sodium atom loses an electron and becomes positively charged with a closed shell of electrons, and the chloride atom gains an electron, leaving it with a full shell of electrons.

Metallic Bonds

Metallic bonds occur when the electrons in the outer shell of an atom become delocalized and free-moving. They become shared by many atoms as they move in all directions around the positively charged metal ions. The free-floating electrons create an environment that allows for easy conduction of heat and electricity between the atoms. They also contribute to the **luster,** or surface reflectivity, that is often characteristic of metals, as well as the high tensile strength of metallic material. Metallic bonds are often seen as a sea of electrons with positive ions floating between them.

Hydrogen Bonds

Hydrogen bonds are different from the previously mentioned bonds because they are formed between a hydrogen atom that is present in one molecule and another atom that is already part of a molecular complex. These types of bonds are intermolecular instead of intramolecular. The hydrogen atom is attracted to an atom that has a high electronegativity in the other molecule. The large difference in electronegativity between the molecules creates a strong electrostatic attraction between the molecules. If a hydrogen atom forms a polar covalent bond with another atom, such as an oxygen atom, the hydrogen end of the molecule remains slightly positively charged, and the oxygen end of the molecule remains slightly negatively charged. The hydrogen of this molecule would then be attracted to other atoms with a slightly negative charge in nearby molecules. Hydrogen bonding is also important in the formation of the DNA double helix molecule. The nitrogenous bases on each strand are situated so they can form hydrogen bonds with the bases that are directly opposite them on the other strand.

Types of Chemical Reactions

Generally, chemical reactions are thought to involve changes in positions of electrons with the breaking and re-forming of chemical bonds, without changes to the nucleus of the atoms. The three main types of chemical reactions are combination, decomposition, and combustion.

In a chemical reaction, two or more reactants interact with each other to produce one or more products. Reactants are what exists before any reactions occur. A reaction begins when the reactants interact with one another to form the products. When a chemical reaction is drawn, the reactants are written on the left side of the reaction arrow and the products are written on the right side of the reaction arrow.

Combination

In combination reactions, two or more reactants are combined to form one more complex, larger product. The bonds of the reactants are broken, the elements rearranged, and then new bonds are formed between all of the elements to form the product. It can be written as $A + B \rightarrow C$, where A and B are the reactants and C is the product. An example of a combination reaction is the creation of iron(II) sulfide from iron and sulfur, which is written as $8\text{Fe} + \text{S}_8 \rightarrow 8\text{FeS}$.

Decomposition

Decomposition reactions are almost the opposite of combination reactions. They occur when one substance is broken down into two or more products. The bonds of the first substance are broken, the elements rearranged, and then the elements bonded together in new configurations to make two or more molecules. These reactions can be written as $C \rightarrow B + A$, where C is the reactant and A and B are the products. An example of a decomposition reaction is the electrolysis of water to make oxygen and hydrogen gas, which is written as $2\text{H}_2\text{O} \rightarrow 2\text{H}_2 + \text{O}_2$.

Combustion

Combustion reactions are a specific type of chemical reaction that involves oxygen gas as a reactant. This mostly involves the burning of a substance. The combustion of hexane in air is one example of a combustion reaction. The hexane gas combines with oxygen in the air to form carbon dioxide and water. The reaction can be written as:

$$2C_6H_{14} + 17O_2 \rightarrow 12CO_2 + 14H_2O$$

Balancing Chemical Reactions

The way the hexane combustion reaction is written above ($2C_6H_{14} + 17O_2 \rightarrow 12CO_2 + 14H_2O$) is an example of a chemical equation. Chemical equations describe how the molecules are changed when the chemical reaction occurs. The "+" sign on the left side of the equation indicates that those molecules are reacting with each other, and the arrow, "→," in the middle of the equation indicates that the reactants are producing something else. The coefficient before a molecule indicates the quantity of that specific molecule that is present for the reaction.

The subscript next to an element indicates the quantity of that element in each molecule. In order for the chemical equation to be balanced, the quantity of each element on both sides of the equation should be equal. For example, in the hexane equation above, there are twelve carbon elements, twenty-eight hydrogen elements, and thirty-four oxygen elements on each side of the equation. Even though they are part of different molecules on each side, the overall quantity is the same. The state of matter of the reactants and products can also be included in a chemical equation and would be written in parentheses next to each element as follows: gas (g), liquid (l), solid (s), and dissolved in water, or aqueous (aq).

Mole Concept, Avogadro's Number N_A

The **mole** (mol) refers to a particular number of items. For example, one mole of donuts is equal to 6.022×10^{23} donuts. The number 6.022×10^{23} is known as **Avogadro's number** (N_A). One mole of carbon atoms is equivalent to N_A atoms. If you weighed out 12.01 grams of charcoal, you would have one mole of carbon atoms equal to N_A. For compounds, one mole of carbon dioxide (CO_2) contains N_A CO_2 CO_2 molecules. For every one mole of CO_2, there are 44.01 grams of CO_2.

Conditions Effect on Chemical Reactions

Reaction Rate

The rate of a chemical reaction or **reaction rate** is the decrease in reactant or the increase in product molar concentration per unit of time. The reaction rate has units of moles over liter second expressed as $\text{moles} \cdot \text{Liter}^{-1} \cdot \text{second}^{-1}$ or $\text{mol}/(\text{L} \cdot \text{s})$.

Dependence of Reaction Rate on Concentration of Reactants

Rate Law, Rate Constant

In the decomposition reaction of hydrogen peroxide, the rate of the forward reaction is proportional to the concentration of hydrogen peroxide. If the $[H_2O_2]$ is doubled, the rate will double. A **rate law** for the chemical reaction can be expressed as:

$$\text{Rate} = k[H_2O_2]$$

The rate law relates the rate of reaction to the reactant and catalyst (if used) concentrations raised to a power. The **rate constant**, *k*, is a proportionality constant that has units of liters per moles second ($\text{L}/(\text{mol} \cdot \text{s})$).

Reaction Order

The general form of a rate law, where C is the catalyst, is:

$$\text{Rate} = k[A]^m[B]^n$$

$$aA + bB \overset{C}{\rightarrow} dD + eE$$

If there is no catalyst in the reaction, then the rate would be $\text{Rate} = k[A]^m[B]^n$. The superscripts may be integers and are determined experimentally and have no relationship to the coefficients in the balanced equation. The value of the exponents for a particular species is the **reaction order**. For example, $\text{Rate} = k[\text{H}_2\text{O}_2]^1$, is first order because $m = 1$. When the concentration is double, the rate doubles. If the reaction rate given by $\text{Rate} = k[\text{NO}]^2[\text{H}_2]$, the reaction is second order for NO and first order with respect to H_2. Because $m = 2$ for NO, if the concentration of NO is doubled, the reaction rate increases by a factor of four. The overall reaction order is $m + n = 2 + 1 = 3$.

Rate-Determining Step

Consider the following reaction:

$$\text{NO}_2(\text{g}) + \text{NO}_2(\text{g}) + \text{F}_2(\text{g}) \rightarrow \text{NO}_2\text{F}(\text{g}) + \text{NO}_2\text{F}(\text{g})$$

The predicted reaction rate would be $\text{Rate} = k[NO_2]^2[F_2]$. Suppose the reaction mechanism occurred in two steps:

$$(1)\quad \text{NO}_2 + \text{F}_2 \overset{\text{k}_1}{\rightarrow} \text{NO}_2\text{F} + \text{F} \qquad \text{(Slow step)}$$

$$(2)\quad \text{F} + \text{NO}_2 \overset{\text{k}_2}{\rightarrow} \text{NO}_2\text{F} \qquad \text{(Fast step)}$$

The rate law would now be determined by the rate-determining step, which is the slowest step for the shown 2-step reaction mechanism: $\text{Rate} = k[\text{NO}_2][\text{F}_2]$.

Dependence of Reaction Rate upon Temperature

Reaction rates speed up with temperature and show up in the rate constant. Generally, the rate of reaction doubles for every 10°C. As the temperature increases, molecules acquire more kinetic energy and will react to surmount an energy barrier.

Le Chatelier's Principle

Le Chatelier's principle is utilized to describe how chemical equilibrium of a system is maintained. Le Chatelier's principle states that changes in variables of a system, such as pressure, temperature, concentration, and volume, result in opposite changes in the system to maintain equilibrium. Le Chatelier's principle is commonly used to describe whether the formation of products in a chemical reaction will be favored. For example, if one were to have a surplus of reactants added to a chemical reaction, the reaction will favor forming the product. If the concentration of products within a system is high and the concentration of reactants is very low, the reverse reaction (where the products become the reactants) will be favored. With this being said, Le Chatelier's principle implies that adding heat to a reaction will cause it to favor the endothermic direction to limit the amount of heat produced and maintain balance. In a scientific lab, scientists utilize this principle to manipulate what they get from a reaction. Scientists can push a reaction towards a desired product by adjusting all of the variables, like concentration of reactants, temperature, pressure, and more.

Catalysts

The rate of a chemical reaction can be increased by adding a catalyst to the reaction. Catalysts are substances that lower the activation energy required to go from the reactants to the products of the reaction but are not consumed in the process. The **activation energy** of a reaction is the minimum amount of energy that is required to make the reaction move forward and change the reactants into the products. When catalysts are present, less energy is required to complete the reaction. For example, hydrogen peroxide will eventually decompose into two water molecules and one oxygen molecule. If potassium permanganate is added to the reaction, the decomposition happens at a much faster rate. Similarly, increasing the temperature or pressure in the environment of the reaction can increase the rate of the reaction. Higher temperatures increase the number of high-energy collisions that lead to the products. The same happens when increasing pressure for gaseous reactants, but not with solid or liquid reactants.

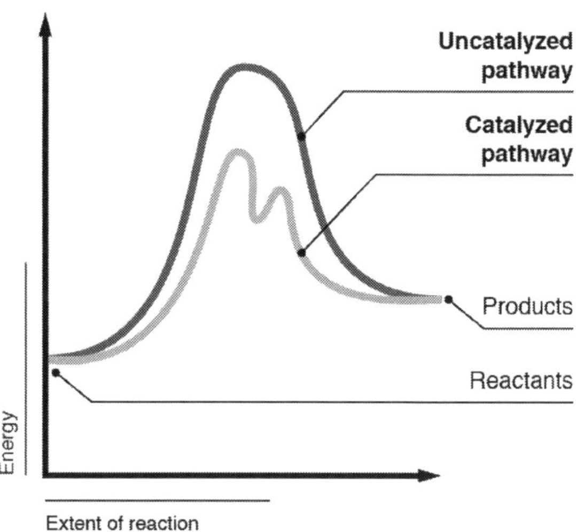

Enzymes

Enzymes are a type of biological catalyst that accelerate chemical reactions. They work like other catalysts by lowering the activation energy of the reaction to increase the reaction rate. They bind to substrates and change them into the products of the reaction without being consumed by the reaction. Enzymes differ from other catalysts by their increased specificity to their substrate. They can also be affected by other molecules. Enzyme inhibitors can decrease their activity, whereas enzyme activators increase their activity. Their activity also decreases dramatically when the environment is not in their optimal pH and temperature range.

An enzyme can encounter several different types of inhibitors. In biological systems, inhibitors are many times expressed as part of a feedback loop where the enzyme is producing too much of a substance too quickly and the reaction needs to be stopped. **Competitive inhibitors** and substrates cannot bind to the enzyme at the same time. These inhibitors often resemble the substrate of the enzyme. Noncompetitive inhibitors bind to the enzyme at a different location than the substrate. The substrate can still bind with the same affinity, but the efficiency of the enzyme is decreased. **Uncompetitive inhibitors** cannot bind to the enzyme alone and can only bind to the enzyme–substrate complex. Once an uncompetitive inhibitor binds to the complex, the complex becomes inactive. An **irreversible inhibitor** binds to the enzyme and permanently inactivates it. It usually does so by forming a covalent bond with the enzyme.

Properties of Solutions

Properties of Water

Water is a polar compound formed from one oxygen atom bonded to two hydrogen atoms. It has many unique properties, such as its ability to exist as a solid, liquid, and gas on Earth's surface. It is the only common substance that can exist in all three forms in this environment. Water is also self-ionizing, breaking itself up into H^+ and OH^- ions, which also makes it both an acid and a base.

The polarity of water and its attraction to other polar molecules is an important characteristic. **Cohesion** is the attraction of water molecules to each other. The slight negative charge of the oxygen atom in one molecule attracts the slightly positively charged hydrogen atoms of other water molecules. This attraction allows water to have surface tension. Insects, such as water striders, can actually walk across the surface of a pool of water. **Adhesion** is the attraction of water molecules to other molecules with which it can form hydrogen bonds. This attraction creates capillary action. **Capillary action** is the ability of water to "climb" up the side of a tube as it is attracted to the material of the tube. Its polarity also helps it break up ions in salts and bond to other polar substances, such as acids and alcohols. It is used to dissolve many substances and is often described as a **universal solvent** because of its polar attraction to other atoms and ions.

While most compounds become denser when they become solid, ice, the solid form of water, is actually less dense than the liquid form of water. The hydrogen bonds that form between the water molecules become ice crystals and more stable. The bonds remain spaced apart as the liquid freezes, creating a low density in the solid structure. Ice, therefore, floats to the top of a glass of liquid water.

Water is also a great moderator of temperature because of its high specific heat and high heat of vaporization. **Specific heat** is the amount of energy that is needed to change the temperature of one gram of a substance 1°C. When a substance has a high specific heat, it requires a lot of energy to change the temperature. Since water molecules form a lot of hydrogen bonds, it takes a lot of energy to break up the bonds. Since there are a lot of hydrogen bonds to absorb and release heat as they break and form, respectively, temperature changes are minimized. Similarly, **heat of vaporization** is the amount of energy needed to change 1 gram of liquid into gas. It takes a lot of energy to break the hydrogen bonds between liquid water molecules and turn them into water vapor.

Solvents and Solutes

In chemistry, a solution is made when a solute is added to a solvent. Many times, small amounts of a reactant are required for a reaction, but they must be a larger mass to react with the other reactant. Therefore, solutions are made to disperse a small amount of a chemical over a larger space to allow reactions to occur. A solute is the reactive material that will be dissolved into something else to make a solution. A solute may exist in any state of matter: a solid, liquid or gas. The quantity of a solute used in creating a solution is less than the quantity of the solvent used. A solvent is the material that the solute dissolves into. The solvent separates the molecules of the solute to disperse them evenly. Solvents are almost always a liquid because liquids allow solutes to dissolve without losing large amounts of material to the atmosphere. A common example of a solvent/solute relationship seen in everyday life is when salt (the solute) is added to water (the solvent) to make a saltwater solution. Solutes must always be soluble in a solvent for a solution to be made.

Concentration and Dilution of Solutions

The concentration of a solution is the number of dissolved solute particles in a specific amount of solvent. When more solute is added to a set volume of solvent, the concentration of the solution will increase. Within chemistry, concentration is typically measured in molarity (moles per liter), molality (moles per kilogram), or parts per million (milligrams per liter). If a solution contains a higher concentration of solute than desired, it can be diluted by adding more of the solvent to the solution. Common lab chemical solutions, such as hydrochloric acid and sodium hydroxide, are often stored as higher concentration solutions to save space in lab storage. When they are used, a portion of the high concentration solution can be taken and diluted to the desired concentration for a specific reaction. When making dilutions, it is very important to know the exact amount of solvent that is needed to create the desired concentration. To aid in making this calculation, the following equation is needed: $M_1V_1 = M_2V_2$, where M_1 is initial molarity, V_1 is initial volume, M_2 is final molarity, and V_2 is final volume. Rearranging to solve for the unknown quantity yields the needed volume.

Osmosis and Diffusion

Osmosis is when particles of a solvent pass through a semipermeable membrane. The direction that solvent particles move is always from higher concentration to lower concentration to reach a balance. Osmosis is an important aspect of biology. A common example of osmosis within a human body is found in the kidneys. Within the nephrons of the kidneys, particles pass through its semi permeable membranes to separate wastes from water and other substances that can be further utilized. Diffusion also describes the movement of particles and occurs in the direction of high concentration to low concentration. However, diffusion does not describe particles passing through a semipermeable membrane but describes the dispersion of particles through available space. An example of diffusion would be a smell spreading throughout a room until it appears to be balanced throughout the air of the room.

Solute Transport Across Membranes

Solutes can be transported across a plasma membrane through diffusion, which moves the solute from an area of higher concentration to an area of lower concentration, producing energy and increasing the entropy of the system. This is a thermodynamically spontaneous process.

Osmosis

Osmosis is a type of diffusion that involves the movement of water molecules, specifically, across a semipermeable membrane. Water molecules move from an area of high water concentration, or low solvent concentration, to an area of low water concentration, or high solvent concentration, until the concentrations are equal in the two areas.

Colligative Properties, Osmotic Pressure

The pressure created by the movement of the water molecules is called the **osmotic pressure**. The more water that moves across the membrane, the higher the osmotic pressure. The colligative properties of a solution include the vapor pressure lowering, the boiling point increasing, the freezing point lowering, and osmotic pressure. They are determined only by the concentration of the solute molecules.

Passive Transport

Passive transport across a membrane happens without any energy and is caused by a concentration gradient. The solute moves from high concentration areas to lower concentration areas.

Active Transport

Active transport requires an energy input and involves the use of a membrane protein. Some solutes require a transporter protein to carry them across the membrane. The relationship between the solute and the transporter protein is similar to an enzyme–substrate relationship except that the solute molecule is not modified by the transporter. When the transporter's binding sites are saturated, the rate of transport is maximized.

Sodium/Potassium Pump

Sodium/potassium pumps hydrolyze ATP and use the energy released to pump sodium out of the cell while pumping potassium into the cell, both against their concentration gradients.

Acids And Bases

pH

In chemistry, **pH** stands for the potential of hydrogen. It is a numeric scale ranging from 0 to 14 that determines the acidity and basicity of an aqueous solution. Solutions with a pH of greater than 7 are considered basic, those with a pH of less than 7 are considered acidic, and solutions with a pH equal to 7 are considered neutral. Pure water is considered neutral with a pH equal to 7. It is important to remember that the pH of solutions can change at different temperatures. While the pH of pure water is 7 at 25°C, at 0°C it is 7.47, and at 100°C it is 6.14. pH is calculated as the negative of the base 10 logarithm of the activity of the hydrogen ions in the solution and can be written as:

$$\mathrm{pH} = -\log 10(\mathrm{a_H}+) = \log 10(\frac{1}{\mathrm{a_H}+})$$

One of the simplest ways to measure the pH of a solution is by performing a litmus test. Litmus paper has a mixture of dyes on it that react with the solution and display whether the solution is acidic or basic depending on the resulting color. Red litmus paper turns blue when it reacts with a base. Blue litmus paper turns red when it reacts with an acid. Litmus tests are generally crude measurements of pH and not very precise. A more precise way to measure the pH of a solution is to use a pH meter. These specialized meters act like voltmeters and measure the electrical potential of a solution. Acids have a lot of positively charged hydrogen ions in solutions that have greater potential than bases to produce an electric current. The voltage measurement is then compared with a solution of known pH and voltage. The difference in voltage is translated into the difference in pH.

Acids and Bases

Acids and bases are two types of substances with differing properties. In general, when acids are dissolved in water, they can conduct electricity, have a sour taste, react with metals to free hydrogen ions, and react with bases to neutralize their properties. Bases, in general, when dissolved in water, conduct electricity, have a slippery feel, and react with acids to neutralize their properties.

The Brønsted-Lowry acid–base theory is a commonly accepted theory about how acid–base reactions work. **Acids** are defined as substances that dissociate in aqueous solutions and form hydrogen ions. **Bases** are defined as substances that dissociate in aqueous solutions and form hydroxide ($\mathrm{OH^-}$) ions. The basic idea behind the theory is that when an acid and base react with each other, a proton is exchanged, and the acid forms its conjugate base, while the base forms its conjugate acid. The acid is the proton donor, and the base is the proton acceptor. The reaction is written as $\mathrm{HA + B \leftrightarrow A^- + HB^+}$, where HA is the acid, B is the base, $\mathrm{A^-}$ is the conjugated base, and $\mathrm{HB^+}$ is the conjugated acid. Since the reverse of the reaction is also possible, the reactants and products are always in equilibrium. The equilibrium of acids and bases in a chemical reaction can be determined by finding the acid dissociation constant, K_a, and the base dissociation constant, K_b. These dissociation constants determine how strong the acid or base is in the aqueous solution. Strong acids and bases dissociate quickly to create the products of the reaction.

In other cases, acids and bases can react to form a neutral salt. This happens when the hydrogen ion from the acid combines with the hydroxide ion of the base to form water, and the remaining ions combine to form a neutral salt. For example, when hydrochloric acid and sodium hydroxide combine, they form salt and water, which can be written as:

$$HCl + NaOH \rightarrow NaCl + H_2O$$

Buffers

Definition and Concepts (Common Buffer Systems)

Buffers can resist changes in pH when small amounts of acids or bases are added to a solution. Sodium citrate ($NaC_6H_7O_7$) is basic salt that acts as a buffer:

$$C_6H_7O_7^-(aq) + H_2O(l) \rightleftarrows C_6H_7O_7H(aq) + OH^-(aq)$$

Addition of an acid, H^+, pushes the equilibrium to the right. Addition of OH^- pushes the equilibrium to the left.

Scientific Reasoning

Scientific Measurement Using Laboratory Tools

Measuring Force

A Newton meter or force meter is a standardized instrument for measuring the force exerted by different elements in the universe that cause movement when they act upon objects by pulling, pushing, rotating, deforming, or accelerating them, such as gravity, friction, or tension. Force is measured in units called Newtons (N), named after Sir Isaac Newton, who defined the laws of motion, including forces. One common example of a force meter is a bathroom scale. When someone steps on the scale, the force exerted on the platform is measured in the form of units of weight. Force meters contain springs, rubber bands, or other elastic materials that stretch in proportion to force applied. A Newton meter displays 50-Newton increments, with four 10-Newton marks in between. Thus, if a Newton meter's needle rests on the third mark between 100 and 150, this indicates 130N.

Measuring Temperature

As those familiar with word roots can determine, thermometers measure heat or temperature (*thermo-* is from Greek for heat and *meter* from Greek for measure). Some thermometers measure outdoor or indoor air temperature, and others measure body temperature in humans or animals. Meat thermometers measure temperature in the center of cooked meat to ensure sufficient cooking to kill bacteria. Refrigerator and freezer thermometers measure internal temperatures to ensure sufficient coldness. Although digital thermometers eliminate the task of reading a thermometer scale by displaying a specific numerical reading, many thermometers still use visual scales. In these, increments are typically two-tenths of a degree. However, basal thermometers, which are more sensitive and accurate, and are frequently used to track female ovulation cycles for measuring and planning fertility, display increments of one-tenth of a degree. Whole degrees are marked by their numbers; tenths of degrees are the smallest marks in between.

Measuring Length

Rulers, yardsticks, tape measures, and other standardized instruments are for measuring short distances. Standard rulers and similar measures show distances in increments of feet, inches, and halves, quarters, eights, and sixteenths of an inch. Tape measures have markings indicating one yard or three feet, six feet, and other common multiple-feet measurements. Each inch on a ruler is marked by number from 1 to 12 (or 1 to 36 on a yardstick). Half-inches are the longest of the non-numbered line marks, then quarter-inches, then eighth-inches, then sixteenth-inches. Some American-made rulers also include metric measurements.

Basic Scientific Measurements

Throughout most of the world, including the entire scientific community, the metric system of units is the standard system used. The metric system is used to measure weight in grams, length in meters, volume in liters, and time in seconds. The metric system relies on the decimal system and can use numbers in powers of 10. Additionally, more relevant measurement units for specific amounts or sizes are described with prefixes. For example, 1,000 meters can be described with the prefix kilo- to simplify measurements. This allows something large, such as the length of a country, to be described by a lower number in kilometers than a very large number in meters. Inversely, prefixes exist for very small measurements. For example, if one were to measure the volume of a drop of water, the prefix milli- can be utilized in milliliters to describe $\frac{1}{1,000}$ of a liter.

Value	Prefix	Symbol
1,000,000	Mega-	M
1,000	Kilo-	k
100	Hecta-	h
10	Deca-	da
1		
0.1	Deci-	d
0.01	Centi-	c
0.001	Milli-	m
0.000001	Micro-	µ (Latin mu)

When one makes a model of any variety to provide information beyond text (whether it's an image, diagram, graph, photograph, or illustration), the inclusion of units of measurement are absolutely necessary to portray information. For example, if one were to make an illustration of the displacement between two objects, if they were to write the distance between the without units it would be impossible to know whether the distance is measured in meters, centimeters, kilometers, or any other unit of measurement for distance. Units of measurement are required to provide context to values in any model.

When choosing a device to measure a specific volume, mass, or length of an object, it is important to first determine the correct unit of measurement. For instance, if one were to measure the length of a finger, they should determine that centimeters should be used, as a finger would be too small to measure with kilometers or meters, and too large to measure with micrometers or millimeters. Once a proper unit of measurement is determined, one can determine which measurement tool would be most accurate based on its range of accuracy. For example, one shouldn't use a 100-milliliter pipet to measure a liquid that is clearly several liters.

The scale of a specific unit is important in accurately determining a measurement. For example, when people refer to the length of a football field, it is described in yards. If one were to describe a football field as 0.057 miles, length of the field would not be understood as well as saying it is 100 yards.

Using the Vernier Scale

French mathematician and inventor Pierre Vernier originated the Vernier measurement principle and corresponding scale in 1631. When measuring small increments using other instruments, it can be impossible to determine precisely small fractions within already small divisions. Vernier's invention solved this problem with simple elegance. For example, dividing millimeters in the metric system or 16ths of an inch in the English system into 10ths or smaller portions is impractical, inaccurate, and unreadable without using magnifiers. A metric Vernier caliper features a main scale and a Vernier scale, i.e. a parallel, sliding scale with ten or eleven marks, spaced equally within themselves but differently from the main scale spacing. English Vernier calipers often have $\frac{1}{16}$" main scale divisions and 8 divisions on the Vernier scale, so they can measure lengths as small as $\frac{1}{28}$". To read a Vernier caliper, close its jaws on the object being measured, note the main scale number, rounding down to the next smaller marking, and see which Vernier scale mark aligns with it to obtain the additional fraction.

Using a Micrometer Caliper

A micrometer caliper is similar to a Vernier caliper in that both have a main scale plus a movable scale for measuring fractions of small numbers. Like many medical instruments, micrometer calipers are typically metrical, measuring in millimeters. The main scale markings are in $\frac{1}{2}$ millimeters. A uniform, precise screw moves the micrometer caliper's jaw. It has a rotating thimble on its handle, marked in 50 equal divisions. Rotating the thimble once moves the screw $\frac{1}{2}$ millimeter along the main scale, enabling the user to read measurements as small as one-hundredth of a millimeter. Most micrometers display $\frac{1}{2}$ mm markings on the thimble on the opposite side from the main scale markings on the micrometer sleeve, making it easier to read. Users require some practice, e.g., rounding up $\frac{1}{2}$ mm if a reading is in the top half of a millimeter; only tightening the caliper jaws using the slip clutch to close them snugly without bending them; and making a zero-correction using a special wrench so fully closing the jaws yields a zero reading if it did not already.

Critiquing a Scientific Explanation Using Logic and Evidence

According to the scientific method, one must either observe something as it is happening or as a constant state, or prove it through experimenting, to say it is a fact. Scientific experiments are found reliable when they can be replicated and produce comparable results regardless of who is conducting them or making the observations. However, historically many beliefs have been considered facts at the time, only to be disproven later when objective evidence became accessible. For instance, in ancient times many people believed the Earth was flat based on limited visual evidence. Ancient Greek philosophers Pythagoras in the 6th century BCE and Aristotle in the 4th century BCE believed the earth was spherical. This was eventually borne out by observational evidence. Aristotle estimated the Earth's circumference; Eratosthenes measured it c. 240 BCE; in the 2nd century CE, Ptolemy had mapped the globe and developed the latitude, longitude, and climes system.

While many phenomena have been established by science as facts, technically many others are actually theories, though many people mistakenly consider them facts. As one example, gravity per se is a fact; however, the scientific explanation of how gravity functions is a theory. Though a theory is not the same as a fact, this does not presume theories are merely speculative ideas. A scientific theory must be tested thoroughly and then applied to established facts, hypotheses, and observations. Moreover, for a theory to be accepted or even considered scientifically sound, it must relate and explain a broad scope of observations which would not be related without the theory. People sometimes state opinions as if they were facts to persuade others. For example, advertising might claim a product is the best without concrete supporting evidence. To evaluate information, one must consider both its source and any supporting evidence to ascertain its veracity.

Identifying the Empirical Basis of Scientific Explanations

When viewing any sort of data portrayed in any sort of model or text, it is important to look closely into the data and determine what is trying to be proven. Additionally, it is important to pay attention to the implications of what the data means. This process is referred to as deriving a logical conclusion. Utilizing logic to form a conclusion about information is simply evaluating information and what the information means. Additionally, when deciding the meaning of information, it is important to identify additional variables that could possibly change the information.

The primary purpose of most scientific studies is to determine the cause and effect of something. Cause is described as the reason why something occurs, while effect can be described as a detailed explanation of what happened as a result of something occurring. An example of this could be rainfall causes water to saturate soil, and its effect could be the hydration of plants. To determine cause and effect, one must note that a cause happens before the effect, a cause always produces an effect, and non-contributing factors must be identified and ignored when determining the relationship between a cause and effect.

In scientific experiments, scientists attempt to find an explanation for a process or object through collecting evidence through observation and experimentation. Evidence is recorded as data and analyzed to determine if it is valuable in supporting or disproving a hypothesis. Gathering evidence is a necessary portion of the scientific method, as it is utilized to support a scientific claim. Evidence can be portrayed as either quantitative or qualitative. Quantitative evidence is able to be measured numerically while qualitative cannot be measured and is something that either exists or does not.

Relationships Among Events, Objects, and Procedures

When we determine relationships among events, objects, and procedures, we are better able to understand the world around us and make predictions based on that understanding. With regards to relationships among events and procedures, we will look at cause and effect. For relationships among objects, we will take a look at Newton's Laws.

Cause

The **cause** of a particular event is the thing that brings it about. A causal relationship may be partly or wholly responsible for its effect, but sometimes it's difficult to tell whether one event is the sole cause of another event. For example, lung cancer can be caused by smoking cigarettes. However, sometimes lung cancer develops even though someone does not smoke, and that tells us that there may be other factors involved in lung cancer besides smoking. It's also easy to make mistakes when considering causation. One

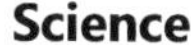

common mistake is mistaking correlation for causation. For example, say that in the year 2008 a volcano erupted in California, and in that same year, the number of infant deaths increased by ten percent. If we automatically assume, without looking at the data, that the erupting volcano *caused* the infant deaths, then we are mistaking correlation for causation. The two events might have happened at the same time, but that does not necessarily mean that one event caused the other. Relationships between events are never absolute; there are a myriad of factors that can be traced back to their foundations, so we must be thorough with our evidence in proving causation.

Effect

An **effect** is the result of something that occurs. For example, the Nelsons have a family dog. Every time the dog hears thunder, the dog whines. In this scenario, the thunder is the cause, and the dog's whining is the effect. Sometimes a cause will produce multiple effects. Let's say we are doing an experiment to see what the effects of exercise are in a group of people who are not usually active. After about four weeks, the group experienced weight loss, rise in confidence, and higher energy. We start out with a cause: exercising more. From that cause, we have three known effects that occurred within the group: weight loss, rise in confidence, and higher energy. Cause and effect are important terms to understand when conducting scientific experiments.

Magnitude

It is important to understand the quantity, scale, and proportions of events, objects, and processes within science. To make scientific observations about real phenomena, it is necessary to understand the dimensions and magnitude of what is being observed. Before any kind of analysis can be made from an observation, one must understand the scale of what is being observed.

Causal relationships between two different events are the relationship between a cause and its direct and indirect effects. Causal relationships can be determined in a relatively simple manner. When determining if two variables are related, if the magnitude of one variable changes and results in the change of a different variable, they have a causal relationship. When determining a causal relationship, it is important to identify if any relationship between two events is the result of a cause or if it is simply a correlation.

To fully understand a scientific process, it is important to be able to identify the logical order of events within the process. This can be done by first identifying the beginning and the end of a series and determining what steps are necessary for beginning to become the end. Given a conclusion, hypothesis, and experiment, a hypothesis is necessary for an experiment to happen, and an experiment is required for a conclusion to be made.

Design of a Scientific Investigation

Scientific investigation is seeking an answer to a specific question using the scientific method. The scientific method is a procedure that is based on an observation. For example, if someone observes something strange, and they want to understand the process, they might ask how that process works. If we were to use the scientific method to understand the process, we would formulate a hypothesis. A hypothesis explains what you expect to happen from the experiment. Then, an experiment is conducted, data from the experiment is analyzed, and a conclusion is reached. Below are steps of the scientific method in a practical situation:

- Observation: One day, a student observes that every time he eats a big lunch, he falls asleep in the next period.
- Experimental Question: The question the student asks is, what is the relationship between eating large meals and energy levels?
- Formulate a Hypothesis: The student hypothesizes that eating a big meal will lead to lower energy due to the body using its energy to digest the food.
- Conduct an Experiment (Materials and Procedure): The student has his whole class eat two meals for lunch for a week, then he measures their energy levels in the next period. The next week, the student has them eat a small lunch, and then measures their energy levels in the next period.
- Analyze Data: The data in the student's experiment showed that in the first week, sixty percent of the students felt sleepy in the next period class and that in the second week, only twenty percent of the students felt sleepy in the next period class.
- Conclusion: The student concluded that the data supported his hypothesis: student energy levels decrease after the consumption of a large meal.

An important component of scientific research after the experiment is conducted is called peer review. This is when the article written about the experiment is sent to other scientists to "review." The reviewers offer feedback so that the editors can decide whether or not to publish the findings in a scholarly or scientific journal.

Dependent Variables, Independent Variables, and Experimental Controls

Within scientific studies, variables can be identified as either dependent or independent. An independent variable is what is adjusted to cause a change in another variable. A dependent variable is what changes as a result of the independent variable. The dependent variable depends on what happens with an independent variable. An experimental control is utilized in experiments to limit unrelated variables and determine if a possible independent variable is actually the cause for the change in the dependent variable. For example, if one were given a medication to decrease their heart rate, the medication is the independent variable and heart rate is the dependent variable because it is changed by the medicine. An experimental control in this situation would be a separate test subject given a faux medication without the active ingredient to determine if the medication is the actual cause for the effect.

Experimental Basis to Support or Reject the Conclusion

The results of any experiment can be used to support or disprove a hypothesis. If results align with a hypothesis, it cannot be said that the hypothesis is proved. However, it can be said that the evidence fails to disprove the hypothesis, which supports its possible validity. If clear evidence contradicts with the hypothesis, it can be concluded that it disproves the hypothesis. From there a hypothesis must either be modified to account for the contradictory evidence or abandoned altogether, as it is incorrect. It is important to note that a large enough sample size, or repetition of an experiment, is necessary to disprove a hypothesis because the contradictory evidence may be due to some form of experimental error.

Science Practice Quiz

1. Which statement is true regarding atomic structure?
   a. Protons orbit around a nucleus.
   b. Neutrons have a positive charge.
   c. Electrons are in the nucleus.
   d. Protons have a positive charge.

2. How is the secondary structure of a protein defined?
   a. By the order of the amino acids
   b. By the coils and folds that form as a result of the hydrogen bonds between the amino acids
   c. By the shape that it takes on due to side-chain interactions
   d. By multiple polypeptide chains binding together

3. In what type of chemical reaction is heat absorbed from the surrounding environment?
   a. Exothermic
   b. Endothermic
   c. Rusting
   d. Freezing

4. What is the largest organ in the human body?
   a. Brain
   b. Large intestine
   c. Skin
   d. Heart

5. Which statement regarding meiosis is correct?
   a. Meiosis produces four diploid cells.
   b. Meiosis contains two cellular divisions separated by interphase II.
   c. Meiosis produces cells with two sets of chromosomes.
   d. Crossing over occurs in the prophase of meiosis I.

See answers on next page.

Answer Explanations

1. D: Protons have a positive charge. An atom is structured with a nucleus in the center that contains neutral neutrons and positive protons. Surrounding the nucleus are orbiting electrons that are negatively charged. Choice *D* is the only correct answer.

2. B: The secondary structure of a protein is defined by the folds and coils formed due to hydrogen bond interactions between the amino acids, Choice *B*. Choice *A* describes the primary structure of a protein, which is defined by the order of the amino acids. Tertiary structure is defined by the geometric shape that forms due to side-chain interactions, which is described by Choice *C*. Choice *D* describes the quaternary structure of a protein, which is defined by multiple polypeptide chains binding together.

3. B: Endothermic reactions consume heat from the surrounding environment to complete the chemical reaction and create a product. For example, holding an ice cube in one's hand and allowing it to melt into water (as a result of body heat) is an example of an endothermic reaction. Exothermic reactions release heat into the environment (i.e., igniting wood to create a fire). Rusting occurs when iron reacts to oxygen over a period of time. Freezing is a type of exothermic reaction.

4. C: The skin is the largest organ of the body, covering every external surface of the body and protecting the body's deeper tissues. The brain performs many complex functions, the large intestine is part of the gastrointestinal system, and the heart keeps blood pumping throughout the body, but none of these is largest organ in the body.

5. D: Choice *A* is incorrect because meiosis produces haploid cells. Choice *B* is incorrect because there is no interphase II (otherwise gametes would be diploid instead of haploid). Choice *C* is incorrect because the resulting cells only have one set of chromosomes. Choice *D* is the only correct answer because each chromosome set goes through a process called crossing over, which jumbles up the genes on each chromatid, during meiosis I.

English and Language Usage

Conventions of Standard English

Conventions of Standard English Spelling

Frequently Misspelled Words

One source of spelling errors is not knowing whether to drop the final letter *e* from a word when its form is changed; some words retain the final *e* when another syllable is added while others lose it. For example, *true* becomes *truly; argue* becomes *arguing; come* becomes *coming; write* becomes *writing;* and *judge* becomes *judging.* In these examples, the final *e* is dropped before adding the ending. But *severe* becomes *severely; complete* becomes *completely; sincere* becomes *sincerely; argue* becomes *argued;* and *care* becomes *careful.* In these instances, the final *e* is retained before adding the ending. Note that some words, like argue in these examples, drops the final e when the –ing ending is added to indicate the participial form, but the regular past tense form keeps the e and adds a –d to make it argued.

Other commonly misspelled English words are those containing the vowel combinations ei and ie. Many people confuse these two. Some examples of words with the ei combination include:

> *ceiling, conceive, leisure, receive, weird, their, either, foreign, sovereign, neither, neighbors, seize, forfeit, counterfeit, height, weight, vein, protein,* and *freight*

Words with *ie* include *piece, believe, chief, field, friend, grief, relief, mischief, siege, niece, priest, fierce, pierce, achieve, retrieve, hygiene, science,* and *diesel.* A rule that also functions as a mnemonic device is "I before E except after C, or when sounded like A as in 'neighbor' or 'weigh'." However, it is obvious from the list above that many exceptions exist.

People often misspell certain words by confusing whether they have the vowel a, e, or i. For example, in the following correctly spelled words, the vowel in boldface is the one people typically get wrong by substituting one of the others for it:

> cem**e**tery, quant**i**ties, ben**e**fit, priv**i**lege, unpleas**a**nt, sep**a**rate, independ**e**nt, excell**e**nt, cat**e**gories, indispens**a**ble, and irrelev**a**nt

Some words with final syllables that sound the same when spoken but are spelled differently include *unpleasant, independent, excellent,* and *irrelevant.* Another source of misspelling is whether or not to double consonants when adding suffixes. For example, double the last consonant before –ed and –ing endings in controlled, beginning, forgetting, admitted, occurred, referred, and hopping; but do not double before the suffix in *shining, poured, sweating, loving, hating, smiling,* and *hoping.*

One final example of common misspellings involves either the failure to include silent letters or the converse of adding extraneous letters. If a letter is not pronounced in speech, it is easy to leave it out in writing. For example, some people omit the silent *u* in *__gu__arantee,* overlook the first *r* in *su__r__prise,* leave out the *z* in *reali__ze__,* fail to double the *m* in *recom__m__end,* leave out the middle *i* from *asp__i__rin,* and exclude the *p* from *tem__p__erature.* The converse error, adding extra letters, is common in words like *until* by adding a second *l* at the end; or by inserting a superfluous syllabic *a* or *e* in the middle of *athletic,* reproducing a common mispronunciation.

Irregular Plurals

While many words in English can become plural by adding –s or –es to the end, there are some words that have irregular plural forms. One type includes words that are spelled the same whether they are singular or plural, such as deer, fish, salmon, trout, sheep, moose, offspring, species, aircraft, etc. The spelling rule for making these words plural is simple: they do not change. Other irregular English plurals change form based on vowel shifts, linguistic mutations, or grammatical and spelling conventions from their languages of origin, like Latin or German. Some examples include *child* and *children; die* and *dice; foot* and *feet; goose* and *geese; louse* and *lice; man* and *men; mouse* and *mice; ox* and *oxen; person* and *people; tooth* and *teeth;* and *woman* and *women.*

Homophones

Homophones are words that have different meanings and spellings, but sound the same. These can be confusing for English Language Learners (ELLs) and beginning students, but even native English-speaking adults can find them problematic unless informed by context. Whereas listeners must rely entirely on context to differentiate spoken homophone meanings, readers with good spelling knowledge have a distinct advantage since homophones are spelled differently. For instance, *their* means belonging to them; *there* indicates location; and *they're* is a contraction of *they are*; despite different meanings, they all sound the same. *Lacks* can be a plural noun or a present-tense, third-person singular verb; either way it refers to absence—*deficiencies* as a plural noun, and *is deficient in* as a verb. But *lax* is an adjective that means loose, slack, relaxed, uncontrolled, or negligent. These two spellings, derivations, and meanings are completely different. With speech, listeners cannot know spelling and must use context; but with print, readers with spelling knowledge can differentiate them with or without context.

Homonyms, Homophones, and Homographs

Homophones are words that sound the same in speech, but have different spellings and meanings. For example, *to, too,* and *two* all sound alike, but have three different spellings and meanings. Homophones with different spellings are also called heterographs. Homographs are words that are spelled identically, but have different meanings. If they also have different pronunciations, they are heteronyms. For instance, *tear* pronounced one way means a drop of liquid formed by the eye; pronounced another way, it means to rip. Homophones that are also homographs are homonyms. For example, *bark* can mean the outside of a tree or a dog's vocalization; both meanings have the same spelling. *Stalk* can mean a plant stem or to pursue and/or harass somebody; these are spelled and pronounced the same. *Rose* can mean a flower or the past tense of *rise.* Many non-linguists confuse things by using "homonym" to mean sets of words that are homophones but not homographs, and also those that are homographs but not homophones.

The word *row* can mean to use oars to propel a boat; a linear arrangement of objects or print; or an argument. It is pronounced the same with the first two meanings, but differently with the third. Because it is spelled identically regardless, all three meanings are homographs. However, the two meanings pronounced the same are homophones, whereas the one with the different pronunciation is a heteronym. By contrast, the word *read* means to peruse language, whereas the word *reed* refers to a marsh plant. Because these are pronounced the same way, they are homophones; because they are spelled differently, they are heterographs. Homonyms are both homophones and homographs—pronounced and spelled identically, but with different meanings. One distinction between homonyms is of those with separate, unrelated etymologies, called "true" homonyms, e.g. *skate* meaning a fish or *skate* meaning to glide over ice/water. Those with common origins are called polysemes or polysemous homonyms, e.g. the *mouth* of an animal/human or of a river.

Contractions

Contractions are formed by joining two words together, omitting one or more letters from one of the component words, and replacing the omitted letter(s) with an apostrophe. An obvious yet often forgotten rule for spelling contractions is to place the apostrophe where the letters were omitted. For example, didn't is a contraction of did not; therefore, the apostrophe replaces the "o" that is omitted from the "not." Another common error is confusing contractions with possessives because both include apostrophes, e.g. spelling the possessive *its* as "it's," which is a contraction of "it is"; spelling the possessive *their* as "they're," a contraction of "they are"; spelling the possessive *whose* as "who's," a contraction of "who is"; or spelling the possessive *your* as "you're," a contraction of "you are."

Conventions of Standard English Punctuation

Commas

Commas separate words or phrases in a series of three or more. The Oxford comma is the last comma in a series. Many people omit this last comma, but many times it causes confusion. Here is an example:

> I love my sisters, the Queen of England and Madonna.

This example without the comma implies that the "Queen of England and Madonna" are the speaker's sisters. However, if the speaker was trying to say that they love their sisters, the Queen of England, as well as Madonna, there should be a comma after "Queen of England" to signify this.

Commas also separate two coordinate adjectives ("big, heavy dog") but not cumulative ones, which should be arranged in a particular order for them to make sense ("beautiful ancient ruins").

A comma ends the first of two independent clauses connected by conjunctions. Here is an example:

> I ate a bowl of tomato soup, and I was hungry very shortly after.

Here are some brief rules for commas:

- Commas follow introductory words like *however, furthermore, well, why,* and *actually*, among others.
- Commas go between city and state: Houston, Texas.
- If using a comma between a surname and Jr. or Sr. or a degree like M.D., also follow the whole name with a comma: "Martin Luther King, Jr., wrote that."
- A comma follows a dependent phrase or clause beginning a sentence: "Although she was very small, . . ."
- Nonessential modifying words/phrases/clauses are enclosed by commas: "Wendy, who is Peter's sister, closed the window."
- Commas introduce or interrupt direct quotations: "She said, 'I hate him.' 'Why,' I asked, 'do you hate him?'"

Quotation Marks

Quotation marks are typically used when someone is quoting a direct word or phrase someone else writes or says. Additionally, quotation marks should be used for the titles of poems, short stories, songs, articles, chapters, and other shorter works. When quotations include punctuation, periods and commas should *always* be placed inside of the quotation marks.

When a quotation contains another quotation inside of it, the outer quotation should be enclosed in double quotation marks and the inner quotation should be enclosed in single quotation marks. For example: "Timmy was begging, 'Don't go! Don't leave!'" When using both double and single quotation marks, writers will find that many word-processing programs may automatically insert enough space between the single and double quotation marks to be visible for clearer reading. But if this is not the case, the writer should write/type them with enough space between to keep them from looking like three single quotation marks. Additionally, non-standard usages, terms used in an unusual fashion, and technical terms are often clarified by quotation marks. Here are some examples:

> My "friend," Dr. Sims, has been micromanaging me again.
>
> This way of extracting oil has been dubbed "fracking."

Correct Sentence Structures

Sentence Types

Four Types of Sentence Structure

When deconstructing sentences grammatically, there are four types of sentence structures: simple, compound, complex, and compound-complex.

Simple sentences contain a subject and a verb, and may contain additional phrases, indirect objects, or direct objects behind the sentence or verb. A simple sentence contains one independent clause only. Simple sentences can be as simple as saying, "Joanie laughed," or they can contain a compound subject, such as "Joanie and Marisa laughed." Simple sentences can also contain prepositional phrases and compound verbs, such as "Joanie and Marisa laughed at the movie and ate chocolate covered pretzels." Here we have a compound subject "Joanie and Marisa" and a compound verb "laughed and ate," yet we still have a single independent clause.

Compound sentences join two independent clauses together by a conjunction (for, and, nor, but, or, so). An example would be, "Zoe wanted to go to the zoo, but it was closed on Sundays." Here, we have two sentences that can stand on their own: "Zoe wanted to go to the zoo." "It was closed on Sundays." We could turn the simple sentence above into a compound sentence: "Joanie and Marisa laughed at the movie, and they ate chocolate covered pretzels." Adding "they" to the second part of the sentence creates two independent clauses. In a compound sentence, the FANBOYS are always separated by commas.

Complex sentences contain one independent clause and one dependent clause. As stated above, dependent clauses are similar to independent clauses; however, they lack some kind of unit that allows them to be a complete sentence. Dependent clauses may look like the following:

- When it started to rain
- After she bought the furniture for her new house
- Until the neighborhood street has a bike lane

In order to make these into complex sentences, we must attach independent clauses to each, either before or after the dependent clause. Here are some examples of a complex sentence:

- When it started to rain, Mazey shut all the windows except the one in the living room.
- Carolynn was ecstatic after she bought the furniture for her new house.
- Until the neighborhood street has a bike lane, I would prefer to take Charlie to the park.

Notice that the independent clauses are able to stand on their own, while the dependent clauses depend on the independent clause to complete the thought.

Compound-complex sentences occur when a complex sentence is merged with a compound sentence. These sentences have two independent clauses and one dependent clause. In the following examples, the dependent clauses are in bold, while the independent clauses are in italics:

- **When it started to rain**, *Mazey shut all the windows except the one in the living room*, and *her brother got out a board game to play.*
- *Carolynn was ecstatic* **after she bought the furniture for her new house**, but *she returned two pieces a day later.*
- **Until the neighborhood street has a bike lane**, *I would prefer to take Charlie to the park to ride his new bike*, for *this road is too busy to ride on.*

For fluent composition, writers must use a variety of sentence types and structures, and also ensure that they smoothly flow together when they are read. One way writers can increase fluency is by varying the beginnings of sentences. Writers do this by starting most of their sentences with different words and phrases rather than monotonously repeating the same ones across multiple sentences. Another way writers can increase fluency is by varying the lengths of sentences. Since run-on sentences are incorrect, writers make sentences longer by also converting them from simple to compound, complex, and compound-complex sentences. The coordination and subordination involved in these also give the text more variation and interest, hence more fluency. Here are a few more ways writers can increase fluency:

- Varying the transitional language and conjunctions used makes sentences more fluent.
- Writing sentences with a variety of rhythms by using prepositional phrases.
- Varying sentence structure adds fluency.

Sentence Fluency

For fluent composition, writers must use a variety of sentence types and structures, and also ensure that they smoothly flow together when they are read. To accomplish this, they must first be able to identify fluent writing when they read it. This includes being able to distinguish among simple, compound, complex, and compound-complex sentences in text; to observe variations among sentence types, lengths, and beginnings; and to notice figurative language and understand how it augments sentence length and imparts musicality. Once students/writers recognize superior fluency, they should revise their own writing to be more readable and fluent. They must be able to apply acquired skills to revisions before being able to apply them to new drafts.

One strategy for revising writing to increase its sentence fluency is flipping sentences. This involves rearranging the word order in a sentence without deleting, changing, or adding any words. For example, the student or other writer who has written the sentence, "We went bicycling on Saturday" can revise it to, "On Saturday, we went bicycling." Another technique is using appositives. An appositive is a phrase or word that renames or identifies another adjacent word or phrase. Writers can revise for sentence fluency by inserting main phrases/words from one shorter sentence into another shorter sentence, combining them into one longer sentence, e.g. from "My cat Peanut is a gray and brown tabby. He loves hunting rats." to "My cat Peanut, a gray and brown tabby, loves hunting rats." Revisions can also connect shorter sentences by using conjunctions and commas and removing repeated words: "Scott likes eggs. Scott is allergic to eggs" becomes "Scott likes eggs, but he is allergic to them."

One technique for revising writing to increase sentence fluency is "padding" short, simple sentences by adding phrases that provide more details specifying why, how, when, and/or where something took place. For example, a writer might have these two simple sentences: "I went to the market. I purchased a cake." To revise these, the writer can add the following informative dependent and independent clauses and prepositional phrases, respectively: "Before my mother woke up, I sneaked out of the house and went to the supermarket. As a birthday surprise, I purchased a cake for her." When revising sentences to make them longer, writers must also punctuate them correctly to change them from simple sentences to compound, complex, or compound-complex sentences.

One way writers can increase fluency is by varying the beginnings of sentences. Writers do this by starting most of their sentences with different words and phrases rather than monotonously repeating the same ones across multiple sentences. Another way writers can increase fluency is by varying the lengths of sentences. Since run-on sentences are incorrect, writers make sentences longer by also converting them from simple to compound, complex, and compound-complex sentences. The coordination and subordination involved in these also give the text more variation and interest, hence more fluency.

Here are a few more ways writers can increase fluency:

- Varying the transitional language and conjunctions used makes sentences more fluent.
- Writing sentences with a variety of rhythms by using prepositional phrases.
- Varying sentence structure adds fluency.

Clauses

A **clause** is the smallest grammatical unit containing a subject and predicate. Two kinds of clauses are the independent clause and the dependent clause.

The **independent clause** can stand by itself as a complete sentence. It must contain a subject and a predicate at minimum, but it must not begin with a subordinating conjunction. The following two sentences are considered independent clauses:

> She swam.
>
> He ran to the edge of the sea and stuck his toe in.

Both of these are considered independent clauses because they express a complete thought. A **dependent clause** begins with a subordinating conjunction and is not considered a complete sentence, because it needs an independent clause to complete it. Let's add subordinating conjunctions to the sentences above and make dependent clauses:

> *Because* she swam.
>
> *Although* he ran to the edge of the sea and stuck his toe in.

These two sentences have become dependent on another idea due to the addition of subordinating conjunctions. Let's make these sentences complete by adding an independent clause:

> Lilo was very healthy because she swam.
>
> Although he ran to the edge of the sea and stuck his toe in, it was too cold to jump in.

Now these sentences consist of an independent clause and a dependent clause, which creates a complete sentence.

Parts of Speech

Nouns

A **noun** identifies a person, animal, place, idea, or thing. The etymology of the word *noun* comes from the Latin *nomen*, which means "name." The two types of nouns are *common* or *proper* nouns. There are also collective nouns, abstract nouns, and concrete nouns.

The term **common noun** refers to nouns that are in a more general category of nouns, and to which **proper nouns** belong. For example, a common noun would be the word *teacher* or *professor*, while *Mrs. Smith* or *Professor Jones* would be considered proper nouns. Proper nouns will usually always be capitalized, so it's easier to tell common nouns from proper nouns. In the sentence below, the common nouns are in **bold**, and the proper nouns are in *italics.*

> *Keegan* wanted to go to a **university**, but she didn't want to go to just any **university**. *Duke University* was a **place** she always set her **eye** on, ever since she was a little **girl**. That was the **place** for her.

Notice how the common nouns like girl, place, and university, become proper nouns once they are specified and capitalized, like Duke University and Keegan.

Abstract nouns are nouns that designate a general concept or idea that is intangible. Below is a list of abstract nouns, expressing emotion, feeling, states, concepts, and events:

- Love
- Hate
- Bravery
- Compassion
- Integrity
- Beauty
- Justice
- Truth
- Thought
- Progress
- Friendship
- Relaxation
- Death

Concrete nouns are things people are capable of experiencing through the five senses. These are opposite of abstract nouns in that you can see, touch, hear, smell, or taste them. Here are some examples of concrete nouns:

- Table
- Student
- Teacher
- Pen
- University
- Storm

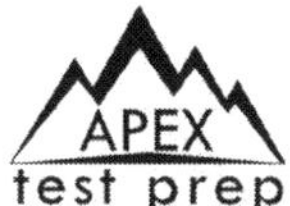

- Fruit
- Cat
- Mountain
- Park
- Gorilla
- Businessman
- Dentist

Collective nouns describe a group of individuals, animals, or things, and in American English, are paired with singular verbs, such as *The family is moving* or *The blue team wins the championship.* A list of collective nouns are as follows:

- Jury
- Team
- Family
- Audience
- Herd
- Band
- Swarm
- Army
- Colony
- Flock
- Group

Pronouns

There are three pronoun cases: subjective case, objective case, and possessive case. Pronouns as subjects are pronouns that replace the subject of the sentence, such as *I, you, he, she, it, we, they* and *who.* Pronouns as objects replace the object of the sentence, such as *me, you, him, her, it, us, them,* and *whom.* Pronouns that show possession are *mine, yours, hers, its, ours, theirs,* and *whose.* The following are examples of different pronoun cases:

- Subject pronoun: *She* ate the cake for her birthday. *I* saw the movie.
- Object pronoun: You gave *me* the card last weekend. She gave the picture to *him.*
- Possessive pronoun: That bracelet you found yesterday is *mine. His* name was Casey.

Verbs

A verb is a word or phrase that expresses action, feeling, or state of being. Verbs explain what their subject is *doing.* Three different types of verbs used in a sentence are action verbs, linking verbs, and helping verbs.

Action verbs show a physical or mental action. Some examples of action verbs are *play, type, jump, write, examine, study, invent, develop,* and *taste.* The following example uses an action verb:

> Kat *imagines* that she is a mermaid in the ocean.

The verb *imagines* explains what Kat is doing: she is imagining being a mermaid.

Linking verbs connect the subject to the predicate without expressing an action. The following sentence shows an example of a linking verb:

The mango *tastes* sweet.

The verb *tastes* is a linking verb. The mango doesn't *do* the tasting, but the word *taste* links the mango to its predicate, sweet. Most linking verbs can also be used as action verbs, such as *smell, taste, look, seem, grow,* and *sound*. Saying something *is* something else is also an example of a linking verb. For example, if we were to say, "Peaches is a dog," the verb *is* would be a linking verb in this sentence, since it links the subject to its predicate.

Helping verbs are verbs that help the main verb in a sentence. Examples of helping verbs are *be, am, is, was, have, has, do, did, can, could, may, might, should,* and *must,* among others. The following are examples of helping verbs:

Jessica *is* planning a trip to Hawaii.

Brenda *does* not like camping.

Xavier *should* go to the dance tonight.

Notice that after each of these helping verbs is the main verb of the sentence: *planning, like,* and *go*. Helping verbs usually show an aspect of time.

Adjectives

Adjectives are descriptive words that modify nouns or pronouns. They may occur before or after the nouns or pronouns they modify in sentences. For example, in "This is a big house," *big* is an adjective modifying or describing the noun *house*. In "This house is big," the adjective is at the end of the sentence rather than preceding the noun it modifies.

A rule of punctuation that applies to adjectives is to separate a series of adjectives with commas. For example, "Their home was a large, rambling, old, white, two-story house." A comma should never separate the last adjective from the noun, though.

Possessive forms indicate possession, i.e. that something belongs to or is owned by someone or something. As such, the most common parts of speech to be used in possessive form are adjectives, nouns, and pronouns. The rule for correctly spelling/punctuating possessive nouns and proper nouns is with -*'s*, like "the woman's briefcase" or "Frank's hat." With possessive adjectives, however, apostrophes are not used: these include *my, your, his, her, its, our,* and *their*, like "my book," "your friend," "his car," "her house," "its contents," "our family," or "their property." Possessive pronouns include *mine, yours, his, hers, its, ours,* and *theirs*. These also have no apostrophes. The difference is that possessive adjectives take direct objects, whereas possessive pronouns replace them. For example, instead of using two possessive adjectives in a row, as in "I forgot my book, so Blanca let me use her book," which reads monotonously, replacing the second one with a possessive pronoun reads better: "I forgot my book, so Blanca let me use hers."

Adverbs

Whereas adjectives modify and describe nouns or pronouns, adverbs modify and describe adjectives, verbs, or other adverbs. Adverbs can be thought of as answers to questions in that they describe when, where, how, how often, how much, or to what extent.

Many (but not all) adjectives can be converted to adverbs by adding *–ly*. For example, in "She is a quick learner," *quick* is an adjective modifying *learner*. In "She learns quickly," *quickly* is an adverb modifying *learns*. One exception is *fast*. *Fast* is an adjective in "She is a fast learner." However, *–ly* is never added to the word *fast*; it retains the same form as an adverb in "She learns fast."

Prepositions

Words that show relationships between a noun or a pronoun and some other word are considered **prepositions**. Prepositional phrases begin with prepositions and end with nouns or pronouns, or the object of the preposition. For example: The cattle ran *over the hill*. The prepositional phrase is *over the hill*. The word *over* is the preposition, and the phrase *the hill* is the object of the preposition. Here is a list of prepositional words, although it is not comprehensive:

about	above	across	after	against	along
among	around	at	because of	before	behind
below	beneath	beside	between	despite	down
during	in front of	inside	into	near	off
onto	outside	over	past	through	toward
under	underneath	until	up	within	without

Prepositional phrases are useful in describing spatial temporal relations, like the following phrases including a box:

- Aside the box
- Under the box
- Inside the box
- Underneath the box
- Through the box
- Onto the box
- Over the box

Conjunctions

A **conjunction** is a word used to connect clauses or sentences, or the words used to connect words to other words. The words *and*, *but*, *or*, *nor*, *yet*, and *so* are conjunctions. Two types of conjunctions are called *coordinating conjunctions* and *subordinating conjunctions*.

Coordinating conjunctions join two or more items of equal linguistic importance. These conjunctions are *for*, *and*, *nor*, *but*, *or*, *yet*, and *so*, also called *FANBOYS* as an acronym. Here are each of the words used as coordinating conjunctions:

- They did not attend the reception that evening, for they were all sick from lunch.
- She bought a chocolate, vanilla, and raspberry cupcake.
- We do not eat pork, nor do we eat fish.
- I would bring her to the circus, but she is afraid of the clowns.

- She went to the grocery store, or she went to the park.
- Grandpa wanted to buy a house, yet he did not want to pay for it.
- We had a baby, so we bought a house on a lake.

Subordinating conjunctions are conjunctions that join an independent clause with a dependent clause. Sometimes they introduce adverbial clauses as well. The most common subordinating conjunctions in the English language are the following: *after, although, as, as far as, as if, as long as, as soon as, as though, because, before, even if, even though, every time, if, in order that, since, so, so that, than, though, unless, until, when, whenever, where, whereas, wherever,* and *while.* Here's an example of the subordinating conjunction, *unless.*

> Theresa was going to go kayaking on the river unless it started to rain.

Notice that "unless it started to rain" is the dependent clause, because it cannot stand by itself as a sentence. "Theresa was going to go kayaking on the river" is the independent clause. Here, *unless* acts as the subordinating conjunction, because the two clauses are not syntactically equal.

Interjections

An interjection is a word or expression that signifies a spontaneous emotion or reaction. Sometimes interjections stand by themselves and precede exclamation marks, such as "Wow!" "Yay!" or "Ouch!" Sometimes, interjections are used as hesitations markers, such as "er" or "um," and sometimes they are used as responses, such as "okay," "uh-huh," and "m-hmm."

Sentence Parts

Subject

The subject of the sentence is the word or phrase that is being discussed or described relating to the verb. The *complete subject* is a subject with all its parts, like the following: *The stormy weather* ruined their vacation. A *simple subject* is the subject with all the modifiers removed. In the previous example the simple subject would be *weather.* There are various forms of subjects listed below:

- Noun (phrase) or pronoun: *The tiny bird* sang all morning long.
- A to-infinitive clause: *To hike the Appalachian Trail* was her lifelong goal.
- A gerund: *Running* was his new favorite sport.
- A that-clause: *That she was old* did not stop her from living her life.
- A direct quotation: *"Here comes the sun"* is a quote from a Beatle's song.
- A free relative clause: *Whatever she said* is none of my business.
- Implied subject: *(You)* Shut the door!

Predicate

In a sentence, the **predicate** contains a verb and all the words that modify the verb. It is the part of the sentence that tells what is done by or done to the subject of the sentence. There are two examples of a predicate below:

> The lady from the bakery *cooked the meal for us tonight.*

> Destiny *wanted to be a surfer.*

A sentence, as a whole, is made up of a subject and a predicate. The predicate will always contain a verb, then any direct objects, indirect objects, or other phrases that come behind that verb.

Complements: Predicate Adjective and Predicate Nominative

Predicate adjectives follow a linking verb and modify the subject of that linking verb. For example, when saying "the lamp is blue," *blue* is the predicate adjective of the sentence because it is an adjective that follows the linking verb *is* and modifies the subject *lamp*. In saying "thunderstorms have become scary," the word *scary* is the predicate adjective, because it modifies the subject *thunderstorms* and follows the linking verbs *have become*.

A **predicate nominative** is the part of a sentence that completes the linking verb and renames the subject. For example, in the sentence "My favorite show is Game of Thrones," *Game of Thrones* is the predicate nominative because it renames "my favorite show" after the linking verb. Another example is saying "The places I have lived have been California, Texas, and Maine." *California, Texas,* and *Maine* are the predicate nominatives because they rename "the places I have lived" after the linking verb *have been*.

Direct Object

A **direct object** is directly affected by the action of the verb. In a sentence, the direct object usually answers the question *what* or *whom* and is the recipient of a transitive verb. The following is a simple sentence:

> Ms. Shephard fed the cat.

Ms. Shephard is the subject, *fed* is the verb, and *the cat* is the direct object. *The cat* answers what Ms. Shephard fed. What did she feed? She fed the cat. Therefore, *the cat* is the direct object of the sentence.

Indirect Object

An **indirect object** refers to someone or something that is affected by the action of a transitive verb, such as the recipient of that action. To identify an indirect object, it is helpful to ask, "to whom was the thing received?" The following sentences contain examples of an indirect object in italics:

- She gave *him* the cat. (To whom did she give the cat? To him.)
- Mom gave *Bobby* a bath. (To whom did she give a bath? To Bobby.)
- Elijah made *Penelope* a cake. (To whom did he give a cake? To Penelope.)

In the above examples, recall the direct objects of each: *the cat, a bath*, and *a cake* are all direct objects of the sentence, while *him, Bobby,* and *Penelope* are the indirect objects of the sentence.

Knowledge of Language

Using Grammar to Enhance Clarity in Writing

Transitional Words and Phrases

In writing, some sentences naturally lead to others, whereas in other cases, a new sentence expresses a new idea. Transitional phrases connect sentences and the ideas they convey, which makes the writing coherent. Transitional language also guides the reader from one thought to the next. For example, when pointing out an objection to the previous idea, starting a sentence with "However," "But," or "On the other hand" is transitional. When adding another idea or detail, writers use "Also," "In addition," "Furthermore," "Further," "Moreover," "Not only," etc. Readers have difficulty perceiving connections between ideas without such transitional wording.

Effective Language

When writing, it's important to use effective language in order to communicate what is desired and to do so well. Communicating using effective language might look like:

- being intentional with word choice
- keeping to the point, not going off on tangents
- using positive, uplifting language rather than passive aggressive or indirect language
- using an appropriate tone for the intended setting or audience
- using specific language so as to avoid any unintended effects

Revising Sentences

Revising and editing are extremely important parts of the writing process. All sentences and paragraphs should be revised for clarity, flow, mood, and tone. The piece of writing should maintain the same mood and tone throughout. Sentence structure, word choices, and punctuation should be consistent with the tone being used. Remove or change any language that does align, and make sure that the clearest possible language and vocabulary are used to convey the meaning of the message. Writing also needs to be edited for grammatical issues that may inhibit comprehension. The following are a few common mistakes that should be checked for and fixed during this process.

Incomplete Sentences

Four types of incomplete sentences are sentence fragments, run-on sentences, subject-verb and/or pronoun-antecedent disagreement, and non-parallel structure.

Sentence fragments are caused by absent subjects, absent verbs, or dangling/uncompleted dependent clauses. Every sentence must have a subject and a verb to be complete. An example of a fragment is "Raining all night long," because there is no subject present. "It was raining all night long" is one correction. Another example of a sentence fragment is the second part in "Many scientists think in unusual ways. Einstein, for instance." The second phrase is a fragment because it has no verb. One correction is "Many scientists, like Einstein, think in unusual ways." Finally, look for "cliffhanger" words like *if, when, because,* or *although* that introduce dependent clauses, which cannot stand alone without an independent clause. For example, to correct the sentence fragment "If you get home early," add an independent clause: "If you get home early, we can go dancing."

Run-On Sentences

A run-on sentence combines two or more complete sentences without punctuating them correctly or separating them. For example, a run-on sentence caused by a lack of punctuation is the following:

> There is a malfunction in the computer system however there is nobody available right now who knows how to troubleshoot it.

One correction is, "There is a malfunction in the computer system; however, there is nobody available right now who knows how to troubleshoot it." Another is, "There is a malfunction in the computer system. However, there is nobody available right now who knows how to troubleshoot it."

An example of a comma splice of two sentences is the following:

Jim decided not to take the bus, he walked home.

Replacing the comma with a period or a semicolon corrects this. Commas that try and separate two independent clauses without a contraction are considered comma splices.

Tense Usage and Consistency

The tense of a sentence indicates when the action in the sentence is completed. The three most common tenses are past, present, and future.

- Past tense: indicates that something happened at a previous time; typically uses helping verbs such as *did, have, had, used to, was, were,* and the suffix *-ed.*
- Present: indicates something happening currently; typically uses helping verbs such as *am, is,* and *are.*
- Future: indicates that something is going to happen at a later time; typically uses helping verbs such as *will* or *shall.*

Writers should be vigilant to maintain consistency in tense as much as possible. Flipping back and forth between different tenses is confusing and almost never necessary.

Subject-Verb Agreement

Lack of subject-verb agreement is a very common grammatical error. One of the most common instances is when people use a series of nouns as a compound subject with a singular instead of a plural verb. Here is an example:

> Identifying the best books, locating the sellers with the lowest prices, and paying for them *is* difficult

instead of saying "*are* difficult." Additionally, when a sentence subject is compound, the verb is plural:

> He and his cousins *were* at the reunion.

However, if the conjunction connecting two or more singular nouns or pronouns is "or" or "nor," the verb must be singular to agree:

> That pen or another one like it is in the desk drawer.

If a compound subject includes both a singular noun and a plural one, and they are connected by "or" or "nor," the verb must agree with the subject closest to the verb: "Sally or her sisters go jogging daily"; but "Her sisters or Sally goes jogging daily."

Simply put, singular subjects require singular verbs and plural subjects require plural verbs. A common source of agreement errors is not identifying the sentence subject correctly. For example, people often write sentences incorrectly like, "The group of students *were* complaining about the test." The subject is not the plural "students" but the singular "group." Therefore, the correct sentence should read, "The group of students *was* complaining about the test." The converse also applies, for example, in this incorrect sentence: "The facts in that complicated court case *is* open to question." The subject of the sentence is not the singular "case" but the plural "facts." Hence the sentence would correctly be written: "The facts in that complicated court case *are* open to question." New writers should not be misled by the distance between the subject and verb, especially when another noun with a different number intervenes as in these examples. The verb must agree with the subject, not the noun closest to it.

Pronoun-Antecedent Agreement

Pronouns within a sentence must refer specifically to one noun, known as the **antecedent.** Sometimes, if there are multiple nouns within a sentence, it may be difficult to ascertain which noun belongs to the pronoun. It's important that the pronouns always clearly reference the nouns in the sentence so as not to confuse the reader. Here's an example of an unclear pronoun reference:

> After Catherine cut Libby's hair, David bought her some lunch.

The pronoun in the examples above is *her*. The pronoun could either be referring to *Catherine* or *Libby*. Here are some ways to write the above sentence with a clear pronoun reference:

> After Catherine cut Libby's hair, David bought Libby some lunch.

> David bought Libby some lunch after Catherine cut Libby's hair.

But many times the pronoun will clearly refer to its antecedent, like the following:

> After David cut Catherine's hair, he bought her some lunch.

Parallel Sentence Structures

Parallel structure in a sentence matches the forms of sentence components. Any sentence containing more than one description or phrase should keep them consistent in wording and form. Readers can easily follow writers' ideas when they are written in parallel structure, making it an important element of correct sentence construction. For example, this sentence lacks parallelism: "Our coach is a skilled manager, a clever strategist, and works hard." The first two phrases are parallel, but the third is not. Correction: "Our coach is a skilled manager, a clever strategist, and a hard worker." Now all three phrases match in form. Here is another example:

> Fred intercepted the ball, escaped tacklers, and a touchdown was scored.

This is also non-parallel. Here is the sentence corrected:

> Fred intercepted the ball, escaped tacklers, and scored a touchdown.

Meeting the Needs of an Audience

Formal and Informal Language

Formal language is less personal than informal language. It is more "buttoned-up" and business-like, adhering to proper grammatical rules. It is used in professional or academic contexts, to convey respect or authority. For example, one would use formal language to write an informative or argumentative essay for school or to address a superior. Formal language avoids contractions, slang, colloquialisms, and first-person pronouns. Formal language uses sentences that are usually more complex and often in passive voice. Punctuation can differ as well. For example, exclamation points (!) are used to show strong emotion or can be used as an interjection but should be used sparingly in formal writing situations.

Informal language is often used when communicating with family members, friends, peers, and those known more personally. It is more casual, spontaneous, and forgiving in its conformity to grammatical rules and conventions. Informal language is used for personal emails and correspondence between coworkers or other familial relationships. The tone is more relaxed. In informal writing, slang, contractions, clichés, and the first- and second-person are often used.

The style and tone of writing should remain consistent throughout a text. Make sure to read through any final draft and revise as necessary to ensure consistency and appropriate formality. When revising, keep the intended audience in mind as well. When writing for diverse audiences, be intentional to use culturally sensitive language as well.

Developing a Well-Organized Paragraph

A **paragraph** is a series of connected and related sentences addressing one topic. Writing good paragraphs benefits writers by helping them to stay on target while drafting and revising their work. It benefits readers by helping them to follow the writing more easily. Regardless of how brilliant their ideas may be, writers who do not present them in organized ways will fail to engage readers—and fail to accomplish their writing goals. A fundamental rule for paragraphing is to confine each paragraph to a single idea. When writers find themselves transitioning to a new idea, they should start a new paragraph. However, a paragraph can include several pieces of evidence supporting its single idea; and it can include several points if they are all related to the overall paragraph topic. When writers find each point becoming lengthy, they may choose instead to devote a separate paragraph to every point and elaborate upon each more fully.

An effective paragraph should have these elements:

- Unity: One major discussion point or focus should occupy the whole paragraph from beginning to end.
- Coherence: For readers to understand a paragraph, it must be coherent. Two components of coherence are logical and verbal bridges. In logical bridges, the writer may write consecutive sentences with parallel structure or carry an idea over across sentences. In verbal bridges, writers may repeat key words across sentences.
- A topic sentence: The paragraph should have a sentence that generally identifies the paragraph's thesis or main idea.
- Sufficient development: To develop a paragraph, writers can use the following techniques after stating their topic sentence:
    - Define terms
    - Cite data
    - Use illustrations, anecdotes, and examples
    - Evaluate causes and effects
    - Analyze the topic
    - Explain the topic using chronological order

A **topic sentence** identifies the main idea of the paragraph. Some are explicit, some implicit. The topic sentence can appear anywhere in the paragraph. However, many experts advise beginning writers to place each paragraph topic sentence at or near the beginning of its paragraph to ensure that their readers understand what the topic of each paragraph is. Even without having written an explicit topic sentence, the writer should still be able to summarize readily what subject matter each paragraph addresses. The writer must then fully develop the topic that is introduced or identified in the topic sentence through supporting details and evidence. Depending on what the writer's purpose is, they may use different methods for developing each paragraph. The concluding sentence of a paragraph should wrap up the topic and fluidly transition into the next.

Two main steps in the process of organizing paragraphs and essays should both be completed after determining the writing's main point, while the writer is planning or outlining the work. The initial step is to give an order to the topics addressed in each paragraph. Writers must have logical reasons for putting one paragraph first, another second, etc. The second step is to sequence the sentences in each paragraph. As with the first step, writers must have logical reasons for the order of sentences. Sometimes the work's main point obviously indicates a specific order.

Topic Sentences

To be effective, a topic sentence should be concise so that readers get its point without losing the meaning among too many words. As an example, in *Only Yesterday: An Informal History of the 1920s* (1931), author Frederick Lewis Allen's topic sentence introduces his paragraph describing the 1929 stock market crash: "The Bull Market was dead." This example illustrates the criteria of conciseness and brevity. It is also a strong sentence, expressed clearly and unambiguously. The topic sentence also introduces the paragraph, alerting the reader's attention to the main idea of the paragraph and the subject matter that follows the topic sentence.

Experts often recommend opening a paragraph with the topic sentences to enable the reader to realize the main point of the paragraph immediately. Application letters for jobs and university admissions also benefit from opening with topic sentences. However, positioning the topic sentence at the end of a paragraph is more logical when the paragraph identifies a number of specific details that accumulate evidence and then culminates with a generalization. While paragraphs with extremely obvious main ideas need no topic sentences, more often—and particularly for students learning to write—the topic sentence is the most important sentence in the paragraph. It not only communicates the main idea quickly to readers; it also helps writers produce and control information.

Revising Paragraphs

During the revision process, writers should carefully read each paragraph and make sure that only relevant information is included. Any extraneous or irrelevant information should be eliminated or moved to a different paragraph. Additionally, writers should make sure that they have clearly and thoroughly covered and supported each of their main points. If any point is lacking evidence or explanation, the writer should develop it further.

Arranging Information

There are several different ways in which writers can organize their paragraphs. The best type of structure will depend on the content and purpose of writing. The following paragraphs describe a few types of text structures.

Problem-Solution Text Structure

The problem-solution text structure organizes textual information by presenting readers with a problem and then developing its solution throughout the course of the text. The author may present a variety of alternatives as possible solutions, eliminating each as they are found unsuccessful, or gradually leading up to the ultimate solution. For example, in fiction, an author might write a murder mystery novel and have the character(s) solve it through investigating various clues or character alibis until the killer is identified. In nonfiction, an author writing an essay or book on a real-world problem might discuss various alternatives and explain their disadvantages or why they would not work before identifying the best solution. For scientific research, an author reporting and discussing scientific experiment results would explain why various alternatives failed or succeeded.

Comparison-Contrast Text Structure

Comparison identifies similarities between two or more things. **Contrast** identifies differences between two or more things. Authors typically employ both to illustrate relationships between things by highlighting their commonalities and deviations. For example, a writer might compare Windows and Linux as operating systems, and contrast Linux as free and open-source vs. Windows as proprietary. When writing an essay, sometimes it is useful to create an image of the two objects or events you are comparing or contrasting. Venn diagrams are useful because they show the differences as well as the similarities between two things. Once you've seen the similarities and differences on paper, it might be helpful to create an outline of the essay with both comparison and contrast. Every outline will look different because every two or more things will have a different number of comparisons and contrasts. Say you are trying to compare and contrast carrots with sweet potatoes.

Here is an example of a compare/contrast outline using those topics:

- Introduction: Talk about why you are comparing and contrasting carrots and sweet potatoes. Give the thesis statement.
- Body paragraph 1: Sweet potatoes and carrots are both root vegetables (similarity)
- Body paragraph 2: Sweet potatoes and carrots are both orange (similarity)
- Body paragraph 3: Sweet potatoes and carrots have different nutritional components (difference)
- Conclusion: Restate the purpose of your comparison/contrast essay.

Of course, if there is only one similarity between your topics and two differences, you will want to rearrange your outline. Always tailor your essay to what works best with your topic.

Descriptive Text Structure

Description can be both a type of text structure and a type of text. Some texts are descriptive throughout entire books. For example, a book may describe the geography of a certain country, state, or region, or tell readers all about dolphins by describing many of their characteristics. Many other texts are not descriptive throughout but use descriptive passages within the overall text. The following are a few examples of descriptive text:

- When the author describes a character in a novel
- When the author sets the scene for an event by describing the setting
- When a biographer describes the personality and behaviors of a real-life individual
- When a historian describes the details of a particular battle within a book about a specific war
- When a travel writer describes the climate, people, foods, and/or customs of a certain place

A hallmark of description is using sensory details, painting a vivid picture so readers can imagine it almost as if they were experiencing it personally.

Cause and Effect Text Structure

When using cause and effect to extrapolate meaning from text, readers must determine the cause when the author only communicates effects. For example, if a description of a child eating an ice cream cone includes details like beads of sweat forming on the child's face and the ice cream dripping down her hand faster than she can lick it off, the reader can infer or conclude it must be hot outside. A useful technique for making such decisions is wording them in "*If...then*" form, e.g. "*If* the child is perspiring and the ice cream melting, *then* it may be a hot day." Cause and effect text structures explain why certain events or actions resulted in particular outcomes. For example, an author might describe America's historical large flocks of dodo birds, the fact that gunshots did not startle/frighten dodos, and that because dodos did not flee, settlers killed whole flocks in one hunting session, explaining how the dodo was hunted into extinction.

Narrative Structure
The structure presented in literary fiction, called **narrative structure**, is the foundation on which the text moves. The narrative structure comes from the plot and setting. The plot is the sequence of events in the narrative that move the text forward through cause and effect. The setting is the place or time period in which the story takes place. Narrative structure has two main categories: linear and nonlinear.

Using Language & Vocabulary to Express Ideas in Writing

Elements of the Writing Process

Skilled writers undergo a series of steps that comprise the writing process. The purpose of adhering to a structured approach to writing is to develop clear, meaningful, coherent work.

The stages are pre-writing or planning, organizing, drafting/writing, revising, and editing. Not every writer will necessarily follow all five stages for every project, but will judiciously employ the crucial components of the stages for most formal or important work. For example, a brief informal response to a short reading passage may not necessitate the need for significant organization after idea generation, but larger assignments and essays will likely mandate use of the full process.

Pre-Writing/Planning

Brainstorming
Before beginning the essay, read the prompt thoroughly and make sure you understand its expectations. Brainstorm as many ideas as you can think of that relate to the topic and list them or put them into a graphic organizer. Refer to this list as you organize your essay outline.

Freewriting
Like brainstorming, freewriting is another prewriting activity to help the writer generate ideas. This method involves setting a timer for two or three minutes and writing down all ideas that come to mind about the topic using complete sentences. Once time is up, writers should review the sentences to see what observations have been made and how these ideas might translate into a more unified direction for the topic. Even if sentences lack sense as a whole, freewriting is an excellent way to get ideas onto the page in the very beginning stages of writing. Using complete sentences can make this a bit more challenging than brainstorming, but overall it is a worthwhile exercise, as it may force the writer to come up with more complete thoughts about the topic.

Take the ideas you generated during pre-writing and organize them in the form of an outline.

Organizing

Although sometimes it is difficult to get going on the brainstorming or prewriting phase, once ideas start flowing, writers often find that they have amassed too many thoughts that will not make for a cohesive and unified essay. During the organization stage, writers should examine the generated ideas, hone in on the important ones central to their main idea, and arrange the points in a logical and effective manner. Writers may also determine that some of the ideas generated in the planning process need further elaboration, potentially necessitating the need for research to gather information to fill the gaps.

Once a writer has chosen their thesis and main argument, selected the most applicable details and evidence, and eliminated the "clutter," it is time to strategically organize the ideas. This is often accomplished with an outline.

Outlining

Outlines are organizational tools that arrange a piece of writing's main ideas and the evidence that supports them. After pre-writing, organize your ideas by topic, select the best ones, and put them into the outline. Be sure to include an introduction, main points, and a conclusion. Typically, it is a good idea to have three main points with at least two pieces of supporting evidence each. The following displays the format of an outline:

I. Introduction
   1. Background
   2. Thesis statement

II. Body
   1. Point A
      a. Supporting evidence
      b. Supporting evidence
   2. Point B
      a. Supporting evidence
      b. Supporting evidence
   3. Point C
      a. Supporting evidence
      b. Supporting evidence

III. Conclusion
   1. Restatement of main points.
   2. Memorable ending.

Drafting/Writing

Now it comes time to actually write the essay. In this stage, writers should follow the outline they developed in the brainstorming process and try to incorporate the useful sentences penned in the freewriting exercise. The main goal of this phase is to put all the thoughts together in cohesive sentences and paragraphs.

It is helpful for writers to remember that their work here does not have to be perfect. This process is often referred to as **drafting** because writers are just creating a rough draft of their work. Because of this, writers should avoid getting bogged down on the small details.

Referencing Sources

Anytime a writer quotes or paraphrases another text, they will need to include a citation. A **citation** is a short description of the work that a quote or information came from. The style manual your teacher wants you to follow will dictate exactly how to format that citation. For example, this is how one would cite a book according to the APA manual of style:

- *Format*: Last name, First initial, Middle initial. (Year Published) *Book Title*. City, State: Publisher.
- *Example*: Sampson, M. R. (1989). *Diaries from an Alien Invasion. Springfield, IL*: Campbell Press.

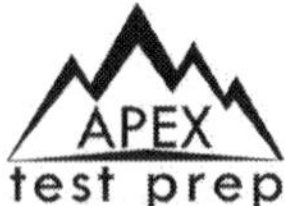

Revising

Revising involves going back over a piece of writing and improving it. Try to read your essay from the perspective of a potential reader to ensure that it makes sense. When revising, check that the main points are clearly stated, logically organized, and directly supported by the sub-points. Remove unnecessary details that do not contribute to the argument.

The main goal of the revision phase is to improve the essay's flow, cohesiveness, readability, and focus. For example, an essay will make a less persuasive argument if the various pieces of evidence are scattered and presented illogically or clouded with unnecessary thought. Therefore, writers should consider their essay's structure and organization, ensuring that there are smooth transitions between sentences and paragraphs. There should be a discernable introduction and conclusion as well, as these crucial components of an essay provide readers with a blueprint to follow.

Additionally, if the writer includes copious details that do little to enhance the argument, they may actually distract readers from focusing on the main ideas and detract from the strength of their work. The ultimate goal is to retain the purpose or focus of the essay and provide a reader-friendly experience. Because of this, writers often need to delete parts of their essay to improve its flow and focus. Removing sentences, entire paragraphs, or large chunks of writing can be one of the toughest parts of the writing process because it is difficult to part with work one has done. However, ultimately, these types of cuts can significantly improve one's essay.

Lastly, writers should consider their voice and word choice. The voice should be consistent throughout and maintain a balance between an authoritative and warm style, to both inform and engage readers. One way to alter voice is through word choice. Writers should consider changing weak verbs to stronger ones and selecting more precise language in areas where wording is vague. In some cases, it is useful to modify sentence beginnings or to combine or split up sentences to provide a more varied sentence structure.

Editing

Rather than focusing on content (as is the aim in the revising stage), the editing phase is all about the mechanics of the essay: the syntax, word choice, and grammar. This can be considered the proofreading stage. Successful editing is what sets apart a messy essay from a polished document.

Look for the following types of errors when checking over your work:

- Spelling
- Tense usage
- Punctuation and capitalization
- Unclear, confusing, or incomplete sentences
- Subject/verb and noun/pronoun agreement

One of the most effective ways of identifying grammatical errors, awkward phrases, or unclear sentences is to read the essay out loud. Listening to one's own work can help move the writer from simply the author to the reader.

During the editing phase, it's also important to ensure the essay follows the correct formatting and citation rules as dictated by the assignment.

Recursive Writing Process

While the writing process may have specific steps, the good news is that the process is recursive, meaning the steps need not be completed in a particular order. Many writers find that they complete steps at the same time such as drafting and revising, where the writing and rearranging of ideas occur simultaneously or in very close order. Similarly, a writer may find that a particular section of a draft needs more development, and will go back to the prewriting stage to generate new ideas. The steps can be repeated at any time, and the more these steps of the recursive writing process are employed, the better the final product will be.

Practice Makes Prepared Writers

Like any other useful skill, writing only improves with practice. While writing may come more easily to some than others, it is still a skill to be honed and improved. Regardless of a person's natural abilities, there is always room for growth in writing. Practicing the basic skills of writing can aid in preparations for the TEAS.

One way to build vocabulary and enhance exposure to the written word is through reading. This can be through reading books, but reading of any materials such as newspapers, magazines, and even social media count towards practice with the written word. This also helps to enhance critical reading and thinking skills, through analysis of the ideas and concepts read. Think of each new reading experience as a chance to sharpen these skills.

Analyzing Word Parts

Readers can learn some etymologies, or origins, of words and their parts, making it easier to break down new words into components and analyze their combined meanings. For example, the root word soph is Greek for "wise" or "knowledge." Knowing this informs the meanings of English words including *sophomore, sophisticated,* and *philosophy.* Those who also know that phil is Greek for "love" will realize that philosophy means "love of knowledge." They can then extend this knowledge of *phil* to understand cognates (related words that come from the same linguistic element(s)), such as *philanthropist* (one who loves people), *bibliophile* (book lover), *philharmonic* (loving harmony), *hydrophilic* (water-loving), and so on. In addition, *phob* derives from the Greek *phobos,* meaning "fear." Words with this root indicate fear of various things *acrophobia* (fear of heights), *arachnophobia* (fear of spiders), *claustrophobia* (fear of enclosed spaces), *ergophobia* (fear of work), and *hydrophobia* (fear of water), among others.

Some English word origins from other languages, like ancient Greek, are found in large numbers and varieties of English words. An advantage of the shared ancestry of these words is that once readers recognize the meanings of some Greek words or word roots, they can determine or at least get an idea of what many different English words mean. As an example, the Greek word *métron* means to measure, a measure, or something used to measure; the English word meter derives from it. Knowing this informs many other English words, including *altimeter, barometer, diameter, hexameter, isometric,* and *metric.* While readers must know the meanings of the other parts of these words to decipher their meaning fully, they already have an idea that they are all related in some way to measures or measuring.

While all English words ultimately derive from a proto-language known as Indo-European, many of them historically came into the developing English vocabulary later, from sources like the ancient Greeks' language, the Latin used throughout Europe and much of the Middle East during the reign of the Roman Empire, and the Anglo-Saxon languages used by England's early tribes. In addition to classic revivals and native foundations, by the Renaissance era other influences included French, German, Italian, and Spanish.

Today we can often discern English word meanings by knowing common roots and affixes, particularly from Greek and Latin.

The following is a list of common prefixes and their meanings:

Prefix	Definition	Examples
a-	Without	atheist, agnostic
ad-	to, toward	advance
ante-	Before	antecedent, antedate
anti-	Opposing	antipathy, antidote
auto-	Self	autonomy, autobiography
bene-	well, good	benefit, benefactor
bi-	Two	bisect, biennial
bio-	Life	biology, biosphere
chron-	Time	chronometer, synchronize
circum-	Around	circumspect, circumference
com-	with, together	commotion, complicate
contra-	against, opposing	contradict, contravene
cred-	belief, trust	credible, credit
de-	From	depart
dem-	People	demographics, democracy
dis-	away, off, down, not	dissent, disappear
equi-	equal, equally	equivalent
ex-	from, out of	extract
for-	away, off, from	forget, forswear
fore-	before, previous	foretell, forefathers
homo-	same, equal	homogenized
hyper-	excessive, over	hypercritical, hypertension
in-	in, into	intrude, invade
inter-	among, between	intercede, interrupt
mal-	bad, poorly, not	malfunction
micr(o)-	Small	microbe, microscope
mis-	bad, poorly, not	misspell, misfire
mono-	one, single	monogamy, monologue
mor-	die, death	mortality, mortuary
neo-	New	neolithic, neoconservative
non-	not	nonentity, nonsense
omni-	all, everywhere	omniscient
over-	above	overbearing
pan-	all, entire	panorama, pandemonium
para-	beside, beyond	parallel, paradox
phil-	love, affection	philosophy, philanthropic
poly-	many	polymorphous, polygamous
pre-	before, previous	prevent, preclude
prim-	first, early	primitive, primary

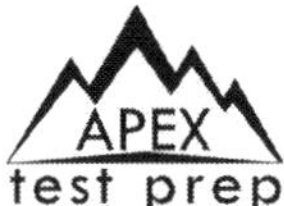

Prefix	Definition	Examples
pro-	forward, in place of	propel, pronoun
re-	back, backward, again	revoke, recur
sub-	under, beneath	subjugate, substitute
super-	above, extra	supersede, supernumerary
trans-	across, beyond, over	transact, transport
ultra-	beyond, excessively	ultramodern, ultrasonic, ultraviolet
un-	not, reverse of	unhappy, unlock
vis-	to see	visage, visible

The following is a list of common suffixes and their meanings:

Suffix	Definition	Examples
-able	likely, able to	capable, tolerable
-ance	act, condition	acceptance, vigilance
-ard	one that does excessively	drunkard, wizard
-ation	action, state	occupation, starvation
-cy	state, condition	accuracy, captaincy
-er	one who does	teacher
-esce	become, grow, continue	convalesce, acquiesce
-esque	in the style of, like	picturesque, grotesque
-ess	feminine	waitress, lioness
-ful	full of, marked by	thankful, zestful
-ible	able, fit	edible, possible, divisible
-ion	action, result, state	union, fusion
-ish	suggesting, like	churlish, childish
-ism	act, manner, doctrine	barbarism, socialism
-ist	doer, believer	monopolist, socialist
-ition	action, result, state,	sedition, expedition
-ity	quality, condition	acidity, civility
-ize	cause to be, treat with	sterilize, mechanize, criticize
-less	lacking, without	hopeless, countless
-like	like, similar	childlike, dreamlike
-ly	like, of the nature of	friendly, positively
-ment	means, result, action	refreshment, disappointment
-ness	quality, state	greatness, tallness
-or	doer, office, action	juror, elevator, honor
-ous	marked by, given to	religious, riotous
-some	apt to, showing	tiresome, lonesome
-th	act, state, quality	warmth, width
-ty	quality, state	enmity, activity

English & Language Usage Practice Quiz

1. Which of these words has an irregular plural that is the same as its singular form?
   a. Louse
   b. Goose
   c. Mouse
   d. Moose

2. Exceptions and variations in rules for capitalization are accurately reflected in which of these?
   a. *Congress* is capitalized and so is *Congressional.*
   b. *Constitution* is capitalized as well as *Constitutional.*
   c. *Caucasian* is capitalized, but *white* referring to race is not.
   d. *African-American* and *Black* as a race are both capitalized.

3. What is the rule for using quotation marks with a quotation inside of a quotation?
   a. Single quotation marks around the outer quotation, double quotation marks around the inner one
   b. Double quotation marks to enclose the outer quotation and also to enclose the inner quotation
   c. Single quotation marks that enclose the outer quotation as well as the inner quotation
   d. Double quotation marks around the outer quotation, single quotation marks around the inner one

4. The underlined portion of the following sentence contains an example of which verb form?
   Sandy <u>will have finished</u> by the end of the second semester.
   a. Present
   b. Past perfect
   c. Future perfect
   d. Present progressive

5. Which of the following sources require a citation when writing? Select all that apply.
   a. Summaries
   b. Paraphrases
   c. Common knowledge
   d. Direct quotations

See answers on next page.

Answer Explanations

1. D: *Moose* is both the singular and plural form of the word. Other words that do not change from singular to plural include *deer, fish,* and *sheep. Louse*, Choice *A*, has an irregular plural, but it is *lice*, not the same as the singular. *Goose*, Choice *B*, has the irregular plural *geese,* also not the same as the singular. *Mouse*, Choice *C*, like *louse,* has the irregular plural *mice*, also different from its singular form.

2. C: While terms like *Caucasian* and *African-American* are capitalized, the words *white*, Choice *C*, and *black*, Choice *D*, when referring to race should NOT be capitalized. While the name *Congress* is capitalized, the adjective *congressional* should NOT be capitalized, Choice *A*. Although the name of the U.S. *Constitution* is capitalized, the related adjective *constitutional* is NOT capitalized, Choice *B*.

3. D: The rule for writing a quotation with another quotation inside it is to use double quotation marks to enclose the outer quotation and use single quotation marks to enclose the inner quotation. Here is an example: "I don't think he will attend, because he said, 'I am extremely busy.'" The correct usage is reversed in Choice *A*. Choices *B* and *C* are incorrect, as this would not distinguish one quotation from the other.

4. C: Future perfect. Choices *A, B*, and *D* are incorrect. Choice *C* is correct because the word *will* in the verb phrase *will have finished* denotes that the action will occur in the future.

5. A, B, and D: Summaries and paraphrases are a condensed version of another person's writing in one's own words. Even though the writer rephrases the original content in their own words, the ideas are not original and therefore require a citation to give credit to the original author. Direct quotations are completely borrowed from someone else and must be attributed to their original author/speaker. Common knowledge is typically considered to be well-known facts that can be found undocumented in five or more scholarly sources. An example of common knowledge is the fact that the boiling point of water is 212° F. Common knowledge does not need to be cited, so Choice *C* is incorrect.

Practice Test

Reading

The next two questions are based on the following passage:

> Rehabilitation, rather than punitive justice, is becoming much more popular in prisons around the world. Prisons in America, especially, where the recidivism rate is 67 percent, would benefit from mimicking prison tactics in Norway, which has a recidivism rate of only 20 percent. In Norway, the idea is that a rehabilitated prisoner is much less likely to offend than one harshly punished. Rehabilitation includes proper treatment for substance abuse, psychotherapy, healthcare and dental care, and education programs.

1. Which of the following best captures the author's purpose?
   a. To show the audience one of the effects of criminal rehabilitation by comparison
   b. To persuade the audience to donate to American prisons for education programs
   c. To convince the audience of the harsh conditions of American prisons
   d. To inform the audience of the incredibly lax system of Norwegian prisons

2. Which of the following describes the word *recidivism* as it is used in the passage?
   a. The lack of violence in the prison system
   b. The opportunity of inmates to receive therapy in prison
   c. The event of a prisoner escaping the compound
   d. The likelihood of a convicted criminal to reoffend

Use the Nutrition Facts label to answer question 3.

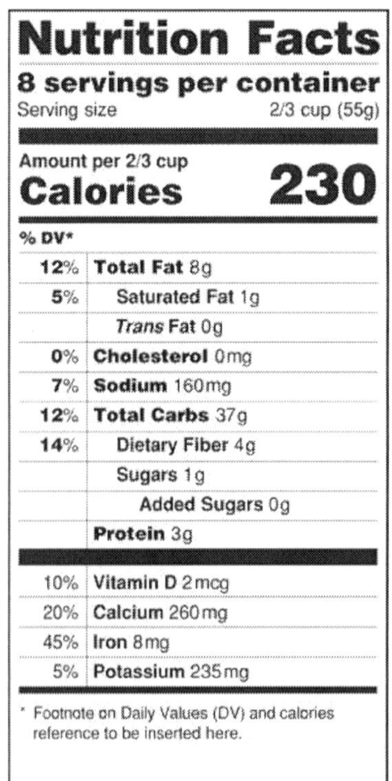

3. A customer who eats two servings of the above food would consume how many carbohydrates? ______

Question 4 is based on the following passage.

Meanwhile the fog and darkness thickened so, that people ran about with flaring links, proffering their services to go before horses in carriages, and conduct them on their way. The ancient tower of a church, whose gruff old bell was always peeping slyly down at Scrooge out of a Gothic window in the wall, became invisible, and struck the hours and quarters in the clouds, with tremulous vibrations afterwards as if its teeth were chattering in its frozen head up there. The cold became intense. In the main street, at the corner of the court, some labourers were repairing the gas-pipes, and had lighted a great fire in a brazier, round which a party of ragged men and boys were gathered: warming their hands and winking their eyes before the blaze in rapture. The water-plug being left in solitude, its overflowings sullenly congealed, and turned to misanthropic ice. The brightness of the shops where holly sprigs and berries crackled in the lamp heat of the windows, made pale faces ruddy as they passed. Poulterers' and grocers' trades became a splendid joke; a glorious pageant, with which it was next to impossible to believe that such dull principles as bargain and sale had anything to do. The Lord Mayor, in the stronghold of the mighty Mansion House, gave orders to his fifty cooks and butlers to keep Christmas as a Lord Mayor's household should; and even the little tailor, whom he had fined five shillings on the previous Monday for being drunk and bloodthirsty in the streets, stirred up to-morrow's pudding in his garret, while his lean wife and the baby sallied out to buy the beef.

Excerpt from *A Christmas Carol* by Charles Dickens

4. Which of the following can NOT be inferred from the passage?
   a. The season of this narrative is in the wintertime.
   b. The majority of the narrative is located in a bustling city street.
   c. This passage takes place during the nighttime.
   d. The Lord Mayor is a wealthy person within the narrative.

Question 5 is based on the following passage.

I trembled excessively; I could not endure to think of, and far less to allude to, the occurrences of the preceding night. I walked with a quick pace, and we soon arrived at my college. I then reflected, and the thought made me shiver, that the creature whom I had left in my apartment might still be there, alive, and walking about. I dreaded to behold this monster; but I feared still more that Henry should see him. Entreating him, therefore, to remain a few minutes at the bottom of the stairs, I darted up towards my own room. My hand was already on the lock of the door before I recollected myself. I then paused; and a cold shivering came over me. I threw the door forcibly open, as children are accustomed to do when they expect a spectre to stand in waiting for them on the other side; but nothing appeared. I stepped fearfully in: the apartment was empty; and my bed-room was also freed from its hideous guest. I could hardly believe that so great a good fortune could have befallen me; but when I became assured that my enemy had indeed fled, I clapped my hands for joy, and ran down to Clerval.

Excerpt from the novel *Frankenstein* by Mary Wollstonecraft Shelley

5. Which of the following can NOT be inferred from the passage?
   a. The creature mentioned is Frankenstein.
   b. Henry does not know of the creature's existence.
   c. The speaker is terrified of the creature.
   d. The speaker is attending a college.

Use the image below to answer question 6.

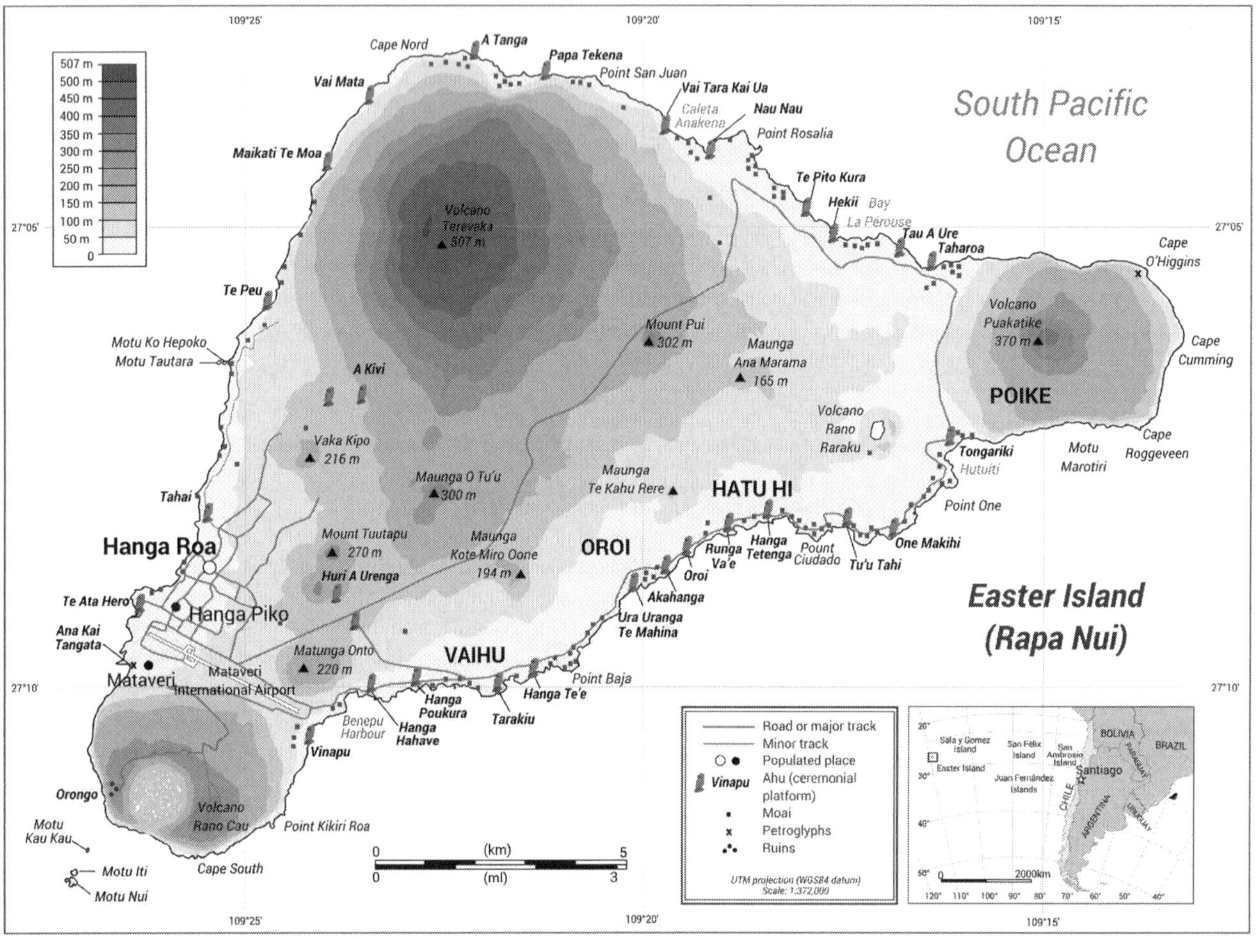

6. According to the map, which of the following is the highest points on the island?
   a. Volcano Terevaka
   b. Maunga Ana Marama
   c. Puakatike Volcano
   d. Vaka Kipo

The next two questions are based on the following passage.

The world war represents not the triumph, but the birth of democracy. The true ideal of democracy—the rule of a people by the *demos*, or group soul—is a thing unrealized. How then is it possible to consider or discuss an architecture of democracy—the shadow of a shade? It is not possible to do so with any degree of finality, but by an intention of consciousness upon this juxtaposition of ideas—architecture and democracy—signs of the times may yield new meanings, relations may emerge between things apparently unrelated, and the future, always existent in every present moment, may be evoked by that strange magic which resides in the human mind.

Architecture, at its worst as at its best, reflects always a true image of the thing that produced it; a building is revealing even though it is false, just as the face of a liar tells the thing his words endeavor to conceal. This being so, let us make such architecture as is ours declare to us our true estate.

The architecture of the United States, from the period of the Civil War, up to the beginning of the present crisis, everywhere reflects a struggle to be free of a vicious and depraved form of feudalism, grown strong under the very ægis of democracy. The qualities that made feudalism endeared and enduring; qualities written in beauty on the cathedral cities of mediaeval Europe—faith, worship, loyalty, magnanimity—were either vanished or banished from this pseudo-democratic, aridly scientific feudalism, leaving an inheritance of strife and tyranny—a strife grown mean, a tyranny grown prudent, but full of sinister power the weight of which we have by no means ceased to feel.

Power, strangely mingled with timidity; ingenuity, frequently misdirected; ugliness, the result of a false ideal of beauty—these in general characterize the architecture of our immediate past; an architecture "without ancestry or hope of posterity," an architecture devoid of coherence or conviction; willing to lie, willing to steal. What impression such a city as Chicago or Pittsburgh might have made upon some denizen of those cathedral-crowned feudal cities of the past we do not know. He would certainly have been amazed at its giant energy, and probably revolted at its grimy dreariness. We are wont to pity the mediaeval man for the dirt he lived in, even while smoke greys our sky and dirt permeates the very air we breathe: we think of castles as grim and cathedrals as dim, but they were beautiful and gay with color compared with the grim, dim canyons of our city streets.

The following is an excerpt from *Architecture and Democracy* by Claude Bragdon

7. By stating that "Architecture, at its worst as at its best, reflects always a true image of the thing that produced it," the author most likely intends to suggest that:
   a. People always create buildings to look like themselves.
   b. Architecture gets more grim, drab, and depressing as the years go by.
   c. Architecture reflects—in shape, color, and form—the attitude of the society which built it.
   d. Modern architecture is a lot like democracy because it is uniform yet made up of more pieces than your traditional architecture.

8. Based on the discussion in paragraph 3, which of the following would be considered architecture from medieval Europe?
   a. Canyon
   b. Castle
   c. Factory
   d. Skyscraper

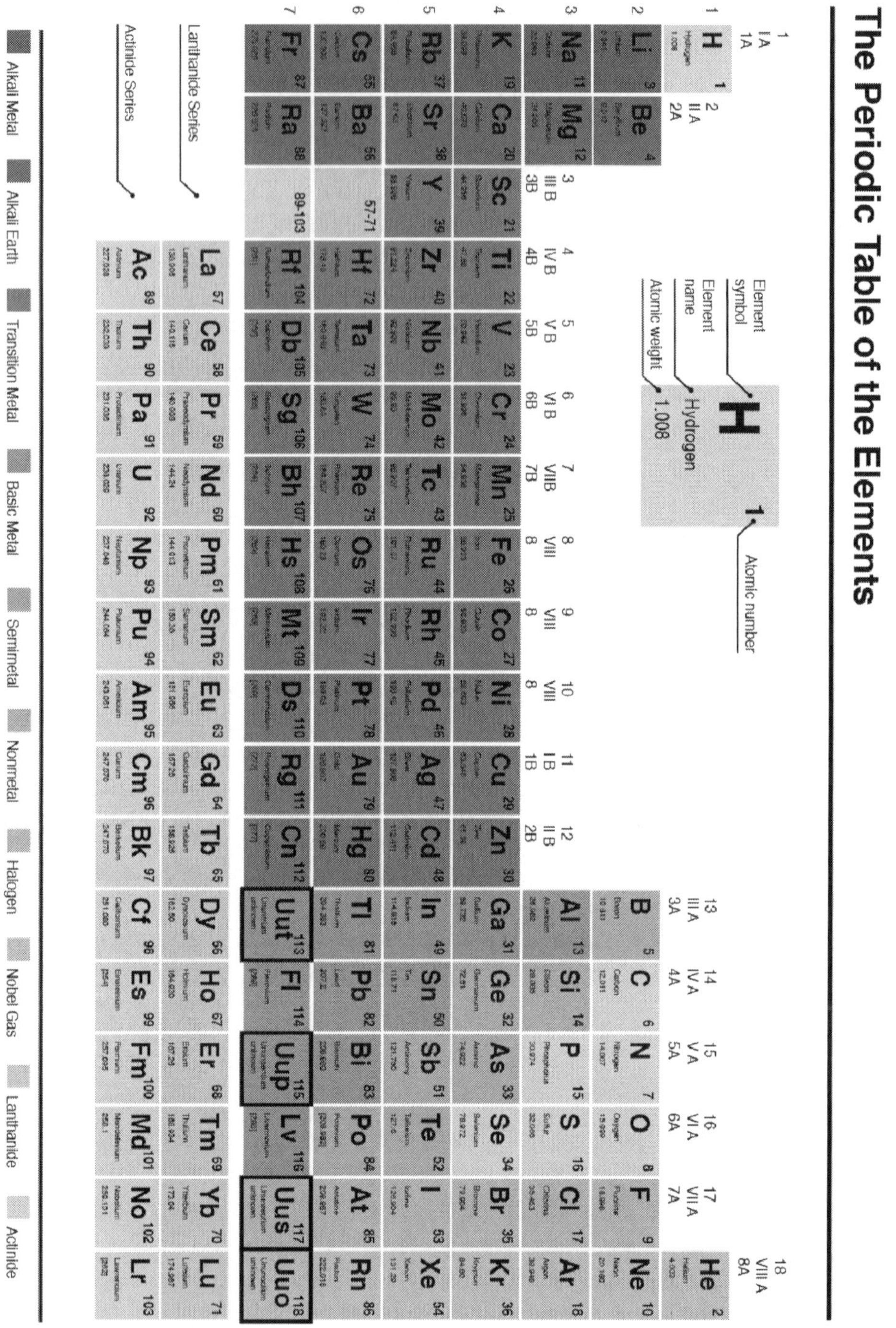

The Periodic Table of the Elements

Element symbol: H; Element name: Hydrogen; Atomic weight: 1.008; Atomic number: 1

Period	1 IA 1A	2 IIA 2A	3 IIIB 3B	4 IVB 4B	5 VB 5B	6 VIB 6B	7 VIIB 7B	8 VIII 8	9 VIII 8	10 VIII 8	11 IB 1B	12 IIB 2B	13 IIIA 3A	14 IVA 4A	15 VA 5A	16 VIA 6A	17 VIIA 7A	18 VIIIA 8A
1	H 1																	He 2
2	Li 3	Be 4											B 5	C 6	N 7	O 8	F 9	Ne 10
3	Na 11	Mg 12											Al 13	Si 14	P 15	S 16	Cl 17	Ar 18
4	K 19	Ca 20	Sc 21	Ti 22	V 23	Cr 24	Mn 25	Fe 26	Co 27	Ni 28	Cu 29	Zn 30	Ga 31	Ge 32	As 33	Se 34	Br 35	Kr 36
5	Rb 37	Sr 38	Y 39	Zr 40	Nb 41	Mo 42	Tc 43	Ru 44	Rh 45	Pd 46	Ag 47	Cd 48	In 49	Sn 50	Sb 51	Te 52	I 53	Xe 54
6	Cs 55	Ba 56	57-71	Hf 72	Ta 73	W 74	Re 75	Os 76	Ir 77	Pt 78	Au 79	Hg 80	Tl 81	Pb 82	Bi 83	Po 84	At 85	Rn 86
7	Fr 87	Ra 88	89-103	Rf 104	Db 105	Sg 106	Bh 107	Hs 108	Mt 109	Ds 110	Rg 111	Cn 112	Uuf 113	Fl 114	Uup 115	Lv 116	Uus 117	Uuo 118

Series														
Lanthanide Series	La 57	Ce 58	Pr 59	Nd 60	Pm 61	Sm 62	Eu 63	Gd 64	Tb 65	Dy 66	Ho 67	Er 68	Tm 69	Yb 70	Lu 71
Actinide Series	Ac 89	Th 90	Pa 91	U 92	Np 93	Pu 94	Am 95	Cm 96	Bk 97	Cf 98	Es 99	Fm 100	Md 101	No 102	Lr 103

Alkali Metal · Alkali Earth · Transition Metal · Basic Metal · Semimetal · Nonmetal · Halogen · Nobel Gas · Lanthanide · Actinide

Use the periodic table to answer question 9.

9. Based on the image above, which element is under Group V, Period 6?
   a. Pb
   b. Bi
   c. Uup
   d. At

The next question is based on the following passage.

To the Greeks and Romans rhetoric meant the theory of oratory. As a pedagogical mechanism it endeavored to teach students to persuade an audience. The content of rhetoric included all that the ancients had learned to be of value in persuasive public speech. It taught how to work up a case by drawing valid inferences from sound evidence, how to organize this material in the most persuasive order, how to compose in clear and harmonious sentences. Thus to the Greeks and Romans rhetoric was defined by its function of discovering means to persuasion and was taught in the schools as something that every free-born man could and should learn.

In both these respects the ancients felt that poetic, the theory of poetry, was different from rhetoric. As the critical theorists believed that the poets were inspired, they endeavored less to teach men to be poets than to point out the excellences which the poets had attained. Although these critics generally, with the exceptions of Aristotle and Eratosthenes, believed the greatest value of poetry to be in the teaching of morality, no one of them endeavored to define poetry, as they did rhetoric, by its purpose. To Aristotle, and centuries later to Plutarch, the distinguishing mark of poetry was imitation. Not until the renaissance did critics define poetry as an art of imitation endeavoring to inculcate morality…

The same essential difference between classical rhetoric and poetics appears in the content of classical poetics. Whereas classical rhetoric deals with speeches which might be delivered to convict or acquit a defendant in the law court, or to secure a certain action by the deliberative assembly, or to adorn an occasion, classical poetic deals with lyric, epic, and drama. It is a commonplace that classical literary critics paid little attention to the lyric. It is less frequently realized that they devoted almost as little space to discussion of metrics. By far the greater bulk of classical treatises on poetics is devoted to characterization and to the technique of plot construction, involving as it does narrative and dramatic unity and movement as distinct from logical unity and movement.

This excerpt is from *Rhetoric and Poetry in the Renaissance: A Study of Rhetorical Terms in English Renaissance Literary Criticism* by D.L. Clark

10. Given the author's description of the content of rhetoric in the first paragraph, shown below, which one of the following is most analogous to what it taught?

It taught how to work up a case by drawing valid inferences from sound evidence, how to organize this material in the most persuasive order, how to compose in clear and harmonious sentences.

a. As a musician, they taught me that the end product of the music is everything—what I did to get there was irrelevant, whether it was my ability to read music or the reliance on my intuition to compose.
b. As a detective, they taught me that time meant everything when dealing with a new case, that the simplest explanation is usually the right one, and that documentation is extremely important to credibility.
c. As a writer, they taught me the most important thing about writing was consistently showing up to the page every single day, no matter where my muse was.
d. As a football player, they taught me how to understand the logistics of the game, how my placement on the field affected the rest of the team, and how to run and throw with a mixture of finesse and strength.

Use the following image to answer question 11.

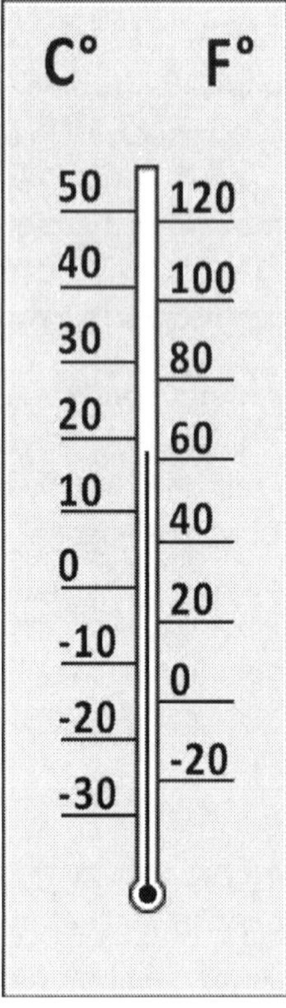

11. According to the image above, what is the temperature in Fahrenheit rounded to the nearest multiple of 5? _______

12. After Sheila recently had a coronary artery bypass, her doctor encouraged her to switch to a plant-based diet to avoid foods loaded with cholesterol and saturated fats. Sheila's doctor has given her a list of foods she can purchase in order to begin making healthy dinners, which excludes dairy (cheese, yogurt, cream), eggs, and meat. The doctor's list includes the following: pasta, marinara sauce, tofu, rice, black beans, tortilla chips, guacamole, corn, salsa, rice noodles, stir-fry vegetables, teriyaki sauce, quinoa, potatoes, yams, bananas, eggplant, pizza crust, cashew cheese, almond milk, bell pepper, and tempeh.

Which of the following dishes can Sheila make that will be okay for her to eat?

a. Eggplant parmesan with a salad
b. Veggie pasta with marinara sauce
c. Egg omelet with no cheese and bell peppers
d. Quinoa burger with cheese and French fries.

13. Maritza wanted to go to the park to swim with her friends, but when she got home, she realized that nobody was there to take her.

Follow the numbered instructions to transform the sentence above into a new sentence.

1. Replace the phrase "wanted to go" with "went."
2. Replace the word "but" with the word "and."
3. Replace the word "home" with "there."
4. Replace the phrase "nobody was there" with "they had thrown."
5. Take out the phrase "to take."
6. Remove the period and add the phrase, "a surprise party!" at the end of the sentence.

a. Maritza went to the park to swim with her friends, and when she got home, she realized they had thrown her a surprise party!
b. Maritza wanted to go to the park to swim with her friends, but when she got home, she realized they had thrown her a surprise party!
c. Maritza went to the park to swim with her friends, and when she got there, she realized that they had thrown her a surprise party!
d. Maritza went to the park to swim with her friends, and when she got there, she realized that nobody had thrown her a surprise party!

Use the pie chart below to answer question 14:

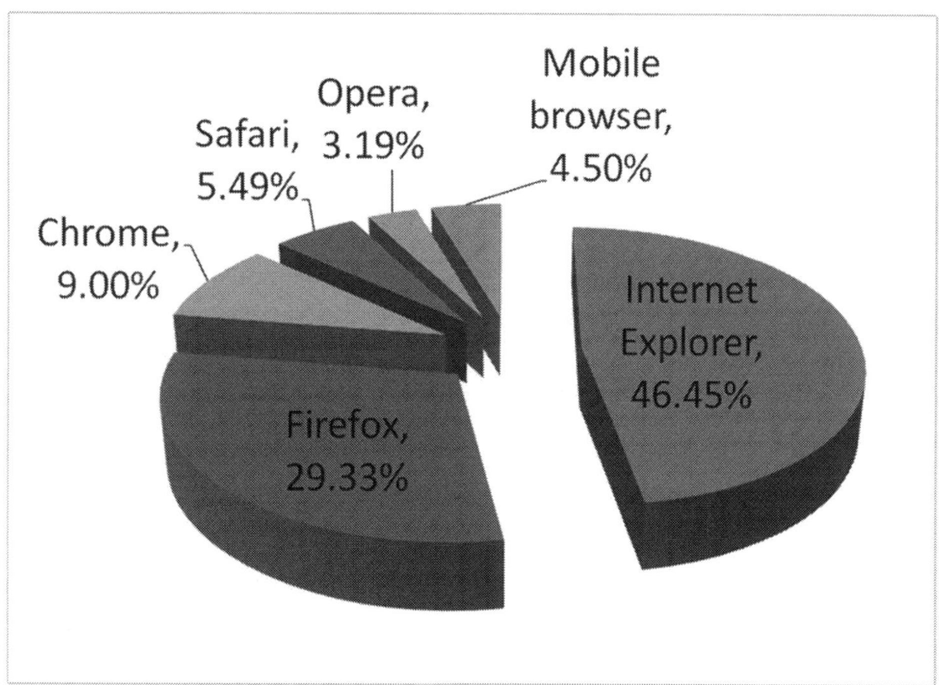

14. According to the pie chart above, which browser is most used on Wikimedia?
   a. Firefox
   b. Chrome
   c. Safari
   d. Internet Explorer

15. A reader comes across a word they do not know in the book they are reading, and they need to find out what the word means in order to understand the context of the sentence. Where should the reader look?
    a. Table of contents
    b. Introduction
    c. Index
    d. Glossary

The next three questions are based on the following passage.

> The old castle soon proved to be too small for the family, and in September 1853 the foundation-stone of a new house was laid. After the ceremony the workmen were entertained at dinner, which was followed by Highland games and dancing in the ballroom.
>
> Two years later they entered the new castle, which the Queen described as "charming; the rooms delightful; the furniture, papers, everything perfection."
>
> The Prince was untiring in planning improvements, and in 1856 the Queen wrote: "Every year my heart becomes more fixed in this dear Paradise, and so much more so now, that *all* has become my dearest Albert's *own* creation, own work, own building, own laying out as at Osborne; and his great taste, and the impress of his dear hand, have been stamped everywhere. He was very busy today, settling and arranging many things for next year."
>
> Excerpt from the biography *Queen Victoria* by E. Gordon Browne, M.A.

16. Which of the following is this excerpt considered?
    a. Primary source
    b. Secondary source
    c. Tertiary source
    d. None of these

17. How many years did it take for the new castle to be built?
    a. One year
    b. Two years
    c. Three years
    d. Four years

18. What does the word *impress* mean in the third paragraph?
    a. To affect strongly in feeling
    b. To urge something to be done
    c. To impose a certain quality upon
    d. To press a thing onto something else

The next three questions are based on the following passage.

> The play proceeded, although "Our American Cousin," without Mr. Sothern, has, since that gentleman's departure from this country, been justly esteemed a very dull affair. The audience at Ford's, including Mrs. Lincoln, seemed to enjoy it very much. The worthy wife of the President

leaned forward, her hand upon her husband's knee, watching every scene in the drama with amused attention. Even across the President's face at intervals swept a smile, robbing it of its habitual sadness.

About the beginning of the second act, the mare, standing in the stable in the rear of the theater, was disturbed in the midst of her meal by the entrance of the young man who had quitted her in the afternoon. It is presumed that she was saddled and bridled with exquisite care.

Having completed these preparations, Mr. Booth entered the theater by the stage door; summoned one of the scene shifters, Mr. John Spangler, emerged through the same door with that individual, leaving the door open, and left the mare in his hands to be held until he (Booth) should return. Booth who was even more fashionably and richly dressed than usual, walked thence around to the front of the theater, and went in. Ascending to the dress circle, he stood for a little time gazing around upon the audience and occasionally upon the stage in his usual graceful manner. He was subsequently observed by Mr. Ford, the proprietor of the theater, to be slowly elbowing his way through the crowd that packed the rear of the dress circle toward the right side, at the extremity of which was the box where Mr. and Mrs. Lincoln and their companions were seated. Mr. Ford casually noticed this as a slightly extraordinary symptom of interest on the part of an actor so familiar with the routine of the theater and the play.

Excerpt from *The Life, Crime, and Capture of John Wilkes Booth* by George Alfred Townsend

19. How is the above passage organized?
    a. Chronological
    b. Cause and effect
    c. Problem to solution
    d. Main idea with supporting details

20. Given the author's description of the play "Our American Cousin," which one of the following is most analogous to Mr. Sothern's departure from the theater?
    a. A ballet dancer who leaves the New York City Ballet just before they go on to their final performance.
    b. A basketball player leaves an NBA team and the next year they make it to the championship but lose.
    c. A lead singer leaves their band to begin a solo career, and the band drops in sales by 50 percent on their next album.
    d. A movie actor who dies in the middle of making a movie and the movie is made anyway by actors who resemble the deceased.

21. Based on your knowledge of history, what is about to happen shortly after the end of the passage?
    a. An asteroid is about to hit the earth.
    b. The best opera of all times is about to premiere.
    c. A playhouse is about to be burned to the ground.
    d. A president is about to be assassinated.

The next five questions are based on the following passage.

> When we study more carefully the effect upon the milk of the different species of bacteria found in the dairy, we find that there is a great variety of changes which they produce when they are allowed to grow in milk. The dairyman experiences many troubles with his milk. It sometimes curdles without becoming acid. Sometimes it becomes bitter, or acquires an unpleasant "tainted" taste, or, again, a "soapy" taste. Occasionally a dairyman finds his milk becoming slimy, instead of souring and curdling in the normal fashion. At such times, after a number of hours, the milk becomes so slimy that it can be drawn into long threads. Such an infection proves very troublesome, for many a time it persists in spite of all attempts made to remedy it. Again, in other cases the milk will turn blue, acquiring about the time it becomes sour a beautiful sky-blue colour. Or it may become red, or occasionally yellow. All of these troubles the dairyman owes to the presence in his milk of unusual species of bacteria which grow there abundantly.

Excerpt from *The Story of Germ Life* by Herbert William Conn

22. What is the tone of this passage?
    a. Excitement
    b. Anger
    c. Neutral
    d. Sorrowful

23. Which of the following reactions occur(s) in the above passage when bacteria infect the milk? Select all that apply.
    a. It can have a soapy taste.
    b. The milk will turn black.
    c. It can become slimy.
    d. The milk will turn blue.

24. What is the meaning of "curdle" as depicted in the following sentence?

    > Occasionally a dairyman finds his milk becoming slimy, instead of souring and curdling in the normal fashion.

    a. Lumpy
    b. Greasy
    c. Oily
    d. Slippery

25. Why, according to the passage, does an infection with slimy threads prove very troublesome?
    a. Because it is impossible to get rid of.
    b. Because it can make the milk-drinker sick.
    c. Because it turns the milk a blue color.
    d. Because it makes the milk taste bad.

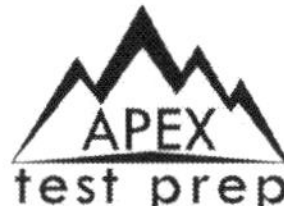

26. Given the author's account of the consequences of milk souring, which of the following is most closely analogous to the author's description of what happens after milk becomes slimy?
    a. The chemical change that occurs when a firework explodes
    b. A rainstorm that overwaters a succulent plant
    c. Mercury inside of a thermometer that leaks out
    d. A child who swallows flea medication

The next two questions are based on the following image.

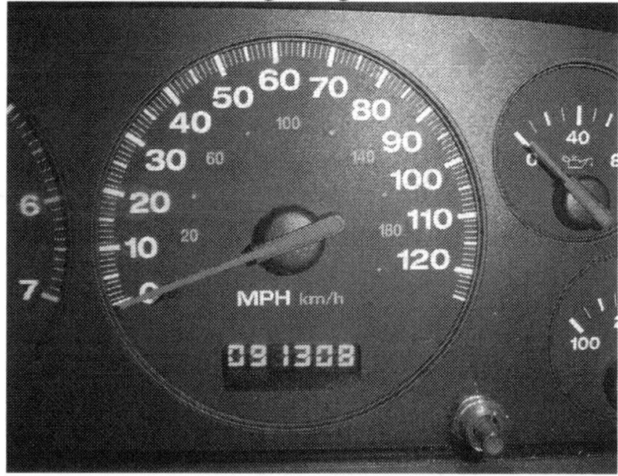

27. According to the image, what's the highest speed you can measure on this odometer? ________

28. According to the image above, how many miles have been driven on this car? ________

29. Although Olivia felt despondent, she knew her sister would be home to cheer her up.

In the sentence above, what is the best definition of the underlined word?

a. Depressed
b. Joyful
c. Pathetic
d. Humorous

The next six questions are based on the following passage.

> Portland is a very beautiful city of 60,000 inhabitants, and situated on the Willamette river twelve miles from its junction with the Columbia. It is perhaps true of many of the growing cities of the West, that they do not offer the same social advantages as the older cities of the East. But this is principally the case as to what may be called boom cities, where the larger part of the population is of that floating class which follows in the line of temporary growth for the purposes of speculation, and in no sense applies to those centers of trade whose prosperity is based on the solid foundation of legitimate business. As the metropolis of a vast section of country, having broad agricultural valleys filled with improved farms, surrounded by mountains rich in mineral wealth, and boundless forests of as fine timber as the world produces, the cause of Portland's growth and prosperity is the trade which it has as the center of collection and distribution of this great wealth of natural resources, and it has attracted, not the boomer and speculator, who find their profits in the wild excitement of the boom, but the merchant, manufacturer, and investor, who seek the surer if slower channels of legitimate business and investment. These have come from the East, most of them within the last few years. They came as seeking a better and wider

field to engage in the same occupations they had followed in their Eastern homes, and bringing with them all the love of polite life which they had acquired there, have established here a new society, equaling in all respects that which they left behind. Here are as fine churches, as complete a system of schools, as fine residences, as great a love of music and art, as can be found at any city of the East of equal size.

Excerpt from *Oregon, Washington, and Alaska. Sights and Scenes for the Tourist* by E.L. Lomax in 1890

30. What is a characteristic of a "boom city," as indicated by the passage?
   a. A city that is built on solid business foundation of mineral wealth and farming
   b. An area of land on the west coast that quickly becomes populated by residents from the east coast
   c. A city that, due to the hot weather and dry climate, catches fire frequently, resulting in a devastating population drop
   d. A city whose population is made up of people who seek quick fortunes rather than building a solid business foundation

31. According to the author, Portland is:
   a. A boom city
   b. A city on the east coast
   c. A capital city
   d. A city of legitimate business

32. What type of passage is this?
   a. A business proposition
   b. A travel guide
   c. A journal entry
   d. A scholarly article

33. What does the word *metropolis* mean in the middle of the passage?
   a. Farm
   b. Country
   c. City
   d. Valley

34. By stating that "they do not offer the same social advantages as the older cities of the East" in the first paragraph, the author most likely intends to suggest that:
   a. Inhabitants who reside in older cities in the East are much more social than inhabitants who reside in newer cities in the West because of background and experience.
   b. Cities in the West have no culture compared to the East because the culture in the East comes from European influence.
   c. Cities in the East are older than cities in the West, and older cities always have better culture than newer cities.
   d. Since cities in the West are newly established, it takes them a longer time to develop cultural roots and societal functions than those cities that are already established in the East.

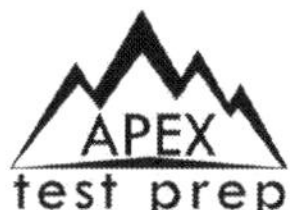

35. Based on the information at the end of the passage, what would the author say of Portland?
    a. It has twice as much culture as the cities in the East.
    b. It has as much culture as the cities in the East.
    c. It doesn't have as much culture as cities in the East.
    d. It doesn't have as much culture as cities in the West.

The next two questions are based on the following passage.

> The other of the minor deities at Nemi was Virbius. Legend had it that Virbius was the young Greek hero Hippolytus, chaste and fair, who learned the art of venery from the centaur Chiron, and spent all his days in the greenwood chasing wild beasts with the virgin huntress Artemis (the Greek counterpart of Diana) for his only comrade.

Excerpt from *The Golden Bough* by Sir James George Frazer.

36. Based on a prior knowledge of literature, the reader can infer this passage is taken from which of the following?
    a. A eulogy
    b. A myth
    c. A historical document
    d. A technical document

37. What is the meaning of the word "comrade" as the last word in the passage?
    a. Friend
    b. Enemy
    c. Brother
    d. Pet

The next question is based on the following passage.

> When I wrote the following passages, or rather the bulk of them, I lived alone, in the woods, a mile from any neighbor, in a house which I had built myself on the shore of Walden Pond, in Concord, Massachusetts, and earned my living by the labor of my hands only. I lived there two years and two months. At present I am a sojourner in civilized life again.

Excerpt from *Walden* by Henry David Thoreau.

38. What does the word *sojourner* most likely mean at the end of the passage?
    a. Illegal immigrant
    b. Temporary resident
    c. Lifetime partner
    d. Farm crop

The following image is for question 39.

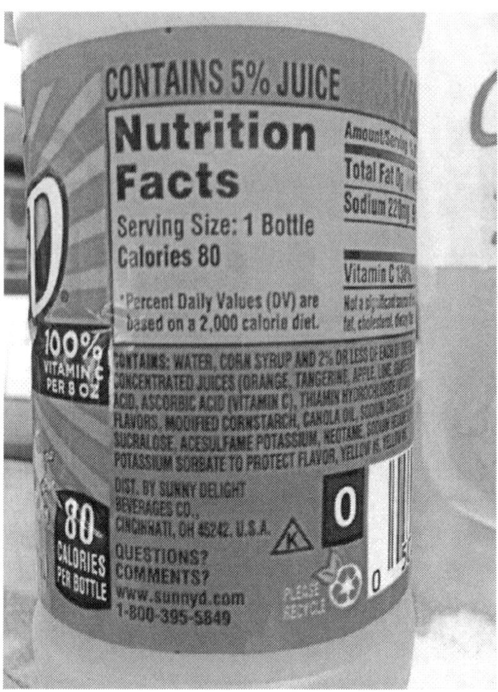

39. Based on the label above, this juice contains the most of which two ingredients?
    a. Vitamin C and cornstarch
    b. Corn syrup and Vitamin C
    c. Water and corn syrup
    d. Water and cornstarch

40. According to the label above, how many calories would you consume if you drank two bottles of this drink? ________

The next two questions are based on the following passage.

I do not believe there are as many as five examples of deviation from the literalness of the text. Once only, I believe, have I transposed two lines for convenience of translation; the other deviations are (*if* they are such) a substitution of an *and* for a comma in order to make now and then the reading of a line musical. With these exceptions, I have sacrificed *everything* to faithfulness of rendering. My object was to make Pushkin himself, without a prompter, speak to English readers. To make him thus speak in a foreign tongue was indeed to place him at a disadvantage; and music and rhythm and harmony are indeed fine things, but truth is finer still. I wished to present not what Pushkin would have said, or should have said, if he had written in English, but what he does say in Russian. That, stripped from all ornament of his wonderful melody and grace of form, as he is in a translation, he still, even in the hard English tongue, soothes and stirs, is in itself a sign that through the individual soul of Pushkin sings that universal soul whose strains appeal forever to man, in whatever clime, under whatever sky.

Excerpt from *Poems by Alexander Pushkin* by Ivan Panin.

41. From clues in this passage, what type of work is the author doing?
    a. Translation work
    b. Criticism
    c. Historical validity
    d. Writing a biography

42. According to the author, what is the most important aim of translation work?
    a. To retain the beauty of the work
    b. To retain the truth of the work
    c. To retain the melody of the work
    d. To retain the form of the work

The next three questions are based on the following passages.

Passage A

In approaching this problem of interpretation, we may first put out of consideration certain obvious limitations upon the generality of all guaranties of free speech. An occasional unthinking malcontent may urge that the only meaning not fraught with danger to liberty is the literal one that no utterance may be forbidden, no matter what its intent or result; but in fact it is nowhere seriously argued by anyone whose opinion is entitled to respect that direct and intentional incitations to crime may not be forbidden by the state. If a state may properly forbid murder or robbery or treason, it may also punish those who induce or counsel the commission of such crimes. Any other view makes a mockery of the state's power to declare and punish offences. And what the state may do to prevent the incitement of serious crimes which are universally condemned, it may also do to prevent the incitement of lesser crimes, or of those in regard to the bad tendency of which public opinion is divided. That is, if the state may punish John for burning straw in an alley, it may also constitutionally punish Frank for inciting John to do it, though Frank did so by speech or writing. And if, in 1857, the United States could punish John for helping a fugitive slave to escape, it could also punish Frank for inducing John to do this, even though a large section of public opinion might applaud John and condemn the Fugitive Slave Law.

Excerpt from *Free Speech in War Time* by James Parker Hall, written in 1921, published in Columbia Law Review, Vol. 21 No. 6

Passage B

The true boundary line of the First Amendment can be fixed only when Congress and the courts realize that the principle on which speech is classified as lawful or unlawful involves the balancing against each other of two very important social interests, in public safety and in the search for truth. Every reasonable attempt should be made to maintain both interests unimpaired, and the great interest in free speech should be sacrificed only when the interest in public safety is really imperiled, and not, as most men believe, when it is barely conceivable that it may be slightly affected. In war time, therefore, speech should be unrestricted by the censorship or by punishment, unless it is clearly liable to cause direct and dangerous interference with the conduct of the war.

Thus our problem of locating the boundary line of free speech is solved. It is fixed close to the point where words will give rise to unlawful acts. We cannot define the right of free speech with the precision of the Rule against Perpetuities or the Rule in Shelley's Case, because it involves national policies which are much more flexible than private property, but we can establish a workable principle of classification in this method of balancing and this broad test of certain danger. There is a similar balancing in the determination of what is "due process of law." And we can with certitude declare that the First Amendment forbids the punishment of words merely for their injurious tendencies. The history of the Amendment and the political function of free speech corroborate each other and make this conclusion plain.

Excerpt from *Freedom of Speech in War Time* by Zechariah Chafee, Jr. written in 1919, published in Harvard Law Review Vol. 32 No. 8

43. Which one of the following questions is central to both passages?
   a. What is the interpretation of the first amendment and its limitations?
   b. Do people want absolute liberty or do they only want liberty for a certain purpose?
   c. What is the true definition of freedom of speech in a democracy?
   d. How can we find an appropriate boundary of freedom of speech during wartime?

44. The authors of the two passages would be most likely to disagree over which of the following?
   a. A man is thrown in jail due to his provocation of violence in Washington D.C. during a riot.
   b. A man is thrown in jail for stealing bread for his starving family, and the judge has mercy for him and lets him go.
   c. A man is thrown in jail for encouraging a riot against the U.S. government for the wartime tactics, although no violence ensues.
   d. A man is thrown in jail because he has been caught as a German spy working within the U.S. army.

45. The relationship between Passage *A* and Passage *B* is most analogous to the relationship between the documents described in which of the following?
   a. A journal article in the Netherlands about the law of euthanasia that cites evidence to support only the act of passive euthanasia as an appropriate way to die; a journal article in the Netherlands about the law of euthanasia that cites evidence to support voluntary euthanasia in any aspect
   b. An article detailing the effects of radiation in Fukushima; a research report describing the deaths and birth defects as a result of the hazardous waste dumped on the Somali Coast.
   c. An article that suggests that labor laws during times of war should be left up to the states; an article that showcases labor laws during the past that have been altered due to the current crisis of war
   d. A research report arguing that the leading cause of methane emissions in the world is from agriculture practices; an article citing that the leading cause of methane emissions in the world is from the transportation of coal, oil, and natural gas

Mathematics

1. What is $\frac{12}{60}$ converted to a percentage?
   a. 0.20
   b. 20%
   c. 25%
   d. 12%

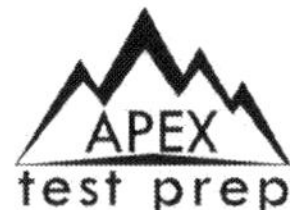

2. Which of the following is the correct decimal form of the fraction $\frac{14}{33}$ rounded to the nearest hundredth place?
   a. 0.41
   b. 0.42
   c. 0.424
   d. 0.141

3. Which of the following represents the correct sum of $\frac{14}{15}$ and $\frac{2}{5}$, in lowest possible terms?
   a. $\frac{20}{15}$
   b. $\frac{4}{3}$
   c. $\frac{16}{20}$
   d. $\frac{4}{5}$

4. What is the product of $\frac{5}{14}$ and $\frac{7}{20}$, in lowest possible terms?
   a. $\frac{1}{8}$
   b. $\frac{35}{280}$
   c. $\frac{12}{34}$
   d. $\frac{1}{2}$

5. What is the result of dividing 24 by $\frac{8}{5}$, in lowest possible terms?
   a. $\frac{5}{3}$
   b. $\frac{3}{5}$
   c. $\frac{120}{8}$
   d. 15

6. Subtract $\frac{5}{14}$ from $\frac{5}{24}$. Which of the following is the correct result?
   a. $\frac{25}{168}$
   b. 0
   c. $-\frac{25}{168}$
   d. $\frac{1}{10}$

7. Which of the following is a correct mathematical statement?
   a. $\frac{1}{3} < -\frac{4}{3}$
   b. $-\frac{1}{3} > \frac{4}{3}$
   c. $\frac{1}{3} > -\frac{4}{3}$
   d. $-\frac{1}{3} \geq \frac{4}{3}$

8. Which of the following is NOT correct?
   a. $-\frac{1}{5} < \frac{4}{5}$
   b. $\frac{4}{5} > -\frac{1}{5}$
   c. $-\frac{1}{5} > \frac{4}{5}$
   d. $\frac{1}{5} > -\frac{4}{5}$

9. What is the solution to the equation $3(x + 2) = 14x - 5$?
   a. $x = 1$
   b. No solution
   c. $x = 0$
   d. All real numbers

10. The following set represents the test scores from a university class: {35, 79, 80, 87, 87, 90, 92, 95, 95, 98, 99}. If the outlier is removed from this set, which of the following is true?
   a. The mean and the median will decrease.
   b. The mean and the median will increase.
   c. The mean and the mode will increase.
   d. The mean and the mode will decrease.

11. Which of the following is the result when solving the equation $4(x + 5) + 6 = 2(2x + 3)$?
   a. Any real number is a solution.
   b. There is no solution.
   c. $x = 6$ is the solution.
   d. $x = 26$ is the solution.

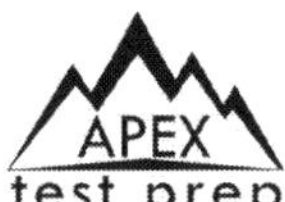

	/	/	
.	.	.	.
0	0	0	0
1	1	1	1
2	2	2	2
3	3	3	3
4	4	4	4
5	5	5	5
6	6	6	6
7	7	7	7
8	8	8	8
9	9	9	9

12. How many cases of cola can Lexi purchase if each case is $3.50 and she has $40? Enter your answer on the number pad.

13. Two consecutive integers exist such that the sum of three times the first and two less than the second is equal to 411. What are those integers?
    a. 103 and 104
    b. 104 and 105
    c. 102 and 103
    d. 100 and 101

14. In a neighborhood, 15 out of 80 of the households have children under the age of 18. What percentage of the households have children under 18?
    a. 0.1875%
    b. 18.75%
    c. 1.875%
    d. 15%

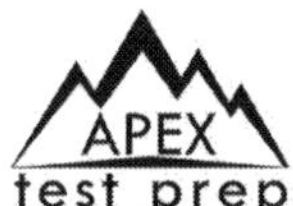

15. Gina took an algebra test last Friday. There were 35 questions, and she answered 60% of them correctly. How many correct answers did she have? Enter your answer in the box.

16. What is the median for the times shown in the chart below?

100 m dash times	
Olivia	11 s
Noah	13 s
Amelia	15 s
Elijah	12 s
Luca	12 s
Chloe	16 s
Asher	19 s

a. 11 s
b. 14 s
c. 12 s
d. 13 s

17. If a car is purchased for $15,395 with a 7.25% sales tax, how much is the total price?
a. $15,395.07
b. $16,511.14
c. $16,411.13
d. $15,402

18. A car manufacturer usually makes 15,412 SUVs, 25,815 station wagons, 50,412 sedans, 8,123 trucks, and 18,312 hybrids a month. About how many cars are manufactured each month?
a. 120,000
b. 200,000
c. 300,000
d. 12,000

19. A family goes to the grocery store every week and spends $105. About how much does the family spend annually on groceries?
a. $10,000
b. $50,000
c. $500
d. $5,000

20. Bindee is having a barbeque on Sunday and needs 12 packets of ketchup for every 5 guests. If 60 guests are coming, how many packets of ketchup should she buy?
a. 100
b. 12
c. 144
d. 60

21. A grocery store sold 48 bags of apples in one day. If 9 of the bags contained Granny Smith apples and the rest contained Red Delicious apples, what is the ratio of bags of Granny Smith to bags of Red Delicious that were sold?
    a. 48:9
    b. 39:9
    c. 9:48
    d. 9:39

22. If Oscar's bank account totaled $4,000 in March and $4,900 in June, what was the rate of change in his bank account total over those three months?
    a. $900 a month
    b. $300 a month
    c. $4,900 a month
    d. $100 a month

23. Erin and Katie work at the same ice cream shop. Together, they always work less than 21 hours a week. In a week, if Katie worked two times as many hours as Erin, how many hours could Erin work?
    a. Less than 7 hours
    b. Less than or equal to 7 hours
    c. More than 7 hours
    d. Less than 8 hours

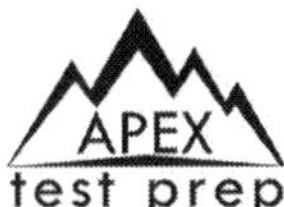

24. From the chart below, which genres are preferred by more men than women? *Select all that apply.*

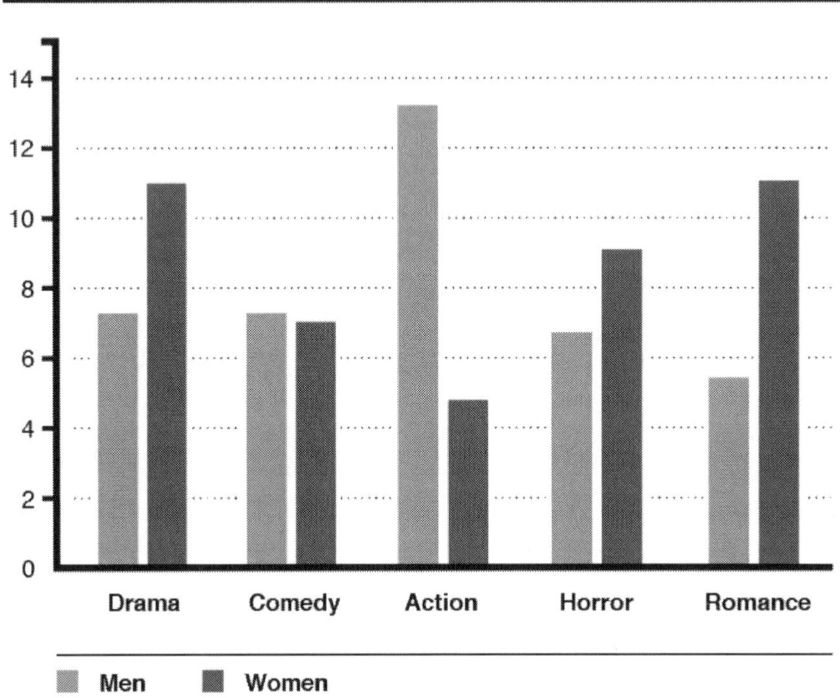

a. Drama
b. Comedy
c. Action
d. Horror

25. Which type of graph best represents a continuous change over a period of time?
a. Bar graph
b. Line graph
c. Pie graph
d. Histogram

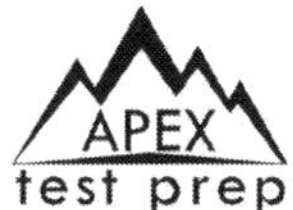

26. Using the graph below, what is the mean number of visitors for the first 4 hours?

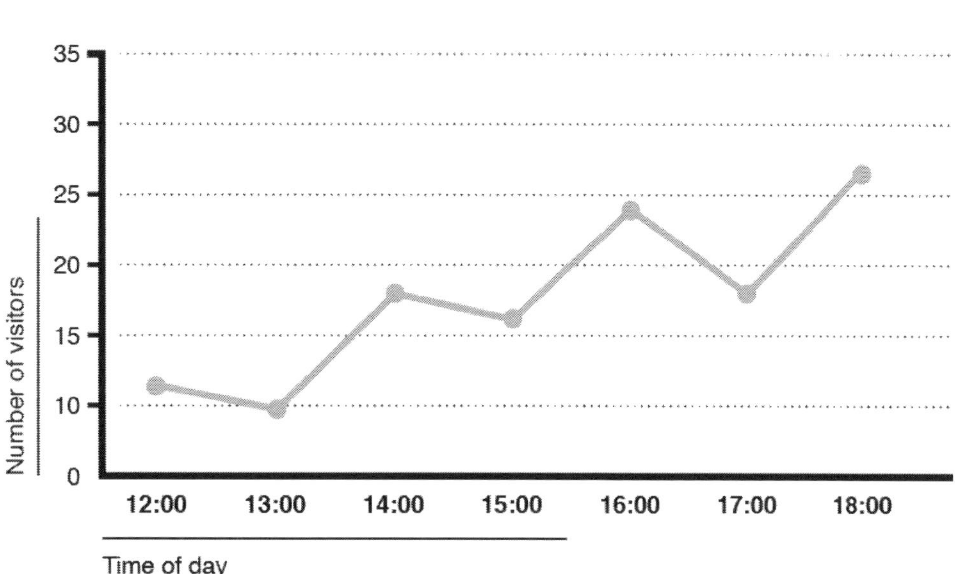

a. 10
b. 12
c. 14
d. 16

27. What is the mode for the grades shown in the chart below?

Science Grades	
Jerry	65
Bill	95
Anna	80
Beth	95
Sara	85
Ben	72
Jordan	98

a. 65
b. 33
c. 95
d. 90

28. What type of relationship is there between age and attention span as represented in the graph below?

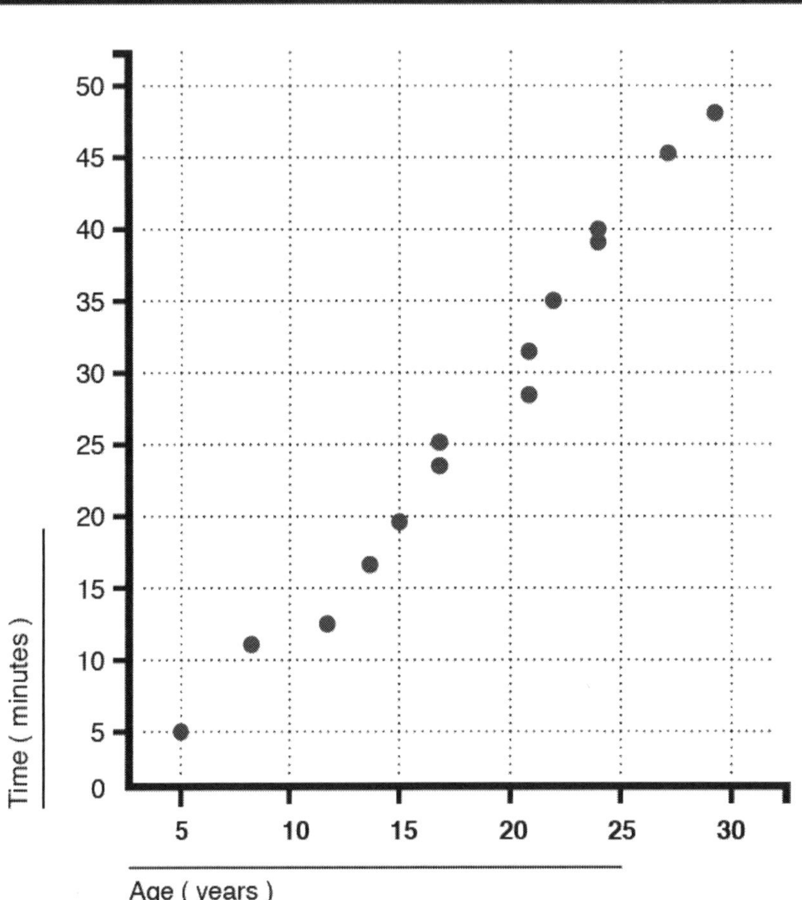

a. No correlation
b. Positive correlation
c. Negative correlation
d. Weak correlation

29. What is the area of the shaded region?

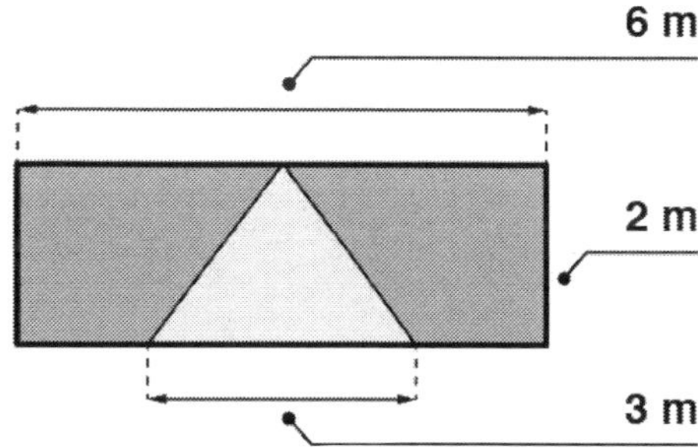

a. $9\ m^2$
b. $12\ m^2$
c. $6\ m^2$
d. $8\ m^2$

30. What is the volume of the cylinder below? Use 3.14 for π.

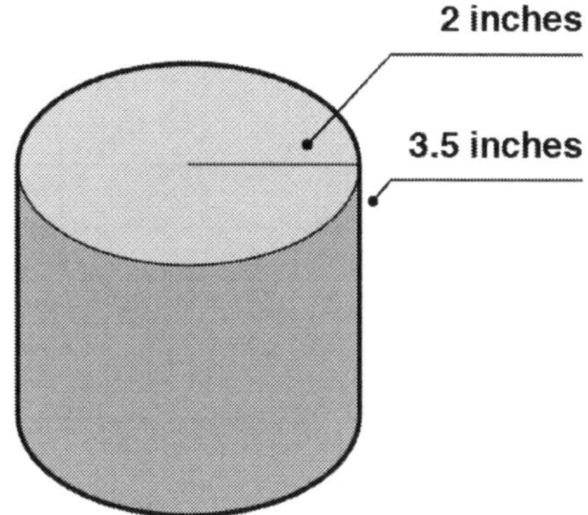

a. $18.84\ in^3$
b. $45.00\ in^3$
c. $70.43\ in^3$
d. $43.96\ in^3$

31. How many kiloliters are in 6 liters?
a. 6,000
b. 600
c. 0.006
d. 0.0006

32. How many centimeters are in 3 feet? (Note: $2.54\text{ cm} = 1\text{ in}$)
a. 0.635
b. 91.44
c. 14.17
d. 7.62

33. The percentage of smokers above the age of 18 in 2000 was 23.2%. The percentage of smokers over the age of 18 in 2015 was 15.1%. Find the average rate of change in the percentage of smokers over the age of 18 from 2000 to 2015.
    a. -0.54%
    b. -54%
    c. -5.4%
    d. -15%

34. What type of units are used to describe surface area?
    a. Square
    b. Cubic
    c. Single
    d. Quartic

35. Which of the following is the equation of a vertical line that runs through the point $(1, 4)$?
    a. $x = 1$
    b. $y = 1$
    c. $x = 4$
    d. $y = 4$

36. What is the area of the following figure?

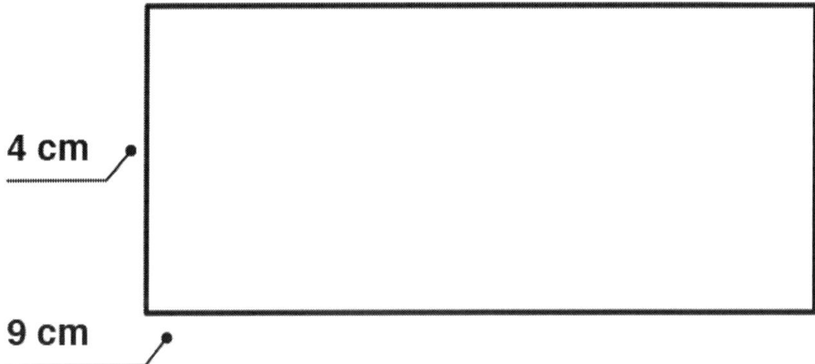

    a. $26\ cm$
    b. $36\ cm$
    c. $13\ cm^2$
    d. $36\ cm^2$

37. Approximately how many pounds are in 5 kilograms?
    a. 5 lbs
    b. 8 lbs
    c. 11 lbs
    d. 14 lbs

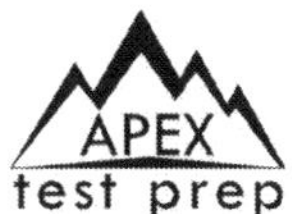

38. Use the graph below entitled "Projected Temperatures for Tomorrow's Winter Storm" to answer the question.

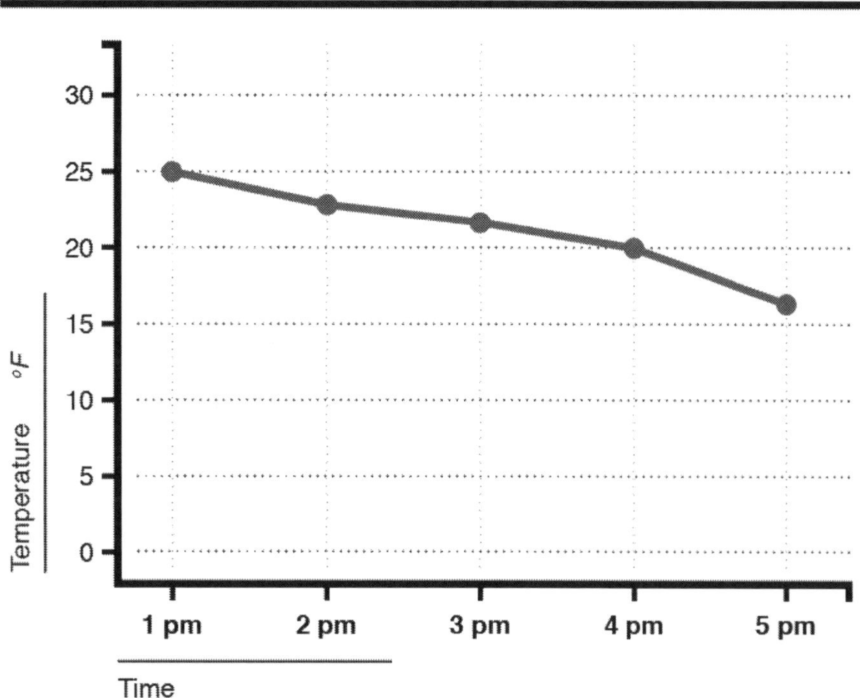

What is the expected temperature at 3:00 p.m.?

a. 25 degrees
b. 22 degrees
c. 20 degrees
d. 16 degrees

Science

1. How many different types of cells are there in the human body?
   a. Two hundred
   b. One thousand
   c. Ten
   d. Twenty-five

2. What type of tissue provides a protective barrier for delicate organs?
   a. Epithelial
   b. Muscle
   c. Connective
   d. Neural

3. What part of the respiratory system is responsible for regulating the temperature and humidity of the air that comes into the body?
   a. Larynx
   b. Lungs
   c. Trachea
   d. Sinuses

4. The following are four of the stages of meiosis 1. Put them in the correct order.

- Anaphase
- Metaphase
- Prophase
- Telophase

- 1. ____________________
- 2. ____________________
- 3. ____________________
- 4. ____________________

5. In which part of the atom is 99 percent of its mass found?
   a. Nucleus
   b. Protons
   c. Neutrons
   d. Electrons

6. What is different between the isotopes of an atom?
   a. The number of protons
   b. The number of orbitals
   c. The number of neutrons
   d. The number of electrons

7. What is another name for the mitral valve?
   a. Bicuspid valve
   b. Pulmonary valve
   c. Aortic valve
   d. Tricuspid valve

8. Which component of blood helps to fight off diseases?
   a. Red blood cells
   b. White blood cells
   c. Plasma
   d. Platelets

9. Viruses belong to which of the following classifications?
   a. Domain Archaea
   b. Kingdom Monera
   c. Kingdom Protista
   d. None of the above

10. There are multiple steps that the gastrointestinal system performs. In which step do chemicals and enzymes break down complex food molecules into smaller molecules?
   a. Digestion
   b. Absorption
   c. Compaction
   d. Ingestion

11. Which accessory organ of the gastrointestinal system is responsible for storing and concentrating bile?
   a. Liver
   b. Pancreas
   c. Stomach
   d. Gallbladder

12. How do prokaryotic cells divide?
   a. Meiosis
   b. Binary fission
   c. Mitosis
   d. They grow exponentially but do not divide

13. How do neuroglia support neurons?
   a. Provide nutrition to them
   b. Provide a framework around them and protect them from the surrounding environment
   c. Relay messages to them from the brain
   d. Connect them to other surrounding cells

14. Which nerve system allows the brain to regulate body functions such as heart rate and blood pressure?
   a. Central
   b. Somatic
   c. Autonomic
   d. Afferent

15. Which of the following organs is NOT considered an accessory organ of the male reproductive system?
   a. Testes
   b. Prostate
   c. Vas deferens
   d. Bulbourethral glands

16. How many gametes do the ovaries produce every month?
    a. One million
    b. One
    c. One-half billion
    d. Two

17. In what part of the female reproductive system do sperm fertilize an oocyte?
    a. Ovary
    b. Mammary gland
    c. Vagina
    d. Fallopian tubes

18. Which of the following is an example of the regenerative capacity of an organism?
    a. A flatworm dies after it is cut into pieces.
    b. A lizard loses its tail and grows a new one.
    c. A five-armed starfish loses an arm and continues life with four arms.
    d. Cardiac tissue is damaged and does not generate new healthy tissue.

19. Which of the following is a function of the skin?
    a. Temperature regulation
    b. Breathing
    c. Ingestion
    d. All of the above

20. Which accessory organ of the integumentary system provides a hard layer of protection over the skin?
    a. Hair
    b. Nails
    c. Sweat glands
    d. Sebaceous glands

21. Which of the following is a distinct characteristic of tissues and glands that are a part of the endocrine system?
    a. Lack a blood supply
    b. Act quickly in response to stimuli
    c. Secrete bile
    d. Ductless

22. Identify the location of the hypothalamus by placing an "X" on the circle at its location:

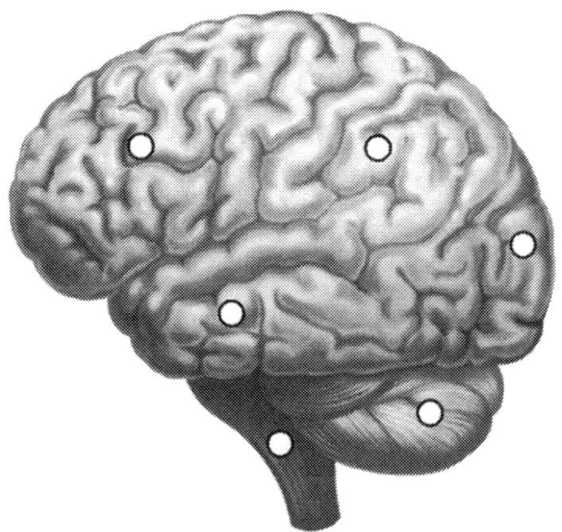

23. How are amino acids classified if they have a positively charged side chain?
    a. Basic
    b. Hydrophilic
    c. Acidic
    d. Hydrophobic

24. Which organ is responsible for filtering waste products out of the bloodstream?
    a. Kidneys
    b. Urinary bladder
    c. Pancreas
    d. Urethra

25. Which of the following statements is true regarding DNA?
    a. DNA is the genetic code.
    b. DNA provides energy.
    c. DNA is single-stranded.
    d. All of the above statements are true.

26. What happens to the urinary bladder as urine enters and is stored until the bladder is emptied?
    a. Blood flow to the organ increases.
    b. It secretes waste into the urine.
    c. Its walls stretch and become thinner.
    d. Its internal pressure increases.

27. Which immune system works in a nonspecific way and does not remember pathogens that it previously fought against?
    a. Innate
    b. Adaptive
    c. Hormonal
    d. B cell

28. How does the adaptive immune system work to fight against previously encountered pathogens?
    a. It sends out all antibodies to inactivate the pathogen.
    b. It sends out target-specific antibodies to inactivate the pathogen.
    c. It uses a mechanical barrier, such as the skin, to protect against pathogens.
    d. It uses a chemical barrier, such as gastric acid, to protect against pathogens.

29. What type of disorder can develop if the immune system is not functioning properly?
    a. Adaptive
    b. Innate
    c. Lymphocytic
    d. Autoimmune

30. In the Periodic Table, what similarity do the elements in columns have with each other?
    a. They have the same atomic number.
    b. They have similar chemical properties.
    c. They have similar electron valence configurations.
    d. They have the same density.

31. Which is a distinct characteristic of spongy bone?
    a. Dense
    b. Filled with organic and inorganic salts
    c. Found inside compact bone
    d. Lightweight

32. What number on the pH scale indicates a neutral solution?
    a. 13
    b. 8
    c. 7
    d. 0

33. Which molecule is the simplest form of sugar?
    a. Monosaccharide
    b. Fatty acid
    c. Polysaccharide
    d. Amino acid

34. Which type of macromolecule contains genetic information that can be passed to subsequent generations?
    a. Carbohydrates
    b. Lipids
    c. Proteins
    d. Nucleic acids

35. What is the primary unit of inheritance between generations of an organism?
    a. Chromosome
    b. Gene
    c. Gamete
    d. Atom

36. Which one of Mendel's laws theorizes that the alleles for different traits are NOT linked and can be inherited independently of one another?
   a. The Law of Dominance
   b. The Law of Segregation
   c. The Law of Independent Assortment
   d. None of the above

37. In which situation is an atom considered neutral?
   a. The number of protons and neutrons are equal.
   b. The number of neutrons and electrons are equal.
   c. The number of protons and electrons are equal.
   d. There are more electrons than protons.

38. Which is an example of a physical property of substances?
   a. Odor
   b. Reactivity
   c. Flammability
   d. Toxicity

39. Which type of matter has molecules that cannot move within its substance and breaks evenly across a plane caused by the symmetry of its molecular arrangement?
   a. Gas
   b. Crystalline solid
   c. Liquid
   d. Amorphous solid

40. What type of reactions involve the breaking and re-forming of bonds between atoms?
   a. Chemical
   b. Physical
   c. Isotonic
   d. Electron

41. When is it helpful to use scientific notation to represent numbers?
   a. When the number is very large or very small
   b. When the number is a multiple of ten
   c. When the number is involved in a scientific experiment
   d. For numbers between 0 and 100 only

42. Which of the following describes an invention used to measure small fractions within already small divisions?
   a. A tape measure
   b. A ruler
   c. A yardstick
   d. Vernier Scale

43. When are scientific experiments found reliable?
    a. When all the materials needed for the experiment are used
    b. When the scientists conducting them are credible
    c. When they prove the hypothesis to be true
    d. When they can be replicated

44. Which of the following scenarios describes mistaking correlation for causation? *Select all that apply.*
    a. In the same year, the drinking water was contaminated by a nearby chicken farm and stomach cancer in the area increased 3 percent. The contaminated water obviously caused stomach cancer to increase.
    b. Victoria notices that every time she turns on the stove burner underneath a pot with water in it, the water boils. Victoria realizes that putting heat under water causes it to boil.
    c. We saw that the thunderstorm that day caused all the neighborhoods in the East Village to flood. The power outage in West Village must have been because of the storm.
    d. Hector learned in school that when tectonic plates shift, it causes earthquakes to happen. There had been many earthquakes when Hector lived in California, and now he knew that the shifting of plates is what caused them.

45. A microscope is particularly useful to visualize which of the following?
    a. Objects that are too big to see as a whole
    b. Objects that are reflected in a mirror
    c. Objects that are too far away to be seen with the human eye
    d. Objects that are too small to see with the human eye

46. In the model of the scientific method, which of the following best explains the step of formulating a hypothesis?
    a. Forming a question that relates to the observation
    b. Writing out an expectation of what's going to happen
    c. Gathering the materials needed for the procedure
    d. Summarizing the results of the experiment

47. When would a peer review be conducted in an experiment?
    a. Before the experiment
    b. During the experiment
    c. After the experiment is over and before it is published
    d. After the experiment is over and published

Questions 48 and 49 are based on the following information:

Soil samples were collected from various locations and analyzed for their composition. Three types of minerals were identified and measured by percentage in each sample. These minerals were sand, silt, and clay. Particle size ranges for each mineral were also measured and recorded for the soil samples.

Soil Sample	Sand (%)	Clay (%)	Silt (%)
1	75	5	20
2	5	80	15
3	20	35	45
4	70	15	15
5	55	25	20

Type of mineral particle	Size range of particles (mm)
Sand	3.0-0.07
Silt	0.07-0.003
Clay	Less than 0.003

48. Which minerals mainly comprised Sample 3?
    a. Sand and silt
    b. Silt and clay
    c. Sand and clay
    d. Sand

49. Which soil sample would MOST likely have particle sizes around 1.7 mm?
    a. Sample 2
    b. Sample 3
    c. Sample 4
    d. Sample 5

50. What is one way to mitigate transmission of communicable disease?
    a. Vaccination
    b. Traveling by car versus traveling by plane
    c. Avoiding people who have traveled abroad in the last 12 months
    d. Following a diet high in biotin

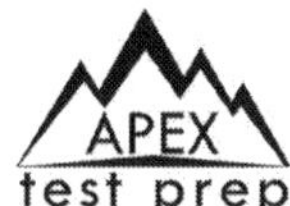

English & Language Usage

1. Which of the following can be used to improve writing style through grammar? Select all that apply.
   a. Alternating among different sentence structures
   b. Using fewer words instead of unnecessary words
   c. Consistently using one-subject and one-verb sentences
   d. Writing in the active voice more than passive voice

2. Of the following statements, which is most accurate about topic sentences?
   a. They are always first in a paragraph.
   b. They are always last in a paragraph.
   c. They are only found once in every essay.
   d. They are explicit or may be implicit.

3. Which of the following is considered criteria for a good paragraph topic sentence?
   a. Clear
   b. Subtle
   c. Lengthy
   d. Ambiguous

4. "We don't go out as much because babysitters, gasoline, and parking is expensive." Which grammatical error does this sentence demonstrate?
   a. It contains a misplaced modifier.
   b. It lacks subject-verb agreement.
   c. It introduces a dangling participle.
   d. It does not have a grammar error.

5. Which of the following versions of a sentence has correct pronoun-antecedent agreement?
   a. Every student must consult their advisor first.
   b. All students must talk with their advisors first.
   c. All students must consult with his advisor first.
   d. Every student must consult their advisors first.

6. Which version of this sentence is grammatically correct? *Select all that apply.*
   a. Give it to Shirley and I.
   b. Give it to both Shirley and I.
   c. Give it to Shirley and me.
   d. Give it to me and Shirley.

7. What parts of speech are modified by adjectives? *Select all that apply.*
   a. Verbs
   b. Nouns
   c. Pronouns
   d. Prepositions

8. What part(s) of speech do adverbs modify? *Select all that apply.*
   a. Verbs
   b. Adverbs
   c. Adjectives
   d. Nouns

9. What accurately reflects expert advice for beginning writers regarding topic sentences?
   a. They should use topic sentences in every two to three paragraphs.
   b. They should vary topic sentence positioning in paragraphs.
   c. They should include a topic sentence in every paragraph.
   d. They should make each topic sentence broad and general.

10. Being familiar with English words such as *claustrophobia, photophobia, arachnophobia, hydrophobia, acrophobia,* etc. could help a reader determine that the Greek *phobos* means which of these?
   a. Love
   b. Fear
   c. Hate
   d. Know

11. Which of the following English words is derived from a Greek source?
   a. Move
   b. Motor
   c. Moron
   d. Mobile

12. Homophones are defined as which of these?
   a. They have the same sounds.
   b. They have the same spelling.
   c. They have the same meaning.
   d. They have the same roots.

13. The word *tear,* pronounced one way, means a drop of eye fluid; pronounced another way, it means to rip. What is this type of word called?
   a. A homograph
   b. A heteronym
   c. A homonym
   d. A synonym

14. Which of these words is considered a plural?
   a. Cactus
   b. Bacteria
   c. Criterion
   d. Elf

15. Which of the following sentences contains an example of passive voice?
   a. The poem was written by a student.
   b. The poem contained two metaphors and a simile.
   c. A student wrote the poem.
   d. A student decided to write a poem yesterday.

16. Which of the following are involved in prewriting? Select all that apply.
    a. Researching
    b. Revising
    c. Publishing
    d. Outlining

17. Which of the following sentences uses the apostrophe(s) correctly?
    a. Please be sure to bring you're invitation to the event.
    b. All of your friends' invitations were sent the same day.
    c. All of your friends parked they're cars along the street.
    d. Who's car is parked on the street leaving it's lights on?

18. Of the following, which word is spelled correctly?
    a. Wierd
    b. Forfeit
    c. Beleive
    d. Concieve

19. "I like writing, playing soccer, and eating" is an example of which grammatical convention?
    a. Appositive
    b. Complement
    c. Verbal
    d. Parallelism

20. Transition words can be used for all EXCEPT which of the following purposes?
    a. To explain
    b. To compare
    c. As conjunctions
    d. To replace a verb

21. Which of the following statements is true about the Oxford comma?
    a. It is the first comma in a series of three or more items.
    b. It is the last comma in a series before *or*, or before *and*.
    c. It is any comma separating items in series of three or more.
    d. It is frequently omitted because it does not serve a purpose.

22. In the following sentence, which version has the correct punctuation?
    a. Delegates attended from Springfield; Illinois, Alamo; Tennessee, Moscow; Idaho, and other places.
    b. Delegates attended from Springfield Illinois, Alamo Tennessee, Moscow Idaho, and other places.
    c. Delegates attended from Springfield, Illinois; Alamo, Tennessee; Moscow, Idaho; and other places.
    d. Delegates attended from Springfield, Illinois, Alamo, Tennessee, Moscow, Idaho, and other places.

23. Which of the following words means "the study of earth?"
    a. Philosophy
    b. Epistemology
    c. Geocentric
    d. Geology

24. Which task would most likely be completed last when writing?
    a. Developing a thesis statement and topic sentences
    b. Revising and editing for clarity and grammar
    c. Brainstorming and researching ideas
    d. Asking for feedback from others

25. Which of the following phrases correctly uses an apostrophe?
    a. Dennis and Pam's house
    b. Dennis's and Pam's house
    c. Dennis' and Pam's house
    d. Dennis's and Pam house

26. To make irregular plural nouns possessive, which of these correctly applies the rule for an apostrophe?
    a. Geeses' honks
    b. Childrens' toys
    c. Teeths' enamel
    d. Women's room

27. Which of the following is a writing technique recommended for attaining sentence fluency?
    a. Varying the endings of sentences
    b. Making sentence lengths uniform
    c. Using consistent sentence rhythm
    d. Varying sentence structures used

28. Among elements of an effective paragraph, the element of coherence is reflected by which of these?
    a. Focus on one main point throughout
    b. The use of logical and verbal bridges
    c. A sentence identifying the main idea
    d. Data, examples, illustrations, analysis

For questions 29-32, select the choice you think best fits the underlined part of the sentence. If the original is the best answer choice, then choose Choice A.

29. After getting a cat, Billy <u>learned the meaning of</u> take care of something other than himself.
    a. learned the meaning of
    b. learned what it meant to
    c. meant to learning the
    d. made to learn of the

30. A toothache does not always denote tooth decay or a cavity; sometimes <u>it was the direct</u> result of having a sinus infection.
    a. it was the direct
    b. it be the direct
    c. it directly was
    d. it is the direct

31. Play baseball, swimming, and dancing are three of Hannah's favorite ways to be active.
    a. Play baseball, swimming, and dancing
    b. Playing baseball; swimming; dancing;
    c. Playing baseball, to swim and to dance,
    d. Playing baseball, swimming, and dancing

32. I was shocked by the sound of the blast muting the television and went outside to see what happened.
    a. I was shocked by the sound of the blast muting
    b. I was shocked by the sound of the blast, muted
    c. Shocked at the sound of the blast, I muted
    d. The sound of the blast shocked me, muting

33. Based on the words *international*, *interaction*, and *intercept*, what does the prefix *inter-* mean?
    a. Through
    b. Between
    c. Across
    d. Behind

34. Samantha gathered research from seven different scholarly sources when writing a research paper on the Great Depression. She concluded her paper with her personal interpretation based on the information she learned from them. Does her conclusion require a citation, and why or why not?
    a. Yes, because she based her interpretation on the writings of other authors.
    b. Yes, because a personal interpretation is not an original idea.
    c. No, because she most likely cited her sources earlier in the paper.
    d. No, because a personal interpretation does not require citation.

35. Which of the following words means *unpleasant*? Select all that apply.
    a. Antipleasant
    b. Unappealing
    c. Distasteful
    d. Disappealing

36. Which of the following steps in the writing process involves gaining feedback from others?
    a. Conferencing
    b. Drafting
    c. Prewriting
    d. Revising

37. A suffix was added to a base word to form each of the following options. Which word with the suffix attached must be a different part of speech than the original word?
    a. Thankful
    b. Characteristic
    c. Talking
    d. Sailed

Answer Explanations

Reading

1. A: Choice *B* is incorrect because although it is obvious the author favors rehabilitation, the author never asks for donations from the audience. Choices *C* and *D* are also incorrect. We can infer from the passage that American prisons are probably harsher than Norwegian prisons. However, the best answer that captures the author's purpose is Choice *A,* because the author compares Norwegian and American prison recidivism rates.

2. D: The passage explains how a Norwegian prison, due to rehabilitation, has a smaller rate of recidivism. Thus, we can infer that recidivism is probably not a positive attribute. Choices *A* and *B* are both positive attributes, the lack of violence and the opportunity of inmates to receive therapy, so Norway would probably not have a lower rate of these two things. Choice *C* is possible, but it does not make sense in context, because the author does not talk about tactics to keep prisoners inside the compound, but ways in which to rehabilitate criminals so that they can live as citizens when they get out of prison.

3. 74 g. One serving contains 37 grams of carbohydrates. Therefore, two servings would be double that amount, or 74 g. Since the question asks how many carbohydrates would be consumed, it is important to include the unit, grams, in your answer.

4. C: Choice *C* is correct; we cannot infer that the passage takes place during the nighttime. While we do have a statement that says that the darkness thickened, this is the only evidence we have. The darkness could be thickening because it is foggy outside. We don't have enough proof to infer this otherwise. Choice *A* is incorrect; some of the evidence here is that "the cold became intense," and people were decorating their shops with "holly sprigs," a Christmas tradition. It also mentions that it's Christmas time at the end of the passage. Choice *B* is incorrect; we *can* infer that the narrative is located in a bustling city street by the actions in the story. People are running around trying to sell things, the atmosphere is busy, there is a church tolling the hours, etc. The scene switches to the Mayor's house at the end of the passage, but the answer says *majority,* so this is still incorrect. Choice *D* is incorrect; we *can* infer that the Lord Mayor is wealthy—he lives in the "Mansion House" and has fifty cooks.

5. A: Choice *A* is correct because, although we know from the title of the work that the passage is from *Frankenstein,* we cannot deduce from the passage itself that the creature mentioned is Frankenstein. In fact, the name Frankenstein in the novel is the name of the doctor, or the speaker of the text, and the creature remains unnamed throughout the entirety of the novel. Choice *B* is incorrect because we see that the speaker fears "that Henry should see him." Choice *C* is incorrect; we see the speaker trembling and terrified to "behold" the creature. Choice *D* is incorrect; we do have proof that the speaker is attending college with the sentence, "and we soon arrived at my college."

6. A: According to the map, Volcano Terevaka is the highest point on the island, reaching 507 m. Volcano Puakatike is the next highest, reaching 307 m. Vaka Kipo is the next highest reaching 216 m. Finally, Maunga Ana Marama is the next highest, reaching 165 m.

7. C: Choice *A* is too specific and is taken too literally. It is not that the architecture represents the builders; it represents the builder's culture. Choice *B* is also incorrect; we do see the words "at its worst as at its best," but the meaning of this is skewed in Choice *B.* Choice *D* is incorrect; the statement does not suggest this analysis.

8. B: The text talks about castles and cathedrals as examples of architecture from medieval Europe. Factories and skyscrapers are considered pre-modern or modern architecture. The term *canyons* is used as a metaphor for city streets, presumably surrounded by tall structures, so Choice *A* is incorrect.

9. B: The element listed under Group V, Period 6 in the table is Bi. The other elements are close by, but they do not fall under this group and period.

10. D: The author's description of the content of rhetoric provides three general principles. Each part parallels Choice *D* by logic, organization, and then style:

1. It taught them how to understand logic and reason (drawing inferences parallels to understanding the logistics of the game).

2. It taught them how to understand structure and organization (organization of material parallels to organization on the field).

3. It taught them how to make the end product beautiful (how to compose in harmonious sentences parallels to how to run with finesse and strength).

11. 60°. To determine this answer, refer to the Fahrenheit scale on the right side of the thermometer. The temperature line ends at about 62° F, so 60° F is the closest multiple of 5 and the correct answer.

12. B: Choices *A* and *D* are incorrect because they both contain cheese, and the doctor gave Sheila a list *without* dairy products. Choice *C* is incorrect because the doctor is also having Sheila stay away from eggs, and the omelet has eggs in it. Choice *B* is the best answer because it contains no meat, dairy, or eggs.

13. C: Following the directions carefully will result in this sentence. All the other sentences are close, but Choices *A, B,* and *D* leave at least one of the steps out.

14. D: According to the pie chart, Internet Explorer (I.E.) is the most used browser on Wikimedia. Following that is Firefox with 23.6% usage, Chrome with 20.6% usage, and Safari with 11.2% usage.

15. D: A glossary is a section in a book that provides brief definitions/explanations for words that the reader may not know. Choice *A* is incorrect because a table of contents shows where each section of the book is located. Choice *B* is incorrect because the introduction is usually a chapter that introduces the book about to be read. Choice *C* is incorrect because an index is usually a list of alphabetical references at the end of a book that a reader can look up to get more information.

16. B: This excerpt is considered a secondary source because it actively interprets primary sources. We see direct quotes from the queen, which would be considered a primary source. But since we see those quotes being interpreted and analyzed, the excerpt becomes a secondary source. Choice *C*, tertiary source, is an index of secondary and primary sources, like an encyclopedia or Wikipedia.

17. B: It took two years for the new castle to be built. The author states this in the first sentence of the second paragraph. In the third year, we see the Prince planning improvements and arranging things for the fourth year.

18. C: The sentence states that "the impress of his dear hand [has] been stamped everywhere". Choice *A* is one definition of *impress*, but this definition is used more as a verb than a noun: "She impressed us as a songwriter." Choice *B* is incorrect because it is also used as a verb: "He impressed the need for something to be done." Choice *D* is incorrect because it is part of a physical act: "the businessman impressed his mark upon the envelope." The phrase in the passage is meant as figurative, since the workmen did most of the physical labor, not the Prince.

19. A: The passage presents us with a sequence of events that happens in chronological order. Choice *B* is incorrect. Cause and effect organization would usually explain why something happened or list the effects of something. Choice *C* is incorrect because problem and solution organization would detail a problem and then present a solution to the audience, and there is no solution presented here. Finally, Choice *D* is incorrect. We are entered directly into the narrative without any main idea or any kind of argument being delivered.

20. C: A lead singer leaves their band to begin a solo career, and the band drops in sales by 50 percent on their next album. The original source of the analogy displays someone significant to an event who leaves, and then the event becomes worse for it. We see Mr. Sothern leaving the theater company, and then the play becoming a "very dull affair." Choice *A* depicts a dancer who backs out of an event before the final performance, so this is incorrect. Choice *B* shows a basketball player leaving an event, and then the team makes it to the championship but then loses. This choice could be a contestant for the right answer; however, we don't know if the team has become the worst for his departure or the better for it. We simply do not have enough information here. Choice *D* is incorrect. The actor departs an event, but there is no assessment of the quality of the movie. It simply states what actors filled in instead.

21. D: The context clues in the passage give hints to what is about to happen. The passage mentions John Wilkes Booth as "Mr. Booth," the man who shot Abraham Lincoln. The passage also mentions a "Mr. Ford," and we know that Lincoln was shot in Ford's theater. Finally, the passage mentions Mr. and Mrs. Lincoln. By adding all the clues together, along with our prior knowledge of history, it is probable that Booth is about to assassinate President Lincoln in Ford's theater.

22. C: The tone of this passage is neutral, since it is written in an academic/informative voice. It is important to look at the author's word choice to determine what the tone of a passage is. We have no indication that the author is excited, angry, or sorrowful at the effects of bacteria on milk, so Choices *A, B,* and *D* are incorrect.

23. A, C, and D: The passage states that the milk may get "soapy," that it can become "slimy," and that it may turn out to be a "beautiful sky-blue colour," making Choices *A, C,* and *D* correct. The milk turning black is not a reaction mentioned in the passage, so Choice *B* is incorrect.

24. A: In the sentence, we know that the word "curdle" means the opposite of "slimy." The words greasy, oily, and slippery are all very similar to the word slimy, making Choices *B, C,* and *D* incorrect. "Lumpy" means clotted, chunky, or thickened.

25. A: The passage mentions milk turning blue or tasting bad, and milk could possibly even make a milk-drinker sick if it has slimy threads. However, we know for sure that the slimy threads prove troublesome because it can become impossible to get rid of from this sentence: "Such an infection proves very troublesome, for many a time it persists in spite of all attempts made to remedy it."

26. A: The chemical change that occurs when a firework explodes. The author tells us that after milk becomes slimy, "it persists in spite of all attempts made to remedy it," which means the milk has gone through a chemical change. It has changed its state from milk to sour milk by changing its odor, color, and material. After a firework explodes, there is little one can do to change the substance of a firework back to its original form—the original substance has combusted and released its energy as heat and light.

Choice *B* is incorrect because, although the rain overwatered the plant, it's possible that the plant is able to recover from this. Choice *C* is incorrect because although mercury leaking out may be dangerous, the actual substance itself stays the same and does not alter into something else. Choice *D* is incorrect; this situation is not analogous to the alteration of a substance.

27. 125 mph. The highest number displayed on the odometer is 120 mph. There are five marks after the 120, making the top speed 125 mph.

28. 91,308 miles. The number of miles driven is shown by the digital numbers underneath the odometer.

29. A: We can guess that the word "despondent" means "depressed" by the end of the sentence. We see that although Olivia feels despondent, her sister can "cheer her up." When someone needs cheering up, they are usually sad or depressed about something. Joyful and humorous, Choices *B* and *D,* have opposite meanings of the word "despondent." Choice *C,* pathetic, is close, but Choice *A* is the best option for the context of the sentence.

30. D: Choice *A* is a characteristic of Portland but not that of a boom city. Choice *B* is close—a boom city is one that becomes quickly populated, but it is not necessarily always populated by residents from the east coast. Choice *C* is incorrect because a boom city is not one that catches fire frequently, but one made up of people who are looking to make quick fortunes from the resources provided on the land.

31. D: A city of legitimate business. We can see the proof in this sentence: "the cause of Portland's growth and prosperity is the trade which it has as the center of collection and distribution of this great wealth of natural resources, and it has attracted, not the boomer and speculator... but the merchant, manufacturer, and investor, who seek the surer if slower channels of legitimate business and investment." Choices *A, B,* and *C* are not mentioned in the passage and are incorrect.

32. B: Our first hint is in the title: *Oregon, Washington, and Alaska. Sights and Scenes for the Tourist.* Although the passage talks about business, there is no proposition included, which makes Choice *A* incorrect. Choice *C* is incorrect because the style of the writing is more informative and formal rather than personal and informal. Choice *D* is incorrect; this could possibly be a scholarly article, but the best choice is that it is a travel guide, due to the title and the details of what the city has to offer at the very end.

33. C: Metropolis means city. Portland is described as having agricultural valleys, but it is not solely a "farm" or "valley," making Choices *A* and *D* incorrect. We know from the description of Portland that it is more representative of a city than a countryside or country, making Choice *B* incorrect.

34. D: Choice *D* is the best answer because of the surrounding context. We can see that the fact that Portland is a "boom city" means that the "floating class" go through, a group of people who only have temporary roots put down. This would cause the main focus of the city to be on employment and industry, rather than society and culture. Choice *A* is incorrect, as we are not told about the inhabitants being social or antisocial. Choice *B* is incorrect because the text does not talk about the culture in the East regarding European influence. Finally, Choice *C* is incorrect; this is an assumption that has no evidence in the text to back it up.

35. B: The author would say that it has as much culture as the cities in the East. The author says that Portland has "as fine churches, as complete a system of schools, as fine residences, as great a love of music and art, as can be found at any city of the East of equal size," which proves that the culture is similar in this particular city to the cities in the East.

36. B: Look for the key words that give away the type of passage this is, such as "deities," "Greek hero," "centaur," and the names of demigods like Artemis. A eulogy is typically a speech given at a funeral, making Choice *A* incorrect. Choices *C* and *D* are incorrect, as "virgin huntresses" and "centaurs" are typically not found in historical or technical documents.

37. A: Based on the context of the passage, we can see that Hippolytus was a friend to Artemis because he "spent all his days in the greenwood chasing wild beasts" with her. The other choices are incorrect.

38. B: Although we don't have much context to go off of, this person is probably not a "lifetime partner" or "farm crop" of civilized life. These two do not make sense, so Choices *C* and *D* are incorrect. Choice *A* is also a bit strange. To be an "illegal immigrant" of civilized life is not a used phrase, making Choice *A* incorrect.

39. C: The list of ingredients on a food or drink label go from the most common ingredient found to the least common ingredient found. Water and corn syrup are both at the very top of the list. Cornstarch is found in the ingredients, but it is not at the top of the list.

40. 160 calories. You would consume 160 calories because one serving of this drink has 80 calories. If you double 80 calories, that gives you 160 calories.

41. A: The author is doing translation work. We see this very clearly in the way the author talks about staying truthful to the original language of the text. The text also mentions "translation" towards the end. Criticism is taking an original work and analyzing it, making Choice *B* incorrect. The work is not being tested for historical validity, but being translated into the English language, making Choice *C* incorrect. The author is not writing a biography, as there is nothing in here about Pushkin himself, only his work, making Choice *D* incorrect.

42. B: The author says that "music and rhythm and harmony are indeed fine things, but truth is finer still," which means that the author stuck to a literal translation instead of changing up any words that might make the English language translation sound better.

43. A: This is a central question to both passages. Choice *B* is incorrect; a quote mentions this at the end of the first passage, but this question is not found in the second passage. Choice *C* is incorrect, as the passages are not concerned with the definition of freedom of speech, but how to interpret it. Choice *D* is incorrect; this is a question for the second passage but is not found in the first passage.

44. C: The authors would most likely disagree over this answer choice. The author of Passage *A* says that "If a state may properly forbid murder or robbery or treason, it may also punish those who induce or counsel the commission of such crimes." This statement tells us that the author of Passage *A* would support throwing the man in jail for encouraging a riot, although no violence ensues. The author of Passage *B* states that "And we can with certitude declare that the First Amendment forbids the punishment of words merely for their injurious tendencies." This is the best answer choice because we are clear on each author's stance in this situation.

Choice *A* is tricky; the author of Passage *A* would definitely agree with this, but it's questionable whether the author of Passage *B* would agree with this. Violence does ensue at the capitol as a result of this man's provocation, and the author of Passage *B* states "speech should be unrestricted by the censorship . . . unless it is clearly liable to cause direct... interference with the conduct of war." This answer is close, but it is not the *best* choice. Choice *B* is incorrect because we have no way of knowing what the authors' philosophies are in this situation. Choice *D* is incorrect because, again, we have no way of knowing what the authors would do in this situation, although it's assumed they would probably both agree with this.

45. A: Choice *A* is the best answer. To figure out the correct answer choice we must find out the relationship between Passage *A* and Passage *B*. Between the two passages, we have a general principle (freedom of speech) that is questioned on the basis of interpretation. In Choice *A*, we see that we have a general principle (right to die, or euthanasia) that is questioned on the basis of interpretation as well. Should euthanasia only include passive euthanasia, or euthanasia in any aspect? Choice *B* is incorrect because it does not question the interpretation of a principle, but rather describes the effects of two events that happened in the past involving contamination of radioactive substances. Choice *C* begins with a principle—that of labor laws during wartime—but in the second option, the interpretation isn't questioned. The second option looks at the historical precedent of labor laws in the past during wartime. Choice *D* is incorrect because the two texts disagree over the cause of something rather than the interpretation of it.

Mathematics

1. B: The fraction $\frac{12}{60}$ can be reduced to $\frac{1}{5}$, in lowest terms. First, it must be converted to a decimal. Dividing 1 by 5 results in 0.2. Then, to convert to a percentage, move the decimal point two units to the right and add the percentage symbol. The result is 20%.

2. B: If a calculator is used, divide 14 into 33 and keep two decimal places. If a calculator is not used, multiply both the numerator and denominator by 3. This results in the fraction $\frac{42}{99}$, and hence a decimal of 0.42.

3. B: Common denominators must be used. The LCD is 15, and $\frac{2}{5} = \frac{6}{15}$. Therefore, $\frac{14}{15} + \frac{6}{15} = \frac{20}{15}$, and in lowest terms, the answer is $\frac{4}{3}$. A common factor of 5 was divided out of both the numerator and denominator.

4. A: A product is found by multiplication. Multiplying two fractions together is easier when common factors are canceled first to avoid working with larger numbers:

$$\frac{5}{14} \times \frac{7}{20} = \frac{5}{2 \times 7} \times \frac{7}{5 \times 4}$$

$$\frac{1}{2} \times \frac{1}{4} = \frac{1}{8}$$

5. D: Division is completed by multiplying by the reciprocal. Therefore:

$$24 \div \frac{8}{5} = \frac{24}{1} \times \frac{5}{8}$$

$$\frac{3 \times 8}{1} \times \frac{5}{8} = \frac{15}{1} = 15$$

6. C: A common denominator must be used to subtract fractions. Remember that in order to find the least common denominator, the least common multiple of both of the denominators must be determined. The smallest multiple that 24 and 14 share is 168, which is 24×7 and 14×12. This means that the LCD is 168, so each fraction must be converted to have 168 as the denominator.

$$\frac{5}{24} - \frac{5}{14} = \frac{5}{24} \times \frac{7}{7} - \frac{5}{14} \times \frac{12}{12}$$

$$\frac{35}{168} - \frac{60}{168} = -\frac{25}{168}$$

7. C: The correct mathematical statement is the one in which the smaller of the two numbers is on the "less than" side of the inequality symbol. It is written in Choice C that $\frac{1}{3} > -\frac{4}{3}$, which is the same as $-\frac{4}{3} < \frac{1}{3}$, a correct statement.

8. C: $-\frac{1}{5} > \frac{4}{5}$ is an incorrect statement. The expression on the left is negative, which means that it is smaller than the expression on the right. As it is written, the inequality states that the expression on the left is greater than the expression on the right, which is not true.

9. A: First, the distributive property must be used on the left side. This results in:

$$3x + 6 = 14x - 5$$

The addition principle is then used to add 5 to both sides, and then to subtract $3x$ from both sides, resulting in $11 = 11x$. Finally, the multiplication principle is used to divide each side by 11. Therefore, $x = 1$ is the solution.

10. B: The outlier is 35. When a small outlier is removed from a data set, the mean and the median increase. The first step in this process is to identify the outlier, which is the number that lies away from the given set. Once the outlier is identified, the mean and median can be recalculated. The mean will be affected because it averages all of the numbers. The median will be affected because it finds the middle number, which is subject to change because a number is lost. The mode will most likely not change because it is the number that occurs the most, which will not be the outlier if there is only one outlier.

11. B: The distributive property is used on both sides to obtain:

$$4x + 20 + 6 = 4x + 6$$

Then, like terms are collected on the left, resulting in:

$$4x + 26 = 4x + 6$$

Next, the addition principle is used to subtract $4x$ from both sides, and this results in the false statement $26 = 6$. Therefore, there is no solution.

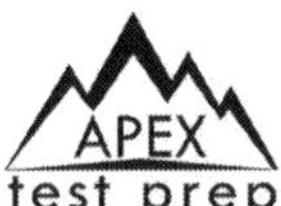

		1	1
	/	/	
.	.	.	.
0	0	0	0
1	1	1	1
2	2	2	2
3	3	3	3
4	4	4	4
5	5	5	5
6	6	6	6
7	7	7	7
8	8	8	8
9	9	9	9

12. This is a one-step, real-world application problem. The unknown quantity is the number of cases of cola to be purchased. Let x be equal to this amount. Because each case costs \$3.50, the total number of cases multiplied by \$3.50 must equal \$40. This translates to the mathematical equation $3.5x = 40$. Divide both sides by 3.5 to obtain $x = 11.4286$, which has been rounded to four decimal places. Because cases are sold whole, and there is not enough money to purchase 12 cases, 11 cases is the correct answer.

13. A: First, the variables have to be defined. Let x be the first integer; therefore, $x + 1$ is the second integer. This is a two-step problem. The sum of three times the first and two less than the second is translated into the following expression:

$$3x + (x + 1 - 2)$$

Set this expression equal to 411 to obtain:

$$3x + (x + 1 - 2) = 411$$

The left-hand side is simplified to obtain:

$$4x - 1 = 411$$

To solve for x, first add 1 to both sides and then divide both sides by 4 to obtain $x = 103$. The next consecutive integer is 104.

14. B: First, the information is translated into the ratio $\frac{15}{80}$. To find the percentage, translate this fraction into a decimal by dividing 15 by 80. The corresponding decimal is 0.1875. Move the decimal point two units to the right to obtain the percentage 18.75%.

15. 21: Gina answered 60% of 35 questions correctly; 60% can be expressed as the decimal 0.60. Therefore, she answered $0.60 \times 35 = 21$ questions correctly.

16. D: The median is the value in the middle of a data set. In the set of 11, 12, 12, 13, 15, 16, and 19 seconds, the value in the middle is 13 seconds, making it the median. 12 seconds represents the mode, as it is the value that occurs the most. 14 seconds represents the mean, as it is the sum of all seven listed times divided by seven.

17. B: If sales tax is 7.25%, the price of the car must be multiplied by 1.0725 to account for the additional sales tax. This is the same as multiplying the initial price by 0.0725 (the tax) and adding that to the initial cost. Therefore,

$$15{,}395 \times 1.0725 = 16{,}511.1375$$

This amount is rounded to the nearest cent, which is $16,511.14.

18. A: Rounding can be used to find the best approximation. All of the values can be rounded to the nearest thousand. 15,412 SUVs can be rounded to 15,000. 25,815 station wagons can be rounded to 26,000. 50,412 sedans can be rounded to 50,000. 8,123 trucks can be rounded to 8,000. Finally, 18,312 hybrids can be rounded to 18,000. The sum of the rounded values is 117,000, which is closest to 120,000.

19. D: There are 52 weeks in a year, and if the family spends $105 each week, that amount is close to $100. A good approximation is $100 a week for 50 weeks, which is found through the product:

$$50 \times \$100 = \$5{,}000$$

20. C: This problem involves ratios and proportions. If 12 packets are needed for every 5 people, this statement is equivalent to the ratio $\frac{12}{5}$. The unknown amount x is the number of ketchup packets needed for 60 people. The proportion $\frac{12}{5} = \frac{x}{60}$ must be solved. Cross-multiply to obtain $12 \times 60 = 5x$. Therefore, $720 = 5x$. Divide each side by 5 to obtain $x = 144$.

21. D: There were 48 total bags of apples sold. If 9 bags were Granny Smith and the rest were Red Delicious, then $48 - 9 = 39$ bags were Red Delicious. Therefore, the ratio of Granny Smith to Red Delicious is 9:39.

22. B: The average rate of change is found by calculating the difference in dollars over the elapsed time. Therefore, the rate of change is equal to $(\$4{,}900 - \$4{,}000) \div 3$ months, which is equal to $\$900 \div 3$, or $300 per month.

23. A: Let x be the unknown, the number of hours Erin can work. We know Katie works $2x$, and the sum of all hours is less than 21. Therefore, $x + 2x < 21$, which simplifies into $3x < 21$. Solving this results in the inequality $x < 7$ after dividing both sides by 3. Therefore, Erin can work less than 7 hours.

24. B, C: The chart is a bar chart showing how many men and women prefer each genre of movies. The dark gray bars represent the number of women, while the light gray bars represent the number of men. The light gray bars are higher and represent more men than women for the genres of Comedy and Action.

25. B: A line graph represents continuous change over time. The line on the graph is continuous and not broken, as on a scatter plot. A bar graph may show change but isn't necessarily continuous over time. A pie graph is better for representing percentages of a whole. Histograms are best used in grouping sets of data in bins to show the frequency of a certain variable.

26. C: The mean for the number of visitors during the first 4 hours is 14. The mean is found by calculating the average for the four hours. Adding up the total number of visitors during those hours gives:

$$12 + 10 + 18 + 16 = 56$$

Dividing total number of visitors by four hours gives the average number of visitors per hour:

$$56 \div 4 = 14$$

27. C: The mode for a set of data is the value that occurs the most. The grade that appears the most is 95. It's the only value that repeats in the set.

28. B: The relationship between age and time for attention span is a positive correlation because the general trend for the data is up and to the right. As the age increases, so does attention span.

29. A: The area of the shaded region is calculated in a few steps. First, the area of the rectangle is found using the formula:

$$A = length \times width = 6\text{ m} \times 2\text{ m} = 12\text{ m}^2$$

Second, the area of the triangle is found using the formula:

$$A = \frac{1}{2} \times base \times height = \frac{1}{2} \times 3\text{ m} \times 2\text{ m} = 3\text{ m}^2$$

The last step is to take the rectangle area and subtract the triangle area. The area of the shaded region is:

$$A = 12\text{ m}^2 - 3\text{ m}^2 = 9\text{ m}^2$$

30. D: The volume for a cylinder is found by using the formula:

$$V = \pi r^2 h = \pi (2\text{ in})^2 \times 3.5\text{ in} = 43.96\text{ in}^3$$

31. C: There are 0.006 kiloliters in 6 liters because 1 liter is 0.001 kiloliters. The conversion comes from the metric prefix, *kilo-*, which has a value of 1,000. Thus, 1 kiloliter is 1,000 liters, and 1 liter is 0.001 kiloliters.

32. B: The conversion between feet and centimeters requires a middle term. Since there are 2.54 centimeters in 1 inch, the conversion between inches and feet must be used first. As there are 12 inches in a foot, the fractions can be set up as follows:

$$3\text{ ft} \times \frac{12\text{ in}}{1\text{ ft}} \times \frac{2.54\text{ cm}}{1\text{ in}}$$

The feet and inches units cancel out to leave only centimeters as units for the answer. The numbers are calculated across the top and bottom to yield:

$$\frac{3 \times 12 \times 2.54}{1 \times 1} = 91.44$$

The number and units used together form the answer of 91.44 cm.

33. A: The formula for the rate of change is the same as slope: change in y over change in x. The y-value in this case is percentage of smokers and the x-value is year. The change in percentage of smokers from 2000 to 2015 was 8.1%. The change in x was $2000 - 2015 = -15$. Therefore:

$$\frac{8.1\%}{-15} = -0.54\%$$

The percentage of smokers decreased 0.54% each year.

34. A: Surface area is a type of area, which means it is measured in square units. Cubic units are used to describe volume, which has three dimensions multiplied by one another. Quartic units describe measurements multiplied in four dimensions.

35. A: A vertical line has the same x-value for any point on the line. Other points on the line would be $(1,3)$, $(1,5)$, $(1,9)$, etc. Mathematically, this is written as $x = 1$. A vertical line is always of the form $x = a$ for some constant a.

36. D: The area for a rectangle is found by multiplying the length by the width. The area is also measured in square units, so the correct answer is Choice *D*. The number 26 in Choice *A* is incorrect because it is the perimeter. Choice *B* is incorrect because the answer must be in centimeters squared. The number 13 in Choice *C* is incorrect because it is the sum of the two dimensions rather than the product of them.

37. C: There are approximately 11 pounds in 5 kilograms, because 1 kilogram is approximately 2.2 pounds (around 2.2046226). Multiplying 5 kg by 2.2 gives 11 lbs; while not exact, 11 lbs is the closest answer provided.

38. B: Look on the horizontal axis to find 3:00 p.m. Move up from 3:00 p.m. to reach the dot on the graph. Move horizontally to the left to the horizontal axis to between 20 and 25; the best answer choice is 22. The answer of 25 is too high above the projected time on the graph, and the answers of 20 and 16 degrees are too low.

Science

1. A: There are only two hundred different types of cells in the human body. While there are trillions of cells that make up the human body, only two hundred different types make up that trillion, each with a specific function.

2. C: Connective tissue is located only on the inside of the body and fills internal spaces. This allows it to protect the organs within the body. Epithelial tissue is found on the outside of the body and as a lining of internal cavities and passageways. Muscle tissue allows for movement of the body. Neural tissue sends information from the brain to the rest of the body through electrical impulses.

3. D: After air enters the nose or mouth, it gets passed on to the sinuses. The sinuses regulate temperature and humidity before passing the air on to the rest of the body. Volume of air can change with varying temperatures and humidity levels, so it is important for the air to be a constant temperature and humidity before being processed by the lungs. The larynx is the voice box of the body, making Choice *A* incorrect. The lungs are responsible for oxygen and carbon dioxide exchange between the air that is breathed in and the blood that is circulating the body, making Choice *B* incorrect. The trachea takes the temperature- and humidity-regulated air from the sinuses to the lungs, making Choice *C* incorrect.

4.

1. **Prophase**
2. **Metaphase**
3. **Anaphase**
4. **Telophase**

Preceded by interphase, the steps of meiosis 1 are prophase, metaphase, anaphase, and telophase.

5. A: The nucleus contains the protons and neutrons of the atom. Together, they make up 99 percent of the atom's mass. Electrons, Choice *D,* are found in the orbitals surrounding the nucleus and do not have as much mass as the protons or neutrons. Protons and neutrons, Choices *B* and *C,* have similar masses, but neither makes up 99 percent of the atom's mass alone.

6. C: The total number of protons and neutrons in an atom is the atom's mass number. The number of protons in an atom is the atomic number. If an atom has a variation in the number of neutrons, the atom's mass number changes, but the atomic number remains the same. This variation creates isotopes of the atom with the same atomic number. The number of protons, Choice *A,* is unique for each atom and does not change. The number of orbitals remains the same for atoms; therefore, Choice *B* is incorrect. The number of electrons, Choice *D,* affects the charge of the atom.

7. A: The mitral valve is also known as the bicuspid valve because it has two leaflets. It is located on the left side of the heart between the atrium and the ventricle. The pulmonary valve, Choice *B,* is located between the right ventricle and the pulmonary artery and has three cusps. The aortic valve, Choice *C,* is located between the left ventricle and the aorta and also has three cusps. The tricuspid valve, Choice *D,* has three leaflets and is located on the right side of the heart between the atrium and the ventricle.

8. B: White blood cells are part of the immune system and help fight off diseases. Red blood cells contain hemoglobin, which carries oxygen through the blood. Plasma is the liquid matrix of the blood. Platelets help with the clotting of the blood.

9. D: Viruses are not classified as living organisms. They are neither prokaryotic or eukaryotic; therefore, they don't belong to any of the answer choices.

10. A: During digestion, complex food molecules are broken down into smaller molecules so that nutrients can be isolated and absorbed by the body. Absorption, Choice *B,* is when vitamins, electrolytes, organic molecules, and water are absorbed by the digestive epithelium. Compaction, Choice *C,* occurs when waste products are dehydrated and compacted. Ingestion, Choice *D,* is when food and liquids first enter the body through the mouth.

11. D: The gallbladder is the organ that is responsible for storing and concentrating bile before secreting it into the small intestine. The liver, Choice *A,* is responsible for producing bile. The pancreas, Choice *B,* is responsible for secreting specific digestive enzymes for different types of food. The stomach, Choice *C,* is where digestion occurs.

12. B: Prokaryotic cells divide by binary fission, Choice *B,* which is a fast process that takes approximately 30 minutes and results in two identical daughter cells. They do not undergo more complex processes, such as meiosis and mitosis, Choices *A* and *C*. For survival, prokaryotic cells must divide and produce daughter cells, so Choice *D* is incorrect.

13. B: Neurons are responsible for transferring and processing information between the brain and other parts of the body. Neuroglia are cells that protect delicate neurons by making a frame around them. They also help to maintain a homeostatic environment around the neurons.

14. C: The autonomic nerve system is part of the efferent division of the peripheral nervous system (PNS). It controls involuntary muscles, such as smooth muscle and cardiac muscle, which are responsible for regulating heart rate, blood pressure, and body temperature. The central nervous system, Choice *A*, includes only the brain and the spinal cord. The somatic nervous system, Choice *B*, is also part of the efferent division of the PNS and controls voluntary skeletal muscle contractions, allowing for body movements. The afferent division of the PNS, Choice *D*, relays sensory information within the body.

15. A: The testes are the main reproductive organ of the male reproductive system. They are the gonads; they secrete androgens and produce and store sperm cells. The prostate, vas deferens, and bulbourethral glands are all accessory organs of the male reproductive system. The prostate provides nourishment to sperm, the vas deferens transports sperm to the urethra, and the bulbourethral glands produce lubricating fluid for the urethra.

16. B: The ovaries produce only one mature gamete each month. If it is fertilized, the result is a zygote that develops into an embryo. The male reproductive system produces one-half billion sperm cells each day.

17. D: Once sperm enter the vagina, they travel through the uterus to the fallopian tubes to fertilize a mature oocyte. The ovaries are responsible for producing the mature oocyte. The mammary glands produce nutrient-filled milk to nourish babies after birth.

18. B: The regenerative capacity of an organism is its ability to generate new body parts after injury. A lizard losing its tail and growing a new one is an example of regenerative capacity, making Choice *B* the correct answer. Choices *A*, *C*, and *D* describe situations where new growth does not occur, with the flatworm dying, the starfish remaining without an arm, and cardiac tissue remaining damaged.

19. A: The skin has three major functions: protection, regulation, and sensation. It has a large supply of blood vessels that can dilate to allow heat loss when the body is too hot and constrict in order to retain heat when the body is cold. The organs of the respiratory system are responsible for breathing, and the mouth is responsible for ingestion.

20. B: The nails on a person's hands and feet provide a hard layer of protection over the soft skin underneath. The hair, Choice *A*, helps to protect against heat loss, provides sensation, and can filter air that enters the nose. The sweat glands, Choice *C*, help to regulate temperature. The sebaceous glands, Choice *D*, secrete sebum, which protects the skin from water loss and bacterial and fungal infections.

21. D: The tissues and glands of the endocrine system are all ductless. They secrete hormones, not bile, into the blood or interstitial fluid of the human body. The endocrine system has a slow, long-lasting response to stimuli, unlike the nervous system, whose response is quick and short termed.

22.

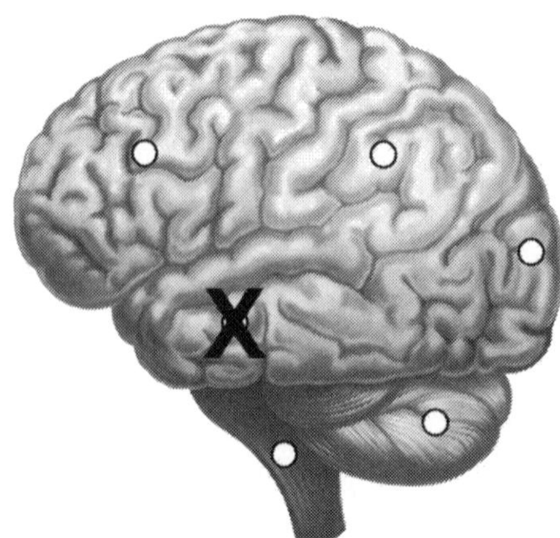

23. C: Acidic amino acids, Choice *C*, have positively charged side chains, whereas basic amino acids, Choice *A*, have negatively charged side chains. Hydrophilic, Choice *B*, and hydrophobic, Choice *D*, describe how the side chains interact with water molecules.

24. A: The kidneys are the main organs responsible for filtering waste products out of the bloodstream. The kidneys have millions of nephrons, which are tiny filtering units that filter 120 to 150 quarts of blood each day and produce waste, approximately one to two quarts of urine daily. The urinary bladder is responsible for storing urine. The pancreas is responsible for regulating blood sugar levels. The urethra is the passageway through which urine exits the body.

25. A: The only true statement provided is that DNA is the genetic code. Choice *B* is incorrect because DNA does not provide energy—that's the job of carbohydrates and glucose. Choice *C* is incorrect because DNA is double-stranded. Because Choices *B* and *C* are incorrect, Choice *D*, all of the above, is also incorrect.

26. C: The urinary bladder is a hollow, elastic muscular organ. As it fills with urine, the walls stretch without breaking—due to their elasticity—and become thinner. When the urine is emptied, the bladder returns to its original size. The urinary bladder does not secrete any fluids into the urine; it is a storage organ for urine. Pressure inside the urinary bladder does not increase as it is filled because the organ grows larger while filling.

27. A: The innate immune system works based on pattern recognition of similar pathogens that have already been encountered. It does not remember specific pathogens or provide an individually-specific response. The responses it provides are short term and do not work toward long-lasting immunity for the body. The adaptive immune system creates a memory of each specific pathogen that has been encountered and provides a pathogen-specific response. This works toward the long-term immunity of the body. Hormones are secreted by the endocrine system in response to stimuli. B cells are lymphocytes that work to provide immunity as part of the adaptive immune system.

28. B: The adaptive immune system provides target-specific antibodies to fight against individual pathogens that are encountered. It does not send out a broad range of antibodies because it has memory of the previously encountered pathogens. Mechanical and chemical barriers are part of the innate immune system and do not provide target-specific immunity.

29. D: If the immune system is not functioning properly, it may begin to attack its own healthy cells, which can result in an autoimmune disorder, such as celiac disease, type I diabetes, or rheumatoid arthritis. The adaptive and innate immune systems are the two parts of the body's immune system that need to be working properly to protect the body from pathogens. Lymphocytes are specialized cells that help the adaptive immune system provide target-specific responses to pathogens.

30. B: The elements are arranged such that the elements in columns have similar chemical properties, such as appearance and reactivity. Each element has a unique atomic number, not the same one, so Choice *A* is incorrect. Elements are arranged in rows, not columns, with similar electron valence configurations, so Choice *C* is incorrect. Density is a physical property, not a chemical one, so elements in columns do not necessarily have the same density. Furthermore, the density of an element depends on the state it is in.

31. D: Spongy bone is porous and lightweight, but also very strong. It covers the outside of dense, compact bone and has a shiny, white appearance. Compact bone is densely filled with organic and inorganic salts, leaving only tiny spaces for osteocytes within the matrix.

32. C: The pH scale goes from 0 to 14. A neutral solution falls right in the middle of the scale at 7. Choice *A,* a value of 13, indicates a strong base. Choice *B,* a value of 8, indicates a solution that is weakly basic. Choice *D,* 0, indicates a strong acid.

33. A: Monosaccharides are the simplest sugars that make up carbohydrates. They are important for cellular respiration. Fatty acids, Choice *B,* make up lipids. Polysaccharides, Choice *C,* are larger molecules with repeating monosaccharide units. Amino acids, Choice *D,* are the building blocks of proteins.

34. D: Nucleic acids include DNA and RNA, which are strands of nucleotides that contain genetic information. Carbohydrates, Choice *A,* are made up of sugars that provide energy to the body. Lipids, Choice *B,* are hydrocarbon chains that make up fats. Proteins, Choice *C,* are made up of amino acids that help with many functions for maintaining life.

35. B: Genes are the primary unit of inheritance between generations of an organism. Humans each have twenty-three pairs of chromosomes, Choice *A*, and each chromosome contains hundreds to thousands of genes. Genes each control a specific trait of the organism. Gametes, Choice *C,* are the reproductive cells that contain all of the genetic information of an individual. Atoms, Choice *D,* are the small units that make up all substances.

36. C: The Law of Independent Assortment states that the alleles for different traits are inherited independently of one another. For example, the alleles for eye color are not linked to the alleles for hair color. So, someone could have blue eyes and brown hair or blue eyes and blond hair. The Law of Dominance, Choice *A,* states that one allele has a stronger effect on phenotype than the other allele. The Law of Segregation, Choice *B,* states that each trait has two versions that can be inherited. Each parent contributes one of its alleles, selected randomly, to the daughter offspring.

37. C: Atoms are considered neutral when the number of protons and electrons is equal. Protons carry a positive charge, and electrons carry a negative charge. When they are equal in number, their charges cancel out, and the atom is neutral. If there are more electrons than protons, or vice versa, the atom has an electric charge and is termed an ion. Neutrons do not have a charge and do not affect the electric charge of an atom.

38. A: Physical properties of substances are those that can be observed without changing the substances' chemical composition, such as odor, color, density, and hardness. Reactivity, flammability, and toxicity are all chemical properties of substances. They describe the way in which a substance may change into a different substance. They cannot be observed without chemically changing the substance.

39. B: Solids have molecules that are packed together tightly and cannot move within their substance. Crystalline solids have atoms or molecules that are arranged symmetrically, making all of the bonds of even strength. When they are broken, they break along a plane of molecules, creating a straight edge. Amorphous solids do not have the symmetrical makeup of crystalline solids, so they do not break evenly. Gases and liquids both have molecules that move around freely.

40. A: Chemical reactions are processes that involve the changing of one set of substances to a different set of substances. In order to accomplish this, the bonds between the atoms in the molecules of the original substances need to be broken. The atoms are rearranged, and new bonds are formed to make the new set of substances. Combination reactions involve two or more reactants becoming one product. Decomposition reactions involve one reactant becoming two or more products. Combustion reactions involve the use of oxygen as a reactant and generally include the burning of a substance. Choices *C* and *D* are not discussed as specific reaction types.

41. A: Scientific notation is a useful system for representing numbers that are very large or very small and cannot be written out without having multiple zeros behind a number in the case of large numbers, or behind a decimal point in the case of small numbers. Any number can be written in scientific notation—there are no restrictions on the digits that comprise the number, as suggested in Choice *B*. While scientific notation is often useful in scientific experiments, it is not used exclusively in this context nor is it mandatory in experiments. For example, if the mass of a substance is measured to be 3.5 g, the investigator would likely report this value rather than convert it to scientific notation (in this case, the number of significant figures is more important). Therefore, Choice *C* is incorrect. Scientific notation is most helpful for numbers larger than 100 or much smaller than 0, making Choice *D* incorrect.

42. D: A Vernier Scale is used to measure small fractions within already small divisions. Choices *A*, *B*, and *C* are used for measuring short distances, yet do not go as small as the Vernier Scale.

43. D: Scientific experiments are found reliable when they can be replicated and produce comparable results regardless of who is conducting them or making the observations, making Choice *B* incorrect. Choice *A* is incorrect, although having all the materials needed is ideal for conducting an experiment. Choice *C* is incorrect; a hypothesis is never proven correct, but it can receive credibility if the data supports it in that particular experiment.

44. A, C: It is possible that the increase in stomach cancer was caused by a factor other than the contaminated drinking water. Neither is the power outage necessarily connected to the thunderstorm or flooding. The two events could have just happened at the same time, which is correlation, not causation. The other two choices are very clear examples of cause and effect. We know for a fact that water boils when it becomes hot enough, and we know that earthquakes are caused by tectonic plates shifting.

45. D: Microscopes magnify objects that are too small to see with the human eye. Microscopes do not reduce the size of objects that are too big. Objects that are reflected in a mirror can be seen with the unaided eye. Telescopes allow you to see objects that are far away. Therefore, Choice *A*, *B*, and *C* are incorrect.

46. B: Formulating a hypothesis means writing out an expectation of what's going to happen. The hypothesis comes after the experimental question, which is forming a question that relates to the observation, making Choice *A* incorrect. Gathering the materials needed for the procedure is the step where we actually conduct the experiment, making Choice *C* incorrect. Summarizing the results of the experiment is the conclusion, making Choice *D* incorrect.

47. C: After the experiment is over and before it is published. A peer review is when other scientists review the experiment's findings in order to test its validity and methods. Peer review is an important part of scientific research and is a way for the scientific community to provide feedback for the experiment.

48. B: According to Table 1, Sample 3 is made up of 45 percent silt and 35 percent clay. Sand comprised only 20 percent of the sample. Therefore, Choices *A, C,* and *D* are incorrect.

49. C: According to Table 2, sand particles can have a size of 1.7 mm. Of the options listed, sample 4 has the highest percent of sand, so Choice *C* is the best option. Choice *D,* Sample 5, also has a higher percent of sand, but still less than Sample 4.

50. A: Vaccinations introduce and encourage immunity to specific contagious diseases. When large populations are vaccinated and develop immunity, this mitigates the presence of specific communicable diseases within that population. It protects the few who may not have been vaccinated through the practice of herd immunity (the larger vaccinated group is able to prevent introduction and spread of the specific disease for which the group has been vaccinated). Car travel and avoiding persons who travel do not necessarily limit interactions that would prevent the spread of communicable disease. Biotin is a vitamin that promotes hair, nail, and skin strength; it is not involved in immunity or disease prevention.

English & Language Usage

1. A, B, and D: Good ways to improve writing style through grammatical choices include alternating among simple, complex, compound, and compound-complex sentence structures Choice *A* to prevent monotony and ensure variety; using fewer words when more words are unnecessary Choice *B*; and writing in the active voice more often than in the passive voice Choice *D*. Active voice uses fewer words and also emphasizes action more strongly. Writing all simple sentences with only one subject and one verb each is NOT a good way to improve writing style, so Choice *C* is incorrect.

2. D: The topic sentence in a paragraph may be stated explicitly, or it may only be implied Choice *D*, requiring the reader to infer what the topic is rather than identify it as an overt statement. The topic sentence of a paragraph is often at or near the beginning, but not always Choice *A*. Some topic sentences are at the ends of paragraphs but not always Choice *B*. There is more than one topic sentence in an essay, especially if the essay is built on multiple paragraphs Choice *C*.

3. A: Criteria for a good paragraph topic sentence include clarity, emphasis rather than subtlety Choice *B*, brevity rather than length Choice *C*, and straightforwardness rather than ambiguousness Choice *D*.

4. B: The sentence lacks subject-verb agreement. Three nouns require the plural "are," not the singular "is." A misplaced modifier Choice *A* is incorrectly positioned, modifying the wrong part. For example, in Groucho Marx's famous joke, "One morning I shot an elephant in my pajamas. How he got into my pajamas I don't know" (*Animal Crackers,* 1930), he refers in the second sentence to the misplaced modifier in the first. A dangling participle Choice *C* leaves a verb participle hanging by omitting the subject it describes; e.g. "Walking down the street, the house was on fire."

5. B: Choice *A* lacks pronoun-antecedent agreement: "Every student" is singular but "their" is plural. Choice *B* correctly combines plural "All students" with plural "their advisors." Choice *C* has plural "All students" but singular "his advisor." Choice *D* has singular "Every student" but plural "their advisors."

6. C: When compounding subjects by adding nouns including proper nouns (names) to pronouns, the pronoun's form should not be changed by the addition. Since "Give it to me" is correct, not "Give it to I," we would not write "Give it to Shirley and I" Choice *A* or "Give it to both Shirley and I" Choice *B*. "Shirley" and "me" is correct, Choice *C*. "Give it to" requires an object. Only "me," "us," "him," "her," and "them" can be objects; "I," "we," "he," "she," and "they" are used as subjects but never as objects. Choice *D* is wrong because the "I" or "me" always goes last in a list.

7. B and C: Adjectives modify nouns Choice *B* or pronouns Choice *C* by describing them. For example, in the phrase "a big, old, red house," the noun "house" is modified and described by the adjectives "big," "old," and "red." Adjectives do not modify prepositions Choice *D* or verbs Choice *A*.

8. A, B, and C: Adverbs modify verbs Choice *A*, other adverbs Choice *B*, or adjectives Choice *C*. For example, in "She slept soundly," the verb is "slept" and the adverb modifying it is "soundly." In "He finished extremely quickly," the adverb "extremely" modifies the adverb "quickly." In "She was especially enthusiastic," the adverb "especially" modifies the adjective "enthusiastic." Adjectives, not adverbs, modify nouns Choice *D*.

9. C: Experts advise students/beginning writers to include a topic sentence in every paragraph. Although professional writers do not always do this, beginners should, to learn how to write good topic sentences and paragraphs, rather than include a topic sentence in only every second or third paragraph Choice *A*. Although experienced writers can also vary the positioning of topic sentences within paragraphs, experts advise new/learning writers to start paragraphs with topic sentences Choice *B*. A topic sentence should be narrow and restricted, not broad and general Choice *D*.

10. B: *Phobos* means "fear" in Greek. From it, English has derived the word *phobia*, meaning an abnormal or exaggerated fear and a multitude of other words ending in *-phobia*, whose beginnings specify the object of the fear, as in the examples given. Another ubiquitous English word part deriving from Greek is *phil* as a prefix or suffix, meaning love Choice *A*, such as *philosophy*, *hydrophilic*, *philanthropist*, and *philharmonic*. The Greek word for hate Choice *C* is *miseo*, found in English words like *misogyny* and *misanthrope*. The Greek word meaning wise or knowledge Choice *D* is *sophos*, found in English words such as *sophisticated* and *philosophy*.

11. C: The English word *moron* is derived from the Greek *mor-* meaning dull or foolish. *Sophomore* also combines *soph* from Greek *sophos*, meaning wise, with *mor*—i.e. literally "wise fool." The words *move* Choice *A*, *motor* Choice *B*, *mobile* Choice *D*, and many others are all derived from the Latin *mot-* or *mov-*, from the Latin words *movere*, to move and *motus*, motion.

12. A: Homophones are words that are pronounced the same way but are spelled differently and have different meanings. For example, *lax* and *lacks* are homophones. Words spelled the same Choice *B* but with different meanings are homographs. Words with the same meaning, Choice *C*, are synonyms, which are spelled and pronounced differently.

13. A and B: Words that are spelled the same way are homographs, Choice *A*; if they are pronounced differently, they are heteronyms, Choice *B*. The example given fits both definitions. But homonyms, Choice *C*, are spelled the same way and also pronounced the same way, not differently. Synonyms, Choice *D*, are words that have similar meanings. Therefore, Choices *A* and *B* both correctly describe *tear*, but Choices *C* and *D* do not.

14. B: Bacteria is considered a plural word. The singular word for "bacteria" is "bacterium." Cactus, criterion, and elf are all considered singular words, making Choices *A, C,* and *D* incorrect.

15. A: Choices *B, C,* and *D* are incorrect. Choice *A* is correct because passive voice occurs when the subject is acted upon by the verb.

16. A and D: Prewriting involves the steps a writer completes before actually starting to write, such as researching, brainstorming, developing the thesis, outlining, etc. Choice *B* is incorrect because revising cannot be accomplished until the writing has occurred. Choice *C* is incorrect because, if a piece or writing is going to be published, that would be the very final step in the process once all prewriting, writing, and revising/editing is finished.

17. B: The plural possessive noun *friends'* is correctly punctuated with an apostrophe following the plural *-s* ending. *Friend's* would indicate a singular possessive noun, i.e. belonging to one friend. *Friends* would indicate a plural noun not possessing anything. In Choice *A*, the second-person possessive is *your*, NOT "you're," a contraction of "you are." In Choice *C*, the third-person plural possessive is *their*, NOT "they're," a contraction of "they are." There are two errors in Choice *D:* the first possessive is *whose*, NOT "who's," a contraction of "who is;" the second is *its*, NOT "it's," a contraction of "it is."

18. B: *Forfeit* is spelled correctly. Choice *A* is misspelled and should be *weird*. Choice *C* is misspelled and should be *believe*. Choice *D* is misspelled and should be *conceive*. Many people confuse the spellings of words with *ie* and *ei* combinations. Some rules that apply to most English words, with 22 exceptions, are: I before E except after C; and before L, P, T, or V; when sounding like A as in weight; when sounding like I as in height; or when an *ei* combination is formed by a prefix or a suffix.

19. D: Choices *A, B,* and *C* are all unrelated. Choice *D* is correct because parallelism refers to the state of being the same or congruent. The present participles *writing, playing,* and *eating* are congruent parts of speech within a list and are thus parallel.

20. D: Choices *A, B,* and *C* are incorrect. Choice *D* is correct. Transition words cannot be used to replace a verb.

21. B: The Oxford comma is the last comma following the last item in a series and preceding the word *or* or *and*. It is NOT the first, Choice *A*, or any comma separating items in a series, Choice *C*, other than the last. While it is true that many people omit this comma, it is NOT true that it serves no purpose, Choice *D*: it can prevent confusion when series include compound nouns.

22. C: A city and its state should always be separated by a comma. When items in a series contain internal commas, they should be separated by semicolons. City and state are never separated by a semicolon, Choice *A*. The city and its state are never named without punctuation between them, Choice *B*. The reason it is incorrect to use all commas, both between each city and its state and also between city-state pairs, Choice *D*, is obvious: some of the names used can refer to multiple places, causing serious confusion without different punctuation marks to identify them.

23. D: The suffix *-ology* means "study of," and the prefix *geo-* means *earth*. Choice *A* is incorrect because the prefix *phil-* means *love*, and the root *soph* means *wisdom*. Therefore, *philosophy* literally means "love of wisdom," and modern English uses the term to refer to the study of wisdom, knowledge, and reality. Choice *B* is incorrect because the Greek root *episteme* means "to know," and the word *epistemology* means "study of knowledge." Choice *C* is incorrect because the suffix *-centric* means *center*, and geocentric means *earth-centered*.

24. B: Revising and editing are typically the last step in the writing process, in which the writer cleans up language, makes sure the content is clearly stated, and makes adjustments based on the feedback of others. Choices *A* and *C* are incorrect because these should be done during the prewriting stage, which is the first step of the writing process. Choice *D* is incorrect because writers should gain feedback before revising and editing, so they can make changes based on the comments received.

25. A: When two people are named and both possess the same object, the apostrophe-*s* indicating possession should be placed ONLY after the second name, NOT after both names, making Choices *B* and *C* incorrect. It is also incorrect to use the apostrophe-*s* after the first name instead of the second, Choice *D*.

26. D: Irregular plurals that do not end in *–s* are always made possessive by adding apostrophe-*s*. A common error people make is to add *–s*-apostrophe instead of vice versa, as in the other three choices. *Geese*, Choice *A*, *children*, Choice *B*, and *teeth*, Choice *C*, are already plural, so adding an *s* before the apostrophe constitutes a double plural. Adding the *–s* after the apostrophe (i.e. *geese's, children's,* and *teeth's*) correctly makes these plurals possessive.

27. D: Some writing techniques recommended for attaining sentence fluency include varying the beginnings of sentences, varying sentence lengths rather than making them all uniform, and varying sentence rhythms rather than consistently using the same rhythm. These techniques are the opposites of Choices *A*, *B*, and *C*. Varying sentence structures Choice *D* among simple, compound, complex, and compound-complex is a valid writing technique for improving sentence fluency.

28. B: Four elements of an effective paragraph are unity, coherence, a topic sentence, and development. Focusing on one main point throughout, Choice *A*, the paragraph reflects the element of unity. Using logical and verbal bridges, Choice *B*, between/across sentences reflects the element of coherence. A sentence identifying the main idea, Choice *C*, of the paragraph reflects the element of a topic sentence. Citing data, giving examples, including illustrations, and analyzing, Choice *D*, the topic all reflect the element of developing the paragraph sufficiently.

29. B: The correct answer is Choice *B*: "Billy learned what it meant to take care of something other than himself." Choice *A* is awkwardly worded and doesn't flow with the rest of the sentence. Choice *C*, "meant to learning" is also incorrect because the verbs are in the wrong order, it is missing a "to" after the phrase, and the word "learning" is also in the wrong verb form. Choice *D* is also worded awkwardly, making the latter part of the sentence unclear.

30. D: The sentence should read: "sometimes it is the direct result of having a sinus infection." Choice *A* is incorrect because "was" is in past tense, and the rest of the sentence is in present tense. Choice *B* is incorrect because "it be" is not proper subject/verb agreement. "Be" should be conjugated to "is" as a being verb. Finally, Choice *C* is incorrect: we have a past tense "was" which is incorrect, we are missing the article "the," and it is poorly worded.

31. D: Choice *D* is the best answer choice because the gerunds are all in parallel structure: "Playing baseball, swimming, and dancing." Choice *A* is incorrect because "Play baseball" does not match the parallel structure of the other two gerunds. Choice *B* is incorrect because the answer uses semicolons instead of commas, which is incorrect. Semicolons are used to separate independent clauses. Choice *C* is incorrect because "to swim" and "to dance" eschew parallel structure.

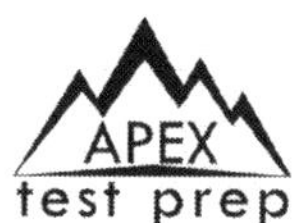

32. C: The correct answer is Choice *C:* "Shocked at the sound of the blast, I muted the television and went outside to see what happened." Choice *A* is incorrect because we're not sure if it is the "I" that's doing the muting or the blast. Choice *B* has incorrect sentence structure. We have "I was shocked" and that carries over to "I was muted," which is incorrect. We need someone doing the muting without the helping verb. Choice *D* is incorrect; we don't have a proper subject to go with the verb "muting." "Me muting" is not correct. In the original sentence, it's the "sound" that's doing the muting, which is incorrect.

33. B: *International* means "occurring between nations," *interaction* means "something that occurs between two or more people," and *intercept* means "come between so as to block something from reaching its destination."

34. D: A personal interpretation does not require citation because it is an original thought. Choice *A* is incorrect because even though she used the writings of others to form her conclusion, her personal interpretation is an original thought and does not need to be cited. Choice *B* is incorrect because a personal interpretation is an original idea. Choice *C* is incorrect because citations are required each time another author's work is quoted or paraphrased, but Samantha did not quote or paraphrase in her conclusion; she used original thoughts.

35. B and C: *Un-* and *dis-* are prefixes meaning *not. Appealing* and *tasteful* are both synonyms of *pleasant. Antipleasant* and *disappealing* are not real words, so Choices *A* and *D* are incorrect.

36. A: Conferencing is the step in the writing process during which writers gain feedback from others in order to improve their content. Choices *B* and *C* are incorrect because these steps take place earlier in the process. Drafting is when the writer puts all of their main points and evidence into paragraph form and fleshes out the concepts in the outline. Prewriting is the step during which the writer researches, brainstorms, and organizes their content. Revising is typically done throughout the writing process and involves making changes to content for clarity and flow.

37. A: The base word of *thankful* is *thanks* (noun) or *to thank* (verb). *Thankful* is an adjective, so it must be a different part of speech than its base word. The base word of *characteristic* is *character* (noun), and *characteristic* can be an adjective or a noun. Therefore, it could be a different part of speech than its base word, but that would need to be determined by context. The base word of *talking* is *to talk* (verb). *Talking* can be a verb or an adjective (gerund), so again, context would have to determine whether it is being used as a different part of speech than its base word. Finally, the base word of *sailed* is *to sail* (verb); both are verbs, so they are not different parts of speech.

Greetings!

First, we would like to give a huge "thank you" for choosing us and this study guide for your **TEAS 7 exam**. We hope that it will lead you to success on this exam and for your years to come.

Our team has tried to make your preparations as thorough as possible by covering all of the topics you should be expected to know. In addition, our writers attempted to create practice questions identical to what you will see on the day of your actual test. We have also included many test-taking strategies to help you learn the material, maintain the knowledge, and take the test with confidence.

We strive for excellence in our products, and if you have any comments or concerns over the quality of something in this study guide, please send us an email so that we may improve.

As you continue forward in life, we would like to remain alongside you with other books and study guides in our library. We are continually producing and updating study guides in several different subjects. If you are looking for something in particular, all of our products are available on Amazon. You may also send us an email!

Sincerely,
APEX Test Prep
info@apexprep.com

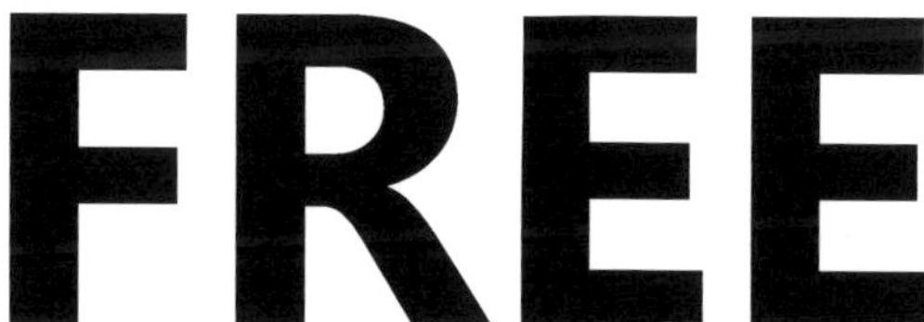

Free Study Tips Videos/DVD

In addition to this guide, we have created a FREE set of videos with helpful study tips. **These FREE videos provide you with top-notch tips to conquer your exam and reach your goals.**

Our simple request is that you give us feedback about the book in exchange for these strategy-packed videos. We would love to hear what you thought about the book, whether positive, negative, or neutral. It is our #1 goal to provide you with quality products and customer service.

To receive your **FREE Study Tips Videos**, scan the QR code or email freevideos@apexprep.com. Please put "FREE Videos" in the subject line and include the following in the email:

a. The title of the book

b. Your rating of the book on a scale of 1-5, with 5 being the highest score

c. Any thoughts or feedback about the book

Thank you!

Made in the USA
Middletown, DE
26 August 2022

72350130R00148